SPRINGER PROTOCOLS HANDBOOKS

For further volumes:
http://www.springer.com/series/8623

Springer Protocols Handbooks collects a diverse range of step-by-step laboratory methods and protocols from across the life and biomedical sciences. Each protocol is provided in the Springer Protocol format: readily-reproducible in a step-by-step fashion. Each protocol opens with an introductory overview, a list of the materials and reagents needed to complete the experiment, and is followed by a detailed procedure supported by a helpful notes section offering tips and tricks of the trade as well as troubleshooting advice. With a focus on large comprehensive protocol collections and an international authorship, Springer Protocols Handbooks are a valuable addition to the laboratory.

Advanced Protocols in Cancer Research

Translational Models for Antitumor and Anticancer Drug Discovery

Karuppusamy Arunachalam

Faculty of Medicine, Federal University of Mato Grosso do Sul, Campo Grande, Mato Grosso do Sul, Brazil

Puthanpura Sasidharan Sreeja

Department of Botany, NSS College Nemmara, Palakkad, Kerala, India

Krishnan Anand

Department of Haematology and Cell Biology, Faculty of Health Sciences, University of the Free State, Bloemfontein, South Africa

Humana Press

Karuppusamy Arunachalam
Faculty of Medicine
Federal University of Mato Grosso do Sul
Campo Grande, Mato Grosso do Sul, Brazil

Puthanpura Sasidharan Sreeja
Department of Botany
NSS College Nemmara
Palakkad, Kerala, India

Krishnan Anand
Department of Haematology and Cell Biology
Faculty of Health Sciences
University of the Free State
Bloemfontein, South Africa

ISSN 1949-2448 ISSN 1949-2456 (electronic)
Springer Protocols Handbooks
ISBN 978-1-0716-5347-0 ISBN 978-1-0716-5348-7 (eBook)
https://doi.org/10.1007/978-1-0716-5348-7

This Humana imprint is published by the registered company Springer Science+Business Media, LLC, part of Springer Nature.
The registered company address is: 1 New York Plaza, New York, NY 10004, U.S.A.

Preface

The landscape of cancer research is defined by its complexity, demanding experimental approaches that are not only innovative but also meticulously reproducible. The journey from a promising chemical entity to a potential therapeutic agent requires a systematic and rigorous evaluation across a spectrum of increasingly sophisticated models. *Advanced Protocols in Cancer Research: Translational Models for Antitumor and Anticancer Drug Discovery* is conceived as a practical guide for navigating this journey. This volume provides a curated collection of detailed protocols, designed to equip researchers with the standardized methodologies needed to generate reliable, translatable data, bridging the gap between in vitro discovery and in vivo application.

This book is built on the premise that robust science is rooted in methodological clarity. Traditional research articles often condense experimental details, leaving critical nuances undocumented. This compendium addresses that gap by offering self-contained, step-by-step protocols. Each chapter is crafted to be a complete resource, guiding the reader through the rationale, materials, precise execution, controls, and data interpretation for a specific technique. Our aim is to empower researchers, whether in academic, clinical, or industrial settings, to implement these sophisticated methods with confidence and to adapt them creatively to their unique hypotheses.

The organization of this book mirrors the logical progression of preclinical and translational cancer research. It begins with foundational in vitro assays, where readers will find established protocols for assessing cytotoxicity and antiproliferative effects using standard methods like the MTT and Alamar Blue assays across a variety of tumor and non-tumor cell lines. Building on these foundational screens, the volume delves into mechanisms of action studies, providing protocols to dissect the biochemical and molecular underpinnings of drug activity, including the evaluation of oxidative stress, DNA interactions, and the delineation of cell death pathways.

Recognizing the limitations of traditional two-dimensional cultures, a significant and distinctive section of this book is dedicated to advanced 2D and 3D culture models. Here, we provide comprehensive guides for establishing and utilizing complex systems, including co-cultures, tumor spheroids, and reconstructed human skin models. These protocols acknowledge the critical importance of the tumor microenvironment and cellular architecture in modulating drug response and resistance, offering a more predictive bridge to in vivo biology.

The transition to living systems is addressed in the in vivo antitumor and efficacy models section. These chapters offer detailed methodologies for evaluating therapeutic efficacy in established murine models, from solid tumor models like Sarcoma 180 to sophisticated syngeneic and xenograft systems for melanoma and colon adenocarcinoma. This in vivo focus is complemented by sections on immunology and inflammation-related assays, providing tools to assess the host response, a key determinant of therapeutic outcome in modern oncology. Finally, the volume concludes with a forward-looking section on clinical studies for cancer research, featuring essential protocols for working with human-derived materials such as lymphocytes, circulating tumor cells, and exosomes, thereby directly connecting laboratory research to clinical specimens.

This book is intended for a diverse audience: from graduate students and technicians seeking to master core techniques, to experienced principal investigators and industry scientists aiming to design comprehensive and rigorous preclinical packages. We are confident that this collection of protocols will serve as a valuable resource, fostering methodological precision and accelerating the translation of scientific discovery into effective cancer therapies. We extend our sincere gratitude to our contributing authors for sharing their expertise and to the research community whose collective efforts drive this field forward. We also acknowledge the institutional support provided by the Federal University of Mato Grosso do Sul (UFMS, Brazil), the University of the Free State (South Africa), and the NSS College Nemmara, Palakkad, India. Finally, we deeply appreciate the Springer Nature team for their professional guidance and support throughout the publication process, with special thanks to David Casey (Senior Editor, Springer Nature) for his exceptional editorial assistance. KA gratefully acknowledges funding support from the Chinese Academy of Sciences (CAS) President's International Fellowship Initiative (PIFI), International Cooperation – International Exchange Program for the visiting scientist (Grant No. 2026PVC0139); the Department of Economic Plants and Biotechnology; and the Yunnan Key Laboratory for Wild Plant Resources, Kunming Institute of Botany, Chinese Academy of Sciences, Kunming - 650201, People's Republic of China.

Mato Grosso do Sul, Brazil — *Karuppusamy Arunachalam*
Palakkad, Kerala, India — *Puthanpura Sasidharan Sreeja*
Bloemfontein, South Africa — *Krishnan Anand*

Contents

Part VII Immuno-Oncology and Inflammation Assays

Part VIII Translational and Clinical Research Protocols

About the Authors

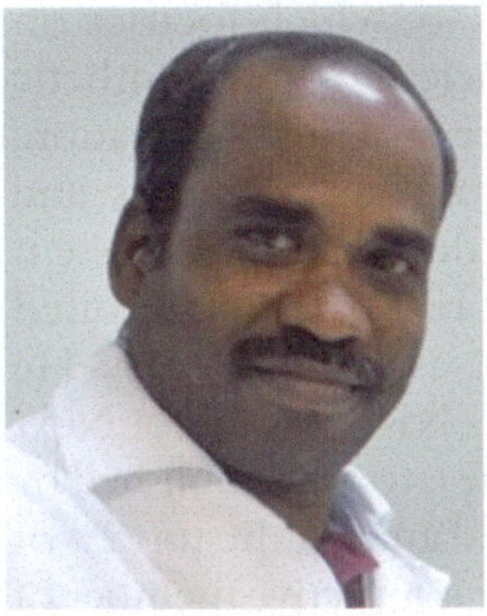

Dr. Karuppusamy Arunachalam, is a visiting professor at the Center for Studies in Stem Cells, Cell Therapy, and Toxicological Genetics (CeTroGen) within the Graduate Program in Health and Development of the Midwest Region, Faculty of Medicine (FAMED), Federal University of Mato Grosso do Sul (UFMS), in Campo Grande, Mato Grosso do Sul, Brazil. In 2020, he was awarded the prestigious President's International Fellowship Initiative (PIFI) by the Chinese Academy of Sciences, during which he conducted research at the Kunming Institute of Botany, Chinese Academy of Sciences. Dr. Arunachalam also completed a 5-year postdoctoral fellowship at the Area Pharmacology Laboratory, Department of Basic Sciences in Health, Faculty of Medicine, Federal University of Mato Grosso (UFMT), Brazil. His research expertise spans a broad spectrum of disciplines, including phytochemistry, biotechnology, ethnopharmacology, and pre-clinical pharmacology, with a primary focus on the development of herbal-based therapies for colorectal cancer. To date, Dr. Arunachalam has published over 65 peer-reviewed journal articles, authored 10 books, and contributed 15 book chapters. He is also the holder of six registered national and international patents (two granted), reflecting his significant contributions to the field of natural product-based drug development.

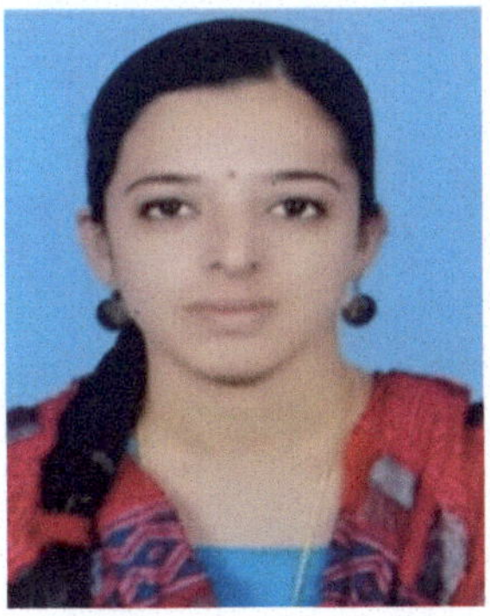

Dr. Puthanpura Sasidharan Sreeja, is an assistant professor (on contract) at NSS College, Nemmara, Palakkad. She completed her undergraduate studies at Calicut University, Kerala, and earned her M.Sc., M.Phil., and PhD from Bharathiar University, Tamil Nadu, India. Dr. Sreeja's current research focuses on the bioprospection of medicinal plants, with an emphasis on phytochemical and pharmacological studies. She has published 16 research articles, which have been cited 330 times according to Google Scholar, as well as six book chapters in renowned international publishers. Additionally, she has authored three books published by Springer Nature. With 5 years of teaching experience and research experience, Dr. Sreeja has made significant contributions to the field of plant-based pharmacology and bioprospecting.

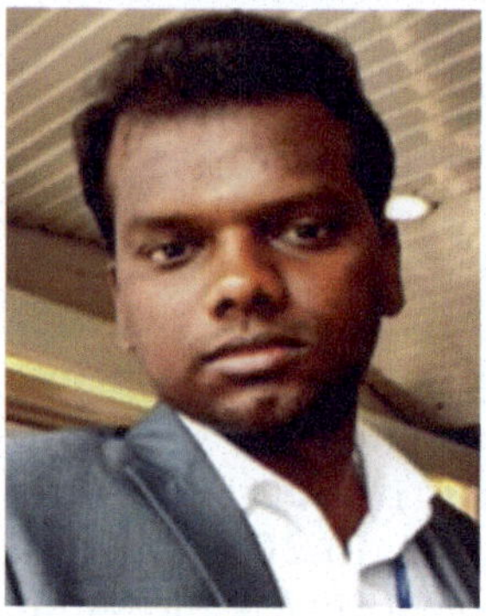

Dr. Krishnan Anand, is a principal investigator in chemical pathology, Department of Haematology and Cell Biology, School of Pathology, Faculty of Health Sciences, University of the Free State, South Africa. He leads the Precision Medicine Integrative Nano Diagnostics (P-MIND) Research Lab, which focuses on the biological functions of extracellular vesicles (EVs) in synthetic biology. His research encompasses cell surface protein modification, biomarker discovery through EVs derived from liquid biopsies, and the role of circulating biomarkers in disease development and stem cell biology. Dr. Krishnan has authored over 150 articles and edited ten books published by Elsevier, Springer Nature, and Wiley. He received the National Research Foundation (NRF) rating for Next Generation Researchers in South Africa. In the latest list published by Stanford University, Dr. Krishnan was named among the top 2% of the most influential scientists worldwide. He is an active member of the International Society of Extracellular Vesicles (ISEV), the African Organisation for Research and Training in Cancer (AORTIC), and the American Association of Cancer Research (AACR). He recently served as an editor for eLife, focusing on the Africa region.

Part I

Foundational Cytotoxicity and Antiproliferative Assays

Chapter 1

In Vitro Cytotoxicity Assays: The MTT Assay

Abstract

This protocol describes a comprehensive set of in vitro assays to evaluate cytotoxicity, cell death mechanisms, and electrophysiological alterations in cancer cell lines, with a focus on the K562 leukemia model. The methodology includes the MTT assay for assessing metabolic activity and cell viability, followed by mechanistic investigations using flow cytometry-based techniques such as propidium iodide exclusion for membrane integrity, TMRM staining for mitochondrial membrane potential, cell cycle analysis, and intracellular ROS detection via H_2-DCFH-DA. Complementary molecular approaches include quantitative real-time PCR to evaluate apoptosis- and cell cycle-related gene expression, as well as whole-cell patch-clamp electrophysiology to examine ion channel modulation. These integrated techniques provide a robust framework for characterizing the cytotoxic and pro-apoptotic effects of test compounds at both the cellular and molecular levels.

Keywords MTT assay, Flow cytometry, Apoptosis, Cell cycle analysis, Patch-clamp electrophysiology

1 Introduction

The MTT assay is a colorimetric method that measures cellular metabolic activity, indirectly reflecting cell viability and proliferation. MTT ([3-(4,5-dimethylthiazol-2-yl)-2,5-diphenyltetrazolium bromide]) is reduced by mitochondrial dehydrogenases to purple formazan crystals, which are solubilized and quantified spectrophotometrically [1].

2 Materials

2.1 Normal and Tumor Cell Lines

A panel of human and murine cell lines, including both normal and tumorigenic types:

- Tumor cell lines: HL-60, MOLT-4, K562, K562-Lucena, MCF-7, HT-29.
- Normal cell lines: L929 (mouse fibroblast), RAW 264.7 (mouse macrophage).

Karuppusamy Arunachalam et al., *Advanced Protocols in Cancer Research*, Springer Protocols Handbooks, https://doi.org/10.1007/978-1-0716-5348-7_1,

2.2 Cell Culture Conditions

All cell lines were cultured under sterile conditions using RPMI 1640 or DMEM culture media (SIGMA, Brazil), supplemented with:

- 10% fetal bovine serum (FBS).
- Penicillin (100 U/mL).
- Streptomycin (100 μg/mL).

Cells were handled under a class II laminar flow hood to avoid contamination, and incubated at 37°C in a humidified atmosphere containing 5% CO_2.

2.3 Cell Culture Maintenance

- Medium was refreshed every 48 h.
- Cultures were monitored daily using an inverted microscope.
- When reaching ~80% confluency, adherent cells were detached with trypsin/EDTA for 5 min.
- Detachment was stopped with 5 mL of complete medium (RPMI + 10% FBS).
- Cells were centrifuged at 500 × g for 5 min, resuspended in 2 mL of medium, and viability was assessed using trypan blue exclusion in a Neubauer chamber.
- Cultures with viability ≥90% were used for assays, and aliquots were subcultured for expansion.

2.4 Cryopreservation

- Detached cells were centrifuged (1500 rpm, 5 min), resuspended in RPMI with 10% FBS and 5% DMSO.
- Cryovials (1 mL) were cooled gradually:
  - 30 min at −20°C.
  - 30 min at −80°C.
  - Then transferred to liquid nitrogen tanks for long-term storage.

3 Methods

3.1 Isolation of Human Peripheral Blood Mononuclear Cells (PBMC) [2]

Isolation Procedure:

1. Mix 3 mL of blood with 3 mL of unsupplemented RPMI in a sterile tube.
2. Carefully layer 4.5 mL of Ficoll-Hypaque solution below the blood–RPMI mixture.
3. Centrifuge at 400 × g for 30 min.

4. Discard plasma and isolate the PBMC layer at the plasma–Ficoll interface.
5. Wash the PBMCs twice in 12 mL of unsupplemented RPMI (400 × *g*, 10 min).
6. Resuspend the pellet in 10 mL of complete RPMI (10% FBS) and vortex.
7. Determine viability using trypan blue exclusion.
8. Samples with ≥90% viable cells proceeded to cytotoxicity assays.

3.2 Cytotoxicity Evaluation by MTT Reduction Assay

1. Seed cells in 96-well plates:
   - Adherent lines (MCF-7, HT-29, L929, RAW264.7, FN1, B16F10): 3×10^4 cells/well.
   - Suspension lines (HL-60, MOLT-4, K562, K562-Lucena): 5×10^4 cells/well.
2. Incubate for 24 h at 37°C, 5% CO_2.
3. Treat with test compounds (AMBH) in concentrations ranging from 1 to 200 μM.
4. After 24 and 72 h, remove part of the supernatant.
5. Centrifuge plates at 200 × *g* for 5 min.
6. Add MTT solution (5 mg/mL in PBS) to each well.
7. Incubate for 3–4 h at 37°C to allow for formazan formation.
8. Solubilize formazan crystals by adding 10% SDS in 0.01 N HCl to each well.
9. Incubate for 16 h to ensure complete dissolution.
10. Measure absorbance at 570 nm using an ELISA plate reader (BIOTEK ELx800, USA).

The absorbance intensity is directly proportional to the number of viable cells.

3.3 Cell Viability Assay—Propidium Iodide (PI)

Objective: Assess cell viability by detecting membrane-compromised (dead) cells.

Materials:

- K562 cells.
- Compound A2CN.
- PI (50 μg/mL; Sigma, USA).
- PBS (ice-cold).
- 24-well culture plates.
- CO_2 incubator (37°C, 5%).
- Flow cytometer (BD FACS Calibur, FL-2 channel, 585 nm).

Protocol:

1. Seed 5×10^5 K562 cells/well in a 24-well plate.
2. Treat cells with A2CN (15, 30, 60 μM) for 24 h at 37°C in 5% CO_2.
3. After incubation, collect cells by centrifugation at 200 × *g* for 5 min.
4. Resuspend the pellet in 998 μL of ice-cold PBS.
5. Just before analysis, add 2 μL of PI (final concentration 50 μg/mL).
6. Incubate samples for 5 min at room temperature protected from light.
7. Analyze samples on a flow cytometer using the FL-2 (585 nm) detector.
8. Record at least 10,000 events per sample.

3.4 Mitochondrial Membrane Potential Assay—TMRM [3]

Objective: Evaluate mitochondrial membrane potential loss, indicative of apoptosis.

Materials:

- K562 cells.
- Compound A2CN.
- TMRM (150 nM; Sigma).
- Etoposide (5 μM; positive control).
- CCCP (100 μM; depolarizing agent).
- DMSO (0.5%; negative control).
- PBS (37°C).
- 24-well plates.
- CO_2 incubator.
- Flow cytometer (FL-2 channel).

Protocol:

1. Seed 5×10^5 K562 cells/well in a 24-well plate.
2. Treat cells for 24 h with:
   - A2CN (15, 30, 60 μM).
   - Etoposide (5 μM) (positive control).
   - DMSO 0.5% (negative control).
3. For CCCP control, treat a separate well with 100 μM CCCP for 15 min.
4. After incubation, centrifuge cells at 200 × *g* for 5 min.
5. Wash cells once with culture medium.

6. Stain cells with 150 nM TMRM and incubate for 30 min at 37°C in the dark.
7. Wash cells once with warm PBS (37°C).
8. Analyze samples immediately by flow cytometry using the FL-2 detector.

3.5 Cell Cycle Analysis—Propidium Iodide (PI) [4]

Objective: Quantify cell distribution in different phases of the cell cycle.

Materials:

- K562 cells.
- Compound A2CN.
- Etoposide (5 μM; positive control).
- PI (50 μg/mL; Sigma).
- Sodium citrate (1%).
- Triton X-100 (0.1%).
- 24-well plates.
- Cold PBS.
- Flow cytometer (FL2-H channel).

Protocol:

1. Seed 5×10^5 K562 cells/well in 24-well plates.
2. Treat cells with A2CN (15, 30, 60 μM) for 24 h.
3. Include Etoposide (5 μM) as a positive control.
4. After incubation, collect cells by centrifugation (200 × *g*, 5 min).
5. Resuspend cells in hypotonic solution:
   - 1% sodium citrate.
   - 0.1% Triton X-100.
   - 50 μg/mL PI.
6. Incubate samples for 30 min at 4°C in the dark.
7. Analyze DNA content by flow cytometry using the FL2-H detector.
8. Record 10,000 events/sample and analyze % of cells in G0/G1, S, G2/M, and Sub-G1 phases.

3.6 Intracellular ROS Assay—H2-DCFH-DA

Objective: Detect reactive oxygen species (ROS) generation in treated cells.

Materials:

- K562 cells.
- Compound A2CN.

- H_2-DCFH-DA (10 μM; Sigma-Aldrich).
- Etoposide (5 μM).
- H_2O_2 (100 μM; positive control).
- DMSO (0.5%; negative control).
- PBS (37°C).
- 24-well plates.
- CO_2 incubator.
- Flow cytometer (FL1-H channel, green fluorescence).

Protocol:

1. Seed 5×10^5 K562 cells/well in 24-well plates.
2. Treat cells with:
   - A2CN (15, 30, 60 μM) for 24 h.
   - Etoposide (5 μM) (positive control).
   - H_2O_2 (100 μM) for 15 min (positive control).
   - DMSO 0.5% (negative control).
3. After treatment, collect cells by centrifugation (200 × *g*, 5 min).
4. Wash cells once with warm PBS (37°C).
5. Incubate cells with 10 μM H2-DCFH-DA for 30 min at 37°C in the dark.
6. Wash cells again with warm PBS.
7. Immediately analyze samples on a flow cytometer using the FL1-H (green) detector.

3.7 Evaluation of Gene Expression Related to the Cell Cycle and Apoptosis [5]

3.7.1 Total RNA Extraction

1. K562 cells will be cultured in six-well plates at a concentration of 1×10^6 cells/mL.
2. Cells will be treated with A2CN (60 μM) for 24 h. Control cells will be maintained in RPMI medium without treatment.
3. Total RNA will be extracted using either 1.0 mL of Trizol reagent (Invitrogen, USA) per 1×10^6 cells or the RNeasy Mini Kit (QIAGEN, Germany), following the manufacturer's protocol.
4. For Trizol extraction:
   - Cells will be centrifuged at 300 × *g* for 4 min.
   - The supernatant will be discarded, and the pellet will be immediately homogenized in 1.0 mL of Trizol.

- 200 μL of chloroform will be added per sample, followed by vigorous mixing for 15 s and incubation at room temperature for 3 min.
- Samples will be centrifuged at 12,000 × *g* for 15 min at 4°C.
- The aqueous phase will be transferred to a new tube, and RNA will be precipitated with 0.5 mL of isopropanol.
- After gentle mixing, samples will be centrifuged at 12,000 × *g* for 15 min at 4°C.
- The RNA pellet will be washed twice with 1 mL of 75% ethanol and centrifuged at 7500 × *g* for 3 min.
- The pellet will be air-dried, resuspended in 30 μL of RNase-free water, and stored at −80°C.

5. RNA concentration will be measured using a Nanodrop spectrophotometer (260 nm), and integrity will be assessed by 1% agarose gel electrophoresis stained with Ez-Vision (Amresco, USA).

3.7.2 cDNA Synthesis

1. Complementary DNA (cDNA) will be synthesized from total RNA using the SuperScript™ III First-Strand Synthesis System (Invitrogen, USA), according to the manufacturer's instructions.
2. Prior to reverse transcription, RNA samples will be treated with RNase-free DNase (RQ1 DNase; Promega, USA).
3. A total of 3 μg of RNA will be mixed with 1 μL of dNTPs and 1 μL of oligo(dT) primers.
4. The mixture will be incubated at 65°C for 5 min and then placed on ice for 1 min.
5. A 2× master mix will be prepared containing:
   - 2 μL RT buffer,
   - 4 μL $MgCl_2$,
   - 2 μL DTT,
   - 1 μL RNaseOUT.
6. The RNA–primer mix will be combined with the master mix and incubated at 42°C for 2 min.
7. Next, 1 μL of SuperScript™ II Reverse Transcriptase will be added, and the mixture will be incubated at:
   - 42°C for 50 min,
   - 70°C for 15 min.
8. Samples will be cooled on ice, and 1 μL of RNase H will be added, followed by incubation at 37°C for 20 min.
9. The synthesized cDNA will either be stored at −20°C or used immediately for qPCR.

3.7.3 Quantitative Real-Time PCR (qPCR)

1. Gene expression levels in treated and untreated K562 cells will be assessed by quantitative real-time PCR (qPCR) using a Bio-Rad CFX96 Touch system (BIO-RAD, USA).
2. Each 25 μL reaction will be prepared using Maxima® SYBR® Green/Fluorescein qPCR Master Mix (2×) (Fermentas, USA) and will contain:
   - 12.5 μL of SYBR Green master mix,
   - 1 μL of cDNA,
   - 10 μM of each specific primer.
   - RNase-free water to adjust volume.
3. GAPDH will serve as the endogenous control.
4. No-template controls will be included in each run to verify specificity.
5. Fluorescence will be recorded at the end of each amplification cycle.
6. Ct (cycle threshold) values will be analyzed using CFX Manager software (BIO-RAD).
7. Relative gene expression will be calculated using the $2^{-\Delta Ct}$ method.
8. Amplification efficiencies for target and reference genes will be verified using standard curves from serial cDNA dilutions (400, 40, 4, and 0.4 ng).
9. Each reaction will be run in duplicate.
10. Specificity will be confirmed through melting curve analysis.
11. All target gene Ct values will be normalized to GAPDH expression.

3.8 Patch-Clamp Electrophysiology [6]

Whole-cell patch-clamp recordings will be performed in voltage-clamp mode using the following setup:

- Recordings will be conducted under an inverted microscope (Carl Zeiss, Germany) mounted on a vibration isolation table (TMC, USA).
- A hydraulic micromanipulator (Narishige, Japan) will be used to position the recording pipette.
- A second micromanipulator will be used to position the perfusion pipette containing the control or test solution.
- Signals will be amplified using a HEKA amplifier (Germany), low-pass filtered at 2.0 kHz, and digitized at 10 kHz.
- Leak subtraction will be performed using the P/4 protocol.
- Cells with series resistance >5 MΩ or unstable seals will be excluded from analysis.

Solutions

- Internal solution (in mM): 140 KCl, 1 $MgCl_2$, 10 EGTA, 10 HEPES, 5 Glucose; pH adjusted to 7.2 with KOH; ~310 mOsm.
- External solution (in mM): 140 NaCl, 5.4 KCl, 1.2 $MgCl_2$, 10 EGTA, 10 HEPES, 10 Glucose; pH adjusted to 7.4 with NaOH; ~330 mOsm.
- All solutions will be filtered through 0.22 μm filters.

Whole-Cell Recording Procedure

1. Patch pipettes (2.5–5 MΩ) will be pulled using a vertical puller (Narishige, Japan) and filled with internal solution.
2. Ag/AgCl electrodes will be placed in the pipettes and connected to the amplifier.
3. A gigaseal (≥1 GΩ) will be formed using light suction, followed by stronger suction to establish whole-cell access.
4. Whole-cell configuration will be verified by the appearance of capacitive transients.
5. Recordings will be performed under constant perfusion (~0.1 mL/min) using a dual-reservoir system connected to a solenoid valve (Dagan, USA).
6. The test compound (A2CN, 120 μM) will be included in one reservoir, and the control solution in the other.

3.9 Cell Preparation for Patch-Clamp

1. Sterile glass coverslips (24 × 24 mm) will be coated with 120 μM poly-D-lysine for 30 min.
2. Coverslips will be rinsed with PBS and dried under sterile conditions.
3. K562 cells (500 μL suspension) will be seeded onto each coverslip.
4. Cells will be allowed to adhere by incubating the plates in a CO_2 incubator for 5 h.
5. Patch-clamp recordings will then be conducted as described.

3.10 Statistical Analysis

- Patch-clamp data: Potassium currents will be normalized to cell capacitance (pA/pF) and reported as mean ± SEM. Comparisons between groups will be made using Student's *t*-test.
- Cell viability assays: Data will be expressed as percent viability relative to control. IC_{50} values will be estimated using non-linear regression in GraphPad Prism v5.01. Statistical significance will be determined using one-way ANOVA followed by Bonferroni post hoc tests. A p-value <0.05 will be considered significant.

- Gene expression data: qPCR results from three independent experiments (each in duplicate) will be analyzed using Student's *t*-test. A *p*-value <0.05 will indicate statistical significance.

References

1. Arunachalam K, Sreeja PS (2025) MTT assay protocol. In: Advanced cell and molecular techniques. Springer protocols handbooks. Humana, New York, NY
2. Chomczynski P, Sacchi N (1987) Single-step method of RNA isolation by acid guanidinium thiocyanate–phenol–chloroform extraction. Anal Biochem 162(1):156–159
3. Bustin SA et al (2009) The MIQE guidelines: minimum information for publication of quantitative real-time PCR experiments. Clin Chem 55(4):611–622
4. Livak KJ, Schmittgen TD (2001) Analysis of relative gene expression data using real-time quantitative PCR and the 2−ΔΔCT method. Methods 25(4):402–408
5. Pfaffl MW (2001) A new mathematical model for relative quantification in real-time RT–PCR. Nucleic Acids Res 29(9):e45
6. Hamill OP, Marty A, Neher E, Sakmann B, Sigworth FJ (1981) Improved patch-clamp techniques for high-resolution current recording from cells and cell-free membrane patches. Pflügers Arch 391(2):85–100

Chapter 2

Alamar Blue Cytotoxicity Assay: Protocol for Tumor Cell Lines and Peripheral Blood Mononuclear Cells (PBMCs)

Abstract

This protocol describes a standardized Alamar Blue (resazurin) reduction assay for evaluating the cytotoxic effects of test compounds against both human tumor cell lines and normal peripheral blood mononuclear cells (PBMCs). The method leverages the metabolic reduction of non-fluorescent blue resazurin to fluorescent pink resorufin by viable cells, providing a quantitative measure of cell viability suitable for high-throughput screening. Detailed procedures are provided for the culture of suspension and adherent tumor cell lines (HL-60, HCT-8, SF-295, MDA-MB-435), the isolation of PBMCs from healthy donors using Ficoll-Hypaque density gradient centrifugation, and the subsequent treatment with test compounds over a 72-h incubation period. By comparing the half-maximal inhibitory concentration (IC_{50}) values obtained from tumor cells versus normal PBMCs, this assay enables the assessment of cytotoxic selectivity, which is crucial for identifying potential anticancer candidates with favorable therapeutic indices.

Keywords Alamar Blue, Resazurin, Cytotoxicity, IC_{50}, PBMC

1 Introduction

The Alamar Blue (resazurin) assay is a colorimetric and fluorometric method for assessing cell viability and cytotoxicity. Metabolically active cells reduce the blue, non-fluorescent resazurin to pink, fluorescent resorufin. The degree of reduction is proportional to the number of viable cells, making it ideal for high-throughput screening of anticancer compounds. This protocol details the assay for human tumor cell lines (e.g., HL-60, HCT-8, SF-295, MDA-MB-435) and normal peripheral blood mononuclear cells (PBMCs), allowing for a comparison of cytotoxic selectivity [1].

2 Aim

To determine the half-maximal inhibitory concentration (IC_{50}) of test compounds against human tumor cell lines and normal PBMCs using the Alamar Blue reduction assay.

Karuppusamy Arunachalam et al., *Advanced Protocols in Cancer Research*, Springer Protocols Handbooks,
https://doi.org/10.1007/978-1-0716-5348-7_2,

3 Materials

3.1 Cell Lines and Biological Material

- Tumor cell lines: HL-60 (promyelocytic leukemia), HCT-8 (colon carcinoma), SF-295 (CNS tumor), MDA-MB-435 (breast cancer).
- Normal cells: Heparinized peripheral blood from healthy donors (18–25 years).

3.2 Reagents and Solutions

- Culture medium: RPMI 1640, supplemented with:
  - For tumor cells: 10% fetal bovine serum (FBS), 1% penicillin–streptomycin.
  - For PBMCs: 20% FBS, 1% penicillin–streptomycin, 4% phytohemagglutinin (PHA).
- Alamar Blue stock: 0.312 mg/mL resazurin in PBS or medium (filter-sterilized).
- Test compounds: Stock solutions (e.g., 10 mg/mL in DMSO). Prepare working dilutions in culture medium.
- Controls: Sterile DMSO (vehicle), doxorubicin or similar (positive control).
- Isolation reagent: Ficoll-Hypaque solution.
- Buffers: Phosphate-buffered saline (PBS, sterile).

3.3 Equipment

- 96-well flat-bottom tissue culture plates.
- CO_2 incubator (37°C, 5% CO_2, humidified).
- Multimode plate reader capable of measuring absorbance at 570 and 595 nm.
- Biological safety cabinet (laminar flow hood).
- Refrigerated centrifuge.
- Micropipettes, sterile filter tips, and sterile tubes.

4 Step-by-Step Protocols [2]

4.1 Cell Preparation

4.1.1 Tumor Cell Culture

1. Maintain tumor cell lines in appropriate culture medium at 37°C, 5% CO_2.
2. For adherent cells (HCT-8, SF-295, MDA-MB-435), detach using trypsin–EDTA when subconfluent. Inactivate trypsin with complete medium.

3. Count cells using a hemocytometer or automated counter.
4. Prepare cell suspensions in complete medium at the following densities:
   - Suspension cells (HL-60): 0.3×10^6 cells/mL.
   - Adherent cells: 0.7×10^5 cells/mL.
5. Seed 100 µL of cell suspension into each well of a 96-well plate. This yields final seeding densities of 30,000 cells/well (HL-60) and 7000 cells/well (adherent lines).

4.1.2 PBMC Isolation and Culture

1. Dilute heparinized blood 1:1 with sterile PBS.
2. Carefully layer the diluted blood over an equal volume of Ficoll-Hypaque in a sterile centrifuge tube. Do not mix.
3. Centrifuge at $400 \times g$ for 30 min at room temperature (20–25°C) with the brake OFF.
4. After centrifugation, aspirate the upper plasma layer. Using a sterile Pasteur pipette, carefully collect the opaque PBMC layer (buffy coat) at the interface.
5. Transfer PBMCs to a new tube, add PBS to wash, and centrifuge at $300 \times g$ for 10 min. Discard supernatant.
6. Repeat the wash step (step 5) once more.
7. Resuspend the cell pellet in complete PBMC medium (RPMI 1640 + 20% FBS + 1% antibiotics + 4% PHA).
8. Count cells and adjust density to 0.3×10^6 cells/mL.
9. Seed 100 µL of PBMC suspension into each well of a 96-well plate (30,000 cells/well).
10. Pre-incubate the PBMC plate for 24 h at 37°C, 5% CO_2 to allow cell stabilization and PHA-induced activation before compound addition.

4.2 Treatment with Test Compounds

1. Prepare serial dilutions of the test compound in culture medium to achieve the desired final concentration range (e.g., 0.78–50 µg/mL). Ensure the final concentration of DMSO is $\leq$0.5% (v/v) to avoid solvent toxicity.
2. **For tumor cells:** Add 100 µL of each compound dilution to the wells immediately after seeding (total well volume = 200 µL). Incubate for 72 h.
3. **For PBMCs:** After the 24-h pre-incubation, gently add 100 µL of each compound dilution to the wells (total well volume = 200 µL). Incubate for an additional 72 h.
4. Include the following controls in each experiment:
   - Negative control: Cells + culture medium only.
   - Vehicle control: Cells + medium + highest equivalent concentration of DMSO used.

- Positive control: Cells + medium + a known cytotoxic agent (e.g., doxorubicin).
- Blank: Medium only (no cells) for background subtraction.

4.3 Alamar Blue Addition and Measurement

1. Four hours before the end of the total 72-h incubation period, add 10 μL of Alamar Blue stock solution (0.312 mg/mL) directly to each well. Gently swirl the plate to mix.
2. Return the plate to the incubator for the final 4 h.
3. After incubation, measure the absorbance using a plate reader at two wavelengths:
   - 570 nm (reduced, pink resorufin).
   - 595 or 600 nm (oxidized, blue resazurin; reference wavelength).

5 Data Analysis

1. **Calculate percent reduction:** Use the formula from the manufacturer or the following derived formula:

   % Alamar Blue reduction

   $$= [(A_{570} - (A_{595} \times R_0))/A_{570}\,(\text{negative control})] \times 100$$

   Where:

   - A_{570} = absorbance of test well at 570 nm.
   - A_{595} = absorbance of test well at 595 nm.
   - R_0 = correction factor (ratio of A_{570}/A_{595} for medium-only *blank* wells). This corrects for background absorbance.

2. **Normalize viability:** Express results as % cell viability relative to the vehicle control (set to 100%).
3. **Determine IC_{50}**: Plot % cell viability versus $\log_{50}$(compound concentration). Use non-linear regression analysis (e.g., log(inhibitor) vs. response—variable slope (four parameters)) in software such as GraphPad Prism to calculate the IC_{50} value (concentration inhibiting 50% of cell viability) with 95% confidence intervals.

References

1. Deb DD, Parimala G, Devi SS, Chakraborty T (2011) Effect of thymol on peripheral blood mononuclear cell PBMC and acute promyelotic cancer cell line HL-60. Chem Biol Interact 193(1):97–106
2. Riedhammer C, Halbritter D, Weissert R (2014) Peripheral blood mononuclear cells: isolation, freezing, thawing, and culture. In: Multiple sclerosis: methods and protocols. Springer New York, New York, NY, pp 53–61

Chapter 3

Protocol for Evaluating the In Vitro Cytotoxicity of Compounds Against LM3 and LP07 Murine Adenocarcinoma Cell Lines Using the MTT Assay

Abstract

This protocol provides a standardized methodology for evaluating the in vitro cytotoxicity of test compounds against LM3 murine breast adenocarcinoma and LP07 murine lung adenocarcinoma cell lines using the MTT colorimetric assay. Detailed procedures are described for cell culture maintenance, harvesting, and seeding in 96-well plates, followed by exposure to serial dilutions of test compounds over a 48-h treatment period. The assay quantifies cellular metabolic activity through the reduction of MTT to insoluble formazan crystals, which are solubilized and measured spectrophotometrically at 570 nm to determine cell viability and calculate half-maximal inhibitory concentration (IC_{50}) values. Additionally, the protocol incorporates an optional co-treatment with the antioxidant N-acetylcysteine (NAC) to investigate the potential involvement of reactive oxygen species (ROS) in compound-mediated cytotoxicity. This approach enables the assessment of cytotoxic potency and provides mechanistic insights into oxidative stress-related cell death pathways in murine adenocarcinoma models.

Keywords MTT assay, Cytotoxicity, LM3 cells, LP07 cells, N-acetylcysteine

1 Introduction

Breast and lung adenocarcinomas represent significant challenges in oncology. The LM3 (murine breast adenocarcinoma) and LP07 (murine lung adenocarcinoma) cell lines, derived from spontaneous tumors in Balb/c mice, are well-established models for studying tumor biology and screening potential chemotherapeutic agents [1]. The MTT (3-(4,5-dimethylthiazol-2-yl)-2,5-diphenyltetrazolium bromide) assay is a standard colorimetric method for assessing cell metabolic activity, which serves as a reliable proxy for cell viability and proliferation in response to therapeutic compounds [2]. This protocol details the methodology for culturing LM3 and LP07 cells, preparing test compounds, and performing the MTT assay to determine the half-maximal inhibitory concentration (IC_{50}) of experimental substances, with provisions for investigating mechanisms involving oxidative stress using the antioxidant N-acetylcysteine [3].

Karuppusamy Arunachalam et al., *Advanced Protocols in Cancer Research*, Springer Protocols Handbooks,
https://doi.org/10.1007/978-1-0716-5348-7_3,

2 Aim

To determine the in vitro cytotoxicity (IC_{50}) of test compounds against LM3 and LP07 murine adenocarcinoma cell lines using the MTT assay, and to evaluate the potential role of reactive oxygen species (ROS) in compound-mediated cytotoxicity by performing parallel assays in the presence of the antioxidant N-acetylcysteine.

3 Materials and Reagents

3.1 Cell Lines and Culture

- Cell lines: LM3 (murine breast adenocarcinoma) and LP07 (murine lung adenocarcinoma). Source: Prof. Dr. Lucas L. Colombo, Angel H. Roffo Institute of Oncology, Buenos Aires, Argentina.
- Basal medium: Minimum Essential Medium (MEM) powder (Gibco, Cat# 41090).
- Complete growth medium (CGM): MEM supplemented with 10% (v/v) fetal bovine serum (FBS, Gibco) and 0.08 mg/mL gentamicin sulfate (Garamycin, Mantecorp).
- Subculturing reagent: 0.25% trypsin–EDTA or equivalent.
- Cell counting: 0.04% (v/v) trypan blue solution (Reagen); phosphate-buffered saline (PBS), pH 7.4.

3.2 Solutions and Reagents for Assay

- Phosphate-buffered saline (PBS), pH 7.4:
  - NaCl: 8.0 g/L.
  - KCl: 0.2 g/L.
  - Na_2HPO_4: 1.44 g/L.
  - KH_2PO_4: 0.24 g/L.
  - Adjust pH to 7.4 with HCl/NaOH, sterilize by autoclaving (121°C, 15 min).
- MTT stock solution (5 mg/mL): Dissolve 10 mg of MTT (Sigma-Aldrich, M2128) in 2.0 mL of sterile PBS. Sonicate for 10 min to ensure complete dissolution. Store protected from light at −20°C for up to 2 weeks.
- MTT working solution (0.5 mg/mL): Immediately before use, dilute the MTT stock solution 1:10 in serum-free MEM (e.g., 1 mL stock + 9 mL MEM). Keep protected from light.
- Solubilization solution: Isopropanol (i-PrOH) or DMSO.
- Positive control: Paclitaxel (Sigma, purity >99%). Prepare a 10 mM stock in DMSO, store at −80°C. Perform serial dilutions in CGM for a final DMSO concentration ≤0.5%.

- Antioxidant solution: N-acetylcysteine (NAC). Dissolve Fluimucil granules (200 mg) directly in CGM to prepare a concentrated stock (e.g., 100 mM). Filter sterilize (0.22 μm). Final working concentration in assay: 0.5 mM (0.5 μmol/mL).
- Test compounds (e.g., pristimerin, tingenone): Prepare a 10 mM stock solution in DMSO. For immediate use, prepare a compound intermediate stock by diluting 2.5 mg of compound in 50 μL DMSO, then adding 9.95 mL CGM (for a ~0.25 mg/mL solution). Aliquot and store all stocks at −80°C. Avoid repeated freeze–thaw cycles.

3.3 Equipment and Consumables

- Laminar flow hood: Class II biological safety cabinet.
- CO_2 incubator: Set at 37°C, 5% CO_2, and 95% humidity.
- Inverted microscope.
- Hemocytometer (Neubauer chamber) or automated cell counter.
- Microplate reader: Capable of reading absorbance at 540 nm (570 nm is also acceptable) with a reference filter of 620–690 nm to reduce background and with plate-shaking capability.
- Centrifuge (for cell preparation).
- Water bath or bead bath (set at 37°C).
- Pipettes and sterile filter tips (multichannel pipette recommended).
- Sterile tissue culture-treated plates: 96-well, flat-bottom (Corning, Cat# 3599).
- Sterile microcentrifuge tubes (1.5 mL and 15/50 mL conical tubes).
- Sterile serological pipettes (5, 10, 25 mL).

4 Methodology [4–6]

4.1 Cell Seeding and Monolayer Formation

1. Cell preparation: Grow LM3 and LP07 cells in T-75 flasks with CGM until 70%–80% confluence.
2. Harvesting: Aspirate medium, wash cells with 5 mL pre-warmed PBS. Detach cells using 2 mL of trypsin–EDTA (37°C, 3–5 min). Neutralize with 4 mL CGM.
3. Counting: Centrifuge cell suspension (300 × *g*, 5 min). Resuspend pellet in 5 mL CGM. Mix 10 μL of cell suspension with 10 μL trypan blue. Count viable (unstained) cells using a hemocytometer.

4. Seeding: Adjust cell density to 2.5×10^4 cells/mL in CGM. Seed 200 μL per well into a 96-well plate (final: 5×10^3 cells/well). Include cell-free control wells (CGM only) for background subtraction.
5. Incubation: Incubate plate for 24 h at 37°C, 5% CO_2 to allow cells to adhere and form a ~70% confluent monolayer.

4.2 Compound Treatment and Incubation

1. Compound dilution: Thaw compound intermediate stocks and prepare a six-point serial dilution (e.g., 1:3 or 1:10 dilutions) in CGM in sterile tubes. Ensure the final concentration of DMSO in any well does not exceed 0.5% (v/v), the predetermined non-toxic threshold.
2. Treatment: After 24 h, carefully aspirate the medium from the cell-seeded plate using a multichannel pipette. Gently add 200 μL of each compound dilution to triplicate wells. Include controls:
   - Negative control: CGM only (100% viability).
   - Vehicle control: CGM + 0.5% DMSO (solvent control).
   - Positive control: Paclitaxel dilutions.
3. Co-treatment with NAC (optional): For ROS investigation, prepare identical compound dilutions in CGM containing 0.5 mM NAC. Add these to a separate plate.
4. Incubation: Incubate the plates for 48 h at 37°C, 5% CO_2.

4.3 MTT Assay and Absorbance Measurement (Fig. 1)

1. MTT addition: After 48 h, carefully aspirate all medium from the wells. Add 100 μL of MTT working solution (0.5 mg/mL) to each well.
2. Formazan formation: Incubate the plate for 3 h at 37°C, 5% CO_2, protected from light.
3. Solubilization: Carefully aspirate the MTT solution. Add 100 μ L of isopropanol to each well to dissolve the formed formazan crystals. Seal the plate and agitate on an orbital shaker for 15 min to ensure complete dissolution.
4. Absorbance reading: Read the absorbance immediately at 570 nm (540–570 nm is acceptable) with a reference wavelength of 620 nm on a plate reader. Program the reader to shake the plate for 10 s prior to reading.

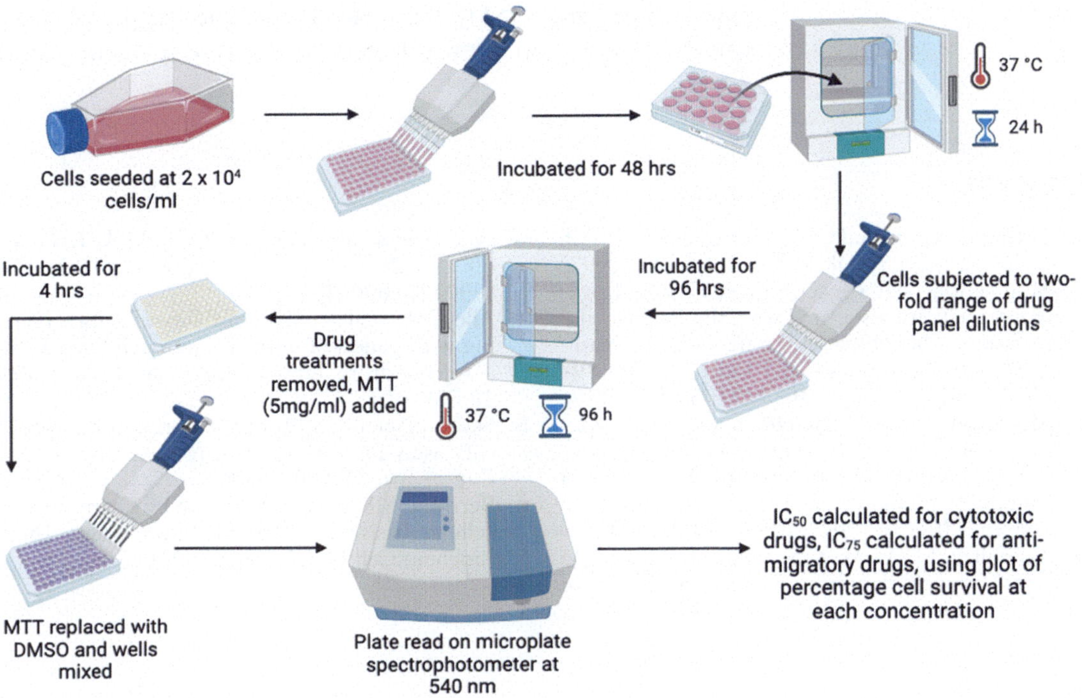

Fig. 1 Experimental representation of MTT assay and absorbance measurement

5 Data Analysis

1. **Background subtraction:** Subtract the average absorbance of the cell-free control wells from all experimental readings.
2. **Viability calculation:** Calculate percent cell viability for each well:

$$\begin{aligned}\%\ \text{Viability} &= (\text{Mean absorbance of treated well} \\ &\quad /\text{Mean absorbance of negative control wells}) \times 100\end{aligned}$$

3. **IC_{50} determination:** Plot % viability (y-axis) against $\log_{10}$[compound concentration] (x-axis). Perform non-linear regression analysis (e.g., log(inhibitor) vs. response—variable slope (four parameters)) using software such as GraphPad Prism. The IC_{50} is the concentration that yields 50% viability.
4. **Statistics:** Perform two to three independent experiments, each with technical triplicates. Report IC_{50} values as mean ±

standard deviation (SD). Compare IC_{50} values with and without NAC using an appropriate statistical test (e.g., unpaired *t*-test).

References

1. Urtreger AJ, Ladeda VE, Puricelli LI, Rivelli A, De Lustig ES, Bal de Kier Joffé ED (1997) Modulation of fibronectin expression and proteolytic activity associated with the invasive and metastatic phenotype in two new murine mammary tumor cell lines. Int J Oncol 11(3):489–496. https://doi.org/10.3892/ijo.11.3.489
2. Mosmann T (1983) Rapid colorimetric assay for cellular growth and survival: application to proliferation and cytotoxicity assays. J Immunol Methods 65(1-2):55–63. https://doi.org/10.1016/0022-1759(83)90303-4
3. Zafarullah M, Li WQ, Sylvester J, Ahmad M (2003) Molecular mechanisms of N-acetylcysteine actions. Cell Mol Life Sci 60(1):6–20. https://doi.org/10.1007/s000180300001
4. Alley MC et al (1988) Feasibility of drug screening with panels of human tumor cell lines using a microculture tetrazolium assay. Cancer Res 48:589–601
5. Skehan P et al (1990) New colorimetric cytotoxicity assay for anticancer-drug screening. J Natl Cancer Inst 82:1107–1112
6. Berridge MV et al (1996) The biochemical and cellular basis of cell proliferation assays. Int J Biochem Cell Biol 29:1019–1030

Check for updates

Chapter 4

Evaluating the Cytotoxic and Anti-Cancer Mechanisms of Peptides on Tumor and Non-Tumor Cell Lines

Abstract

This protocol details a comprehensive methodology for evaluating the anti-cancer potential of peptides. It begins with screening for cytotoxic effects on a panel of tumor and non-tumor cell lines using MTT and trypan blue assays to determine inhibitory concentrations (IC_{50}) and selectivity. Subsequent functional assays are described to investigate the mechanisms of action, specifically focusing on the effects of a lead peptide on B16F10-Nex2 murine melanoma cells. These assays assess changes in cell morphology, proliferation, adhesion, migration, and invasion. Finally, protocols for cell cycle analysis by flow cytometry and protein expression analysis by Western blot are included to elucidate underlying molecular mechanisms.

Keywords Cytotoxicity, Peptides, Melanoma, Cell viability, MTT assay, Cell migration, Invasion assay, Flow cytometry, Western blot

1 Introduction

Melanoma is an aggressive form of skin cancer characterized by its high metastatic potential, making the development of effective therapies a critical challenge. In recent years, bioactive peptides have emerged as promising anti-cancer agents due to their ability to selectively target tumor cells and disrupt key processes involved in cancer progression [1]. While some peptides have demonstrated direct cytotoxic effects, their broader impact on cellular behaviors such as proliferation, adhesion, migration, and invasion—all critical steps in the metastatic cascade—requires further investigation. This protocol is designed to provide a systematic approach for evaluating these multifaceted effects, from initial cytotoxicity screening to in-depth mechanistic studies. The primary aim is to determine the inhibitory concentration (IC_{50}) of peptides on both tumorigenic and non-tumorigenic cell lines to assess their selective cytotoxicity. Subsequently, using B16F10-Nex2 murine melanoma cells as a model, this protocol outlines a series of functional assays to characterize the peptides' impact on cancer cell behavior and to investigate the underlying molecular mechanisms.

Karuppusamy Arunachalam et al., *Advanced Protocols in Cancer Research*, Springer Protocols Handbooks,
https://doi.org/10.1007/978-1-0716-5348-7_4,

2 Aim

To evaluate the anti-cancer potential of peptides by:

1. Determining their inhibitory concentration (IC_{50}) and selective cytotoxicity on a panel of tumor and non-tumor cell lines.
2. Assessing their effects on the morphology, proliferation, adhesion, migration, and invasion of B16F10-Nex2 melanoma cells.
3. Investigating the underlying mechanisms through cell cycle analysis and the expression of key signaling proteins.

3 Materials

- Cell lines: Tumorigenic (B16F10-Nex2, A2058, JurKat, MCF-7, MDA-MB-231, SKBR-3, SiHa, U87) and non-tumorigenic (melan-A, HaCaT).
- Culture media: DMEM, RPMI-1640.
- Supplements: Fetal bovine serum (FBS), heat-inactivated FBS, HEPES, sodium bicarbonate, gentamicin sulfate, trypsin–EDTA.
- Cytotoxicity assay: MTT (3-(4,5-dimethylthiazol-2-yl)-2,5-diphenyltetrazolium bromide), phosphate-buffered saline (PBS), dimethyl sulfoxide (DMSO), 30% SDS solution, trypan blue dye, NaCl, K_2HPO_4.
- Adhesion and invasion assays: Matrigel® (Corning), BioCoat Matrigel invasion chambers (8 μm pore size, BD Biosciences), cotton swabs, glutaraldehyde (5%), Giemsa stain.
- Flow cytometry: Propidium iodide (PI), RNase A, Triton X-100, sodium citrate, BD FACSCanto II flow cytometer, FlowJo software.
- Western blot: SDS sample buffer (62.5 mM Tris-HCl, 2% SDS, 10% glycerol, 50 mM DTT), sonicator, 10% SDS-PAGE gels, nitrocellulose membrane, primary antibodies (e.g., for metastasis/cell cycle proteins), HRP-conjugated secondary antibodies, ECL detection reagent, ImageJ software.
- Equipment: CO_2 incubator, laminar flow hood, inverted microscope with camera, hemocytometer (Neubauer chamber), microplate reader (e.g., SpectraMax M2), electrophoresis and transfer apparatus for Western blot.

4 Detailed Procedures

4.1 Initial Cytotoxicity Screening and IC_{50} Determination

This section outlines the methods to screen peptides for their cytotoxic effects and calculate their half-maximal inhibitory concentration (IC_{50}).

4.1.1 Cell Culture Maintenance

1. Non-tumorigenic cell lines (melan-A, HaCaT): Culture in DMEM supplemented with 10% heat-inactivated FBS, 10 mM HEPES, 24 mM sodium bicarbonate, and 40 µg/mL gentamicin sulfate. Maintain at 37°C in a 5% CO_2 humidified incubator. Subculture at ~80% confluence using trypsin–EDTA.
2. Tumorigenic cell lines (B16F10-Nex2, A2058, JurKat, MCF-7, MDA-MB-231, SKBR-3, SiHa, U87): Culture in RPMI-1640 supplemented with 10% FBS, 10 mM HEPES, 24 mM sodium bicarbonate, and 40 µg/mL gentamicin. Maintain under the same conditions as above.

4.1.2 MTT Assay for Cell Viability [2]

1. MTT solution preparation: Dissolve 50 mg of MTT in 10 mL of PBS to achieve a concentration of 5 mg/mL. Filter-sterilize using a 0.22 µm filter and store at 4°C, protected from light.
2. Cell seeding and treatment: Seed cells at a density of 1×10^4 cells per well in 96-well plates and incubate for 24 h (37°C, 5% CO_2). Treat the cells with the test peptides at a range of concentrations (e.g., 15.6–500 µM) in triplicate. Include untreated controls (cells in medium only) and vehicle controls (cells with the solvent used for peptides). Incubate for 24 h.
3. MTT incubation and measurement: Add 5 µL of the MTT solution (5 mg/mL) to each well and incubate for 3 h (37°C, 5% CO_2). Carefully add 100 µL of 30% SDS to each well to solubilize the formazan crystals. Incubate the plate overnight in the dark at room temperature. Measure the absorbance at 570 nm using a microplate reader. Calculate cell viability as a percentage relative to the untreated control. Use these data to calculate the IC_{50} for each peptide on each cell line.

4.1.3 Trypan Blue Exclusion Assay for IC_{50} Validation [3]

1. Trypan blue solution preparation (0.4% stock): Dissolve 400 mg of trypan blue in 90 mL of Milli-Q water containing 810 mg NaCl and 60 mg K_2HPO_4. Adjust the volume to 100 mL. Heat to fully solubilize and adjust the pH to 7.2 using 1 N NaOH. Before use, dilute the stock to 0.2% with PBS and store at 4°C.
2. Cell viability assessment: Following peptide treatment (as in Sect. 4.1.2), harvest the cells by trypsinization. Mix 10 µL of the cell suspension with 10 µL of 0.2% trypan blue solution. Incubate for 2 min at room temperature. Load the mixture onto a hemocytometer and count the viable (unstained) and

non-viable (blue) cells. Calculate the percentage of viable cells and compare the IC_{50} values with those obtained from the MTT assay.

4.2 Mechanistic Studies on B16F10-Nex2 Melanoma Cells

Based on the IC_{50} results, select a lead peptide and one concentration (e.g., the IC_{50} or a fixed concentration like 500 µM) for the following functional assays. Include appropriate controls (e.g., a scrambled peptide, vehicle control) in all experiments.

4.2.1 Evaluation of Morphological Changes

1. Seed B16F10-Nex2 cells at 1×10^4 cells/well in a 96-well plate.
2. Treat the cells with the selected peptide concentration. Include an untreated control.
3. Incubate the plate at 37°C. For stress control, incubate a separate plate at 4°C.
4. Capture images at 0, 8, and 24 h post-treatment using an inverted microscope (20× magnification).
5. Analyze the images for morphological changes such as cell rounding, shrinkage, membrane blebbing, and detachment from the surface.

4.2.2 Anti-Proliferative Effects (Growth Kinetics)

1. Seed B16F10-Nex2 cells at 1×10^3 cells/well in multiple 96-well plates (one plate per time point). Allow cells to adhere for 4 h.
2. Treat cells with the selected peptide concentration. Include a vehicle control.
3. At 24, 48, and 72 h post-treatment, harvest the cells from one plate by trypsinization.
4. Perform a trypan blue exclusion assay (as in Sect. 4.1.3) to count viable cells.
5. Plot the number of viable cells against time to generate a growth curve. Calculate the population doubling time for treated and control cells.

4.2.3 Cell Adhesion Inhibition Assay [4, 5]

1. Substrate preparation: Coat wells of a 96-well plate with 50 µ L of Matrigel (diluted as per manufacturer's instructions) and allow to polymerize for 2 h at 37°C. For the monolayer condition, seed 1×10^5 cells/well in a separate 96-well plate and incubate overnight to form a confluent monolayer. Uncoated polystyrene wells will serve as the control substrate.
2. Cell pretreatment: Harvest B16F10-Nex2 cells and resuspend at a density suitable for seeding. Pre-incubate the cell suspension (containing 1×10^4 cells per well to be seeded) with the selected peptide concentration for 30 min at 37°C.

3. Adhesion phase: Transfer the pretreated cells (including the peptide) to the prepared wells (Matrigel-coated, monolayer, and uncoated polystyrene). Use 1×10^4 cells per well. Incubate for 4 h (37°C, 5% CO_2).
4. Quantification: Gently wash away non-adherent cells with PBS. Detach the adherent cells by trypsinization and count them using the trypan blue exclusion method.
5. Normalization: Calculate the number of adherent cells in the treated groups and express this as a percentage of the adhesion observed in the control group (RPMI + vehicle) for each substrate.

4.2.4 Wound-Healing Migration Assay

1. Seed B16F10-Nex2 cells at 2.5×10^5 cells/well in a 24-well plate. Incubate for 24 h to obtain a confluent monolayer.
2. Create a scratch ("wound") across the monolayer using a sterile P1000 pipette tip. Gently wash the wells with PBS to remove detached cells and debris.
3. Add fresh medium containing the selected peptide concentration. Include a vehicle control.
4. Capture images of the scratch wound at 0, 4, 8, and 24 h post-scratch, ensuring the same field is imaged each time.
5. Quantify the wound area at each time point using image analysis software (e.g., Wimasis, ImageJ). Calculate the percentage of wound closure relative to the 0-h time point.

4.2.5 Matrigel Invasion Assay [6, 7]

1. Matrigel preparation: Dilute Matrigel in ice-cold PBS according to the manufacturer's instructions (e.g., 1:3 ratio). Add 100 μL of the diluted Matrigel to the upper chamber of each Transwell insert (8 μm pores). Incubate for 30 min at 37°C to allow gelling.
2. Cell preparation and seeding: Harvest B16F10-Nex2 cells and resuspend them in serum-free RPMI. Pre-treat the cell suspension with the selected peptide concentration for 15 min at 37°C. Seed 2.5×10^5 cells in 500 μL of serum-free RPMI (containing the peptide) into the upper chamber of the Matrigel-coated inserts.
3. Chemoattractant: Add 500 μL of RPMI supplemented with 10% FBS to the lower chamber. For the negative control, add RPMI with vehicle to the lower chamber.
4. Incubation and staining: Incubate the plate for 24 h (37°C, 5% CO_2). After incubation, carefully remove the non-invaded cells from the upper surface of the membrane using a cotton swab. Fix the invaded cells on the lower surface of the membrane with 5% glutaraldehyde for 15 min and stain with Giemsa for 10 min.

5. Quantification: Count the stained cells on the membrane under a microscope at 4× magnification. Count at least five random fields per insert. Express the results as the percentage of invasion relative to the control (RPMI + vehicle in both chambers).

4.2.6 Cell Cycle Analysis by Flow Cytometry [8]

1. Cell synchronization: Seed B16F10-Nex2 cells at 2×10^5 cells/well in a 12-well plate. To synchronize the cell cycle, replace the medium with serum-free RPMI for 24 h.
2. Treatment: After synchronization, replace the medium with RPMI containing 10% FBS and the selected peptide concentration. Incubate for 24 h.
3. Staining: Harvest cells by trypsinization, wash with cold PBS, and pellet by centrifugation (240 × *g*, 5 min). Gently resuspend the cell pellet in 300 μL of a hypotonic propidium iodide (PI) staining solution (e.g., 50 μg/mL PI, 10 μg/mL RNase A, 0.1% Triton X-100, and 0.1% sodium citrate in PBS). Incubate for 1 h at 4°C in the dark.
4. Flow cytometry: Acquire the stained cells on a flow cytometer (e.g., BD FACSCanto II) with an excitation wavelength of 488 nm and measure emission at 617 nm. Analyze the DNA content histograms using software such as FlowJo to determine the percentage of cells in the G0/G1, S, and G2/M phases of the cell cycle, applying a model such as Dean–Jett–Fox.

4.2.7 Western Blot for Signaling Pathway Analysis [9]

1. Cell lysis: Treat 1×10^6 B16F10-Nex2 cells with the selected peptide concentration for 24 h. Wash cells with cold PBS and scrape them into 100 μL of ice-cold SDS sample buffer. Sonicate the lysate for 15 s (30% amplitude, pulse mode). Denature the samples by heating at 95°C for 5 min and centrifuge (240 × *g*, 10 min) to pellet debris. Store the supernatant containing proteins at −20°C.
2. Electrophoresis and transfer: Load equal amounts of protein (e.g., 20 μg) per lane onto a 10% SDS-PAGE gel and run at 100 V for 90 min. Transfer the separated proteins from the gel to a nitrocellulose membrane at 100 V for 1 h in transfer buffer (e.g., 1.2 mM Tris/glycine/20% methanol). Confirm transfer with Ponceau S staining.
3. Immunodetection: Block the membrane with 5% skim milk in TTBS (Tris-buffered saline with Tween 20) for 2 h at room temperature. Incubate the membrane with primary antibodies (diluted appropriately, e.g., 1:1000) overnight at 4°C. Wash the membrane three times with TTBS. Incubate with HRP-conjugated secondary antibodies (diluted appropriately, e.g., 1:5000) for 1 h at room temperature. Wash again with TTBS.

4. Detection and analysis: Apply an ECL detection reagent to the membrane and visualize the protein bands. Quantify the band intensities using image analysis software such as ImageJ, and normalize the expression levels of target proteins to a loading control (e.g., β-actin or GAPDH).

References

1. Mosmann T (1983) Rapid colorimetric assay for cellular growth and survival: application to proliferation and cytotoxicity assays. J Immunol Methods 65(1–2):55–63
2. van Meerloo J, Kaspers GJ, Cloos J (2011) Cell sensitivity Assays: The MTT Assay. Cancer cell Culture Methods in Molecular Biology, 731: 237–245. http://dx.doi.org/10.1007/978-1-61779-080-5_20
3. Strober W (2015) Trypan blue exclusion test of cell viability. Curr Protoc Immunol 111:A3.B.1–A3.B.3
4. Kleinman HK, Martin GR (2005) Matrigel: basement membrane matrix with biological activity. Sem Cancer Biol 15(5):378–386
5. Liang CC, Park AY, Guan JL (2007) In vitro scratch assay: a convenient and inexpensive method for analysis of cell migration in vitro. Nat Protoc 2(2):329–333
6. Albini A, Benelli R (2007) The chemoinvasion assay: a method to assess tumor and endothelial cell invasion and its modulation. Nat Protoc 2(3):504–511
7. Darzynkiewicz Z et al (2001). Analysis of cell cycle by flow cytometry. In: Checkpoint controls and cancer. Humana Press, pp 301–311
8. Towbin H, Staehelin T, Gordon J (1979) Electrophoretic transfer of proteins from polyacrylamide gels to nitrocellulose sheets: procedure and some applications. Proc Natl Acad Sci U S A 76(9):4350–4354
9. Schneider CA, Rasband WS, Eliceiri KW (2012) NIH Image to ImageJ: 25 years of image analysis. Nat Methods 9(7):671–675

Chapter 5

Comprehensive Assessment of Antiproliferative Activity and Topoisomerase Inhibition by Test Compounds in Cancer Cell Lines

Abstract

This protocol describes a comprehensive methodological approach for evaluating the antiproliferative activity of test compounds against cancer cell lines and investigating topoisomerase inhibition as a potential mechanism of action. The experimental workflow begins with detailed procedures for cell culture maintenance, including thawing, subculture, and viability assessment of adherent cell lines. Cytotoxicity screening is performed using the sulforhodamine B (SRB) colorimetric assay, which enables quantitative determination of growth inhibition (GI_{50} values) and calculation of selectivity indices by comparing activity against tumor cells versus normal VERO cells. For mechanistic studies, the protocol provides step-by-step instructions for preparing nuclear extracts from HT-29 colon carcinoma cells as a source of topoisomerase enzymes, followed by specific biochemical assays to evaluate topoisomerase I inhibition via DNA relaxation assays using pBR322 plasmid substrate and topoisomerase IIα inhibition via kinetoplast DNA (kDNA) decatenation assays. This integrated approach enables the identification of compounds with selective anticancer activity and elucidation of topoisomerase-mediated mechanisms, supporting rational drug discovery efforts.

Keywords SRB assay, Cytotoxicity, Topoisomerase inhibition, Nuclear extract, Selectivity index

1 Introduction

Cancer remains a leading cause of mortality worldwide, necessitating the discovery of novel chemotherapeutic agents. Topoisomerase enzymes are validated anticancer targets as they regulate DNA topology during replication and transcription. Compounds that inhibit these enzymes can induce DNA damage and apoptosis in rapidly dividing cancer cells [1]. This protocol describes a systematic approach to screen potential anticancer agents, beginning with cytotoxicity evaluation against cancer cell lines, assessing selectivity using normal cells, and subsequently investigating topoisomerase inhibition as a potential mechanism of action. To evaluate the cytotoxic potential and mechanism of action of test compounds/extracts through: (1) determination of growth inhibitory effects on cancer cell lines using the sulforhodamine B (SRB) assay, (2) assessment

Karuppusamy Arunachalam et al., *Advanced Protocols in Cancer Research*, Springer Protocols Handbooks,
https://doi.org/10.1007/978-1-0716-5348-7_5,

of selective cytotoxicity using normal VERO cells, and (3) investigation of topoisomerase I and IIα inhibitory activity as a potential mechanistic pathway.

2 Materials

- **Cell lines:** Cancer cell lines (e.g., HT-29, MCF-7, etc.), African green monkey kidney (VERO) cells.
- **Reagents:** Complete culture medium (e.g., RPMI-1640 with 10% FBS, 1% penicillin–streptomycin), trypsin–EDTA (0.25%), phosphate-buffered saline (PBS), dimethyl sulfoxide (DMSO), trypan blue (0.4%), sulforhodamine B (SRB), trichloroacetic acid (TCA), acetic acid, Tris base, positive controls (cisplatin, doxorubicin, camptothecin, etoposide), agarose, GelRed nucleic acid stain, TBE buffer.
- **Buffers:**
  - **TEMP buffer:** 10 mM Tris-HCl (pH 7.5), 1 mM EDTA, 4 mM $MgCl_2$, 0.5 mM PMSF, 0.5 mM DTT.
  - **TEP buffer:** 10 mM Tris-HCl (pH 7.5), 1 mM EDTA, 0.5 mM PMSF.
  - **Topoisomerase I buffer:** 10 mM Tris-HCl (pH 7.9), 1 mM EDTA, 150 mM NaCl, 0.1% BSA, 0.1 mM spermidine, 5% Glycerol.
  - **Topoisomerase II buffer:** 10 mM Tris-HCl (pH 7.9), 50 mM NaCl, 50 mM KCl, 5 mM $MgCl_2$, 0.1 mM EDTA, 15 μg/mL BSA, 1 mM ATP, 1 mM DTT.
  - **SDS stop solution:** 5% SDS, 0.025% bromophenol blue, 40% glycerol.
  - **Sarkosyl stop solution:** 5% sarkosyl, 0.0025% bromophenol blue, 50% glycerol.
- **DNA substrates:** pBR322 plasmid DNA (for Topo I), kinetoplast DNA (kDNA, for Topo IIα)
- **Equipment:** CO_2 incubator, biological safety cabinet, inverted microscope, centrifuge, water bath, hemocytometer, microplate reader (540 nm), electrophoresis system, UV transilluminator/gel documentation system, −80°C freezer, liquid nitrogen tank, refrigerated microcentrifuge, ultracentrifuge (optional).

3 Detailed Step-by-Step Experimental Procedures [2–5]

3.1 Cell Culture Maintenance and Preparation

3.1.1 Thawing and Revival of Cryopreserved Cells

1. Safety precautions: Wear appropriate PPE. Retrieve the cryovial from liquid nitrogen storage using forceps, wearing cryo-gloves.
2. Rapid thawing: Immediately immerse the vial in a pre-warmed 37°C water bath. Gently agitate until only a small ice crystal remains (~60–90 s). Do not submerge the cap.
3. Decontamination: Wipe the exterior of the vial with 70% ethanol before placing it in the biosafety cabinet.
4. Transfer and dilution: Slowly transfer the thawed cell suspension using a sterile pipette into a 15 mL conical tube containing 9 mL of pre-warmed complete culture medium. This dilutes the cryoprotectant (DMSO).
5. Centrifugation: Centrifuge at 200 × *g* (approximately 1000 rpm) for 4 min at room temperature to pellet cells.
6. Resuspension: Carefully aspirate the supernatant without disturbing the pellet. Gently resuspend the cell pellet in 5 mL of fresh, pre-warmed complete medium by pipetting up and down five to seven times.
7. Seeding: Transfer the entire cell suspension into a labeled T25 culture flask.
8. Incubation: Place the flask in a humidified incubator at 37°C with 5% CO_2.
9. Medium change: After 24 h, aspirate the old medium (which may contain residual DMSO and non-viable cells) and replace it with 5 mL of fresh complete medium. Monitor cells daily under an inverted microscope.

3.1.2 Subculture of Adherent Cells

1. Confirmation: Subculture when cells reach 80%–90% confluence.
2. Washing: Aspirate the spent medium. Gently wash the cell monolayer with 3 mL of sterile PBS to remove serum (which inhibits trypsin).
3. Trypsinization: Add 0.5 mL of pre-warmed 0.25% trypsin–EDTA solution to cover the monolayer. Incubate at 37°C for 3–5 min. Observe under the microscope until cells round up and detach.

4. Neutralization: Add 1.5 mL (3× the trypsin volume) of complete medium to neutralize the trypsin. Gently pipette the liquid over the surface to ensure complete cell detachment.
5. Collection: Transfer the cell suspension to a 15 mL conical tube.
6. Centrifugation and resuspension: Centrifuge at 200 × *g* for 4 min. Aspirate supernatant and resuspend the pellet in an appropriate volume of fresh medium.
7. Seeding: Perform a cell count (Sect. 3.1.3) and seed new flasks/plates at the desired density.

3.1.3 Cell Counting and Viability Assessment(Trypan Blue Exclusion)

1. Prepare sample: Mix 10 μL of the well-resuspended cell suspension with 40 μL of 0.4% trypan blue dye (1:5 dilution).
2. Load hemocytometer: After 1–2 min, pipette 10–15 μL of the mixture into one chamber of a clean hemocytometer.
3. Count cells: Under a microscope at 10× objective, count the live (unstained, bright) and dead (blue-stained) cells in the four large corner squares (each containing 16 smaller squares).
4. Calculation:

- $$\text{Total cells/mL} = (\text{Average count per square}) \cdot \times (\text{Dilution factor, } 5) \times 10^4$$
- $$\%\ \text{Viability} = [\text{Total live cells}/(\text{Total live} \cdot + \text{Total dead cells})] \times 100$$

3.2 Sample Preparation

3.2.1 Reconstitution of Lyophilized Test Samples

1. Weigh the required amount of lyophilized compound/extract in a sterile microcentrifuge tube.
2. Add the calculated volume of sterile, anhydrous DMSO to achieve a primary stock concentration of 100 mg/mL (or as required). Vortex vigorously for 2–3 min until completely dissolved.
3. Critical note: Store primary stocks at −20°C or −80°C in small aliquots to avoid repeated freeze–thaw cycles.

3.2.2 Preparation of Working Concentrations for Cell Treatment

1. Perform serial dilutions of the DMSO stock in complete culture medium to obtain the desired final testing concentrations (e.g., 250, 25, 2.5, 0.25 μg/mL).
2. Crucial control: Ensure the final concentration of DMSO in *any* well does not exceed 0.4% (v/v). Prepare a vehicle control containing the same highest final concentration of DMSO used in treated wells (typically 0.4%).
3. Prepare working solutions fresh on the day of the experiment.

3.3 SRB Cytotoxicity Assay

Day 0: Cell Seeding

1. Cell harvest: Trypsinize and count cells as in Sects. 3.1.2 and 3.1.3.
2. Adjust density: Dilute the cell suspension to the optimal seeding density in complete medium (e.g., 5000–10,000 cells/well for a 48 h assay, determined empirically per cell line).
3. Seed plates: Using a multichannel pipette, add 100 μL of the cell suspension to each well of a 96-well flat-bottom microplate, except for the blank wells (media only).
4. T0 Plate: Prepare an identical "T0" plate, which will be fixed immediately after cell attachment (step 6). This represents the cell mass at the time of treatment.
5. Attachment: Allow cells to settle for 15–30 min at room temperature in the biosafety cabinet to ensure even distribution.
6. Fix T0 plate: Incubate the main plate at 37°C, 5% CO_2. For the T0 plate, after 1–2 h, proceed directly to fixation.
7. Incubate the main plate for a full 24 h.

Day 1: Treatment

8. After 24 h incubation, visually confirm ~60%–70% confluence under a microscope.
9. Prepare treatment plate map: Label the plate to include in triplicate: test compound concentrations, positive control (e.g., 10 μM cisplatin), negative/viable control (0.4% DMSO vehicle), blank (medium only).
10. Aspirate and treat: Carefully aspirate the medium from all wells of the main plate using a multichannel aspirator. Avoid disturbing the monolayer.
11. Immediately add 100 μL of the appropriate test solutions (prepared in Sect. 2.2) to their designated wells.

Day 3: Fixation, Staining, and Solubilization (48 h Post-Treatment)

12. Fixation:
    a. Gently aspirate the treatment medium from all wells.
    b. Add 100 μL of ice-cold 20% (w/v) Trichloroacetic Acid (TCA) to each well to fix the cells.
    c. Incubate the plates at 4°C for 1 h to ensure complete protein precipitation.
13. Washing: Carefully discard the TCA by inverting and flicking the plate over a sink. Wash the plates five times by gently immersing them in a large tub of running tap water. This removes TCA, serum proteins, and low-molecular-weight metabolites. Tap the inverted plate on paper towels to remove

excess water and air-dry completely at room temperature (30–60 min).

14. Staining:
    a. Add 50 μL of 0.1% (w/v) sulforhodamine B dye (in 1% acetic acid) to each dry well.
    b. Incubate at room temperature for 30 min, protected from light.
15. Removal of unbound dye: Quickly aspirate the SRB solution. Wash the plates five times with 1% acetic acid to remove unbound dye. Ensure consistent washing across all wells. Invert, tap, and air-dry.
16. Solubilization:
    a. Add 100 μL of 10 mM unbuffered Tris base solution (pH ~10.5) to each well to solubilize the protein-bound dye.
    b. Place the plate on an orbital shaker for 15–20 min at room temperature to ensure complete and uniform solubilization.

Day 3: Absorbance Measurement and Data Analysis

a. Add 100 μL of 10 mM unbuffered Tris base solution (pH ~10.5) to each well to solubilize the protein-bound dye.
b. Place the plate on an orbital shaker for 15–20 min at room temperature to ensure complete and uniform solubilization.

17. Read the absorbance of each well at 540 nm using a microplate reader. Blank the reader against the "media-only" wells.
18. Data processing:
    - Calculate the mean absorbance for each test condition (triplicates).
    - Percent growth inhibition (GI%) is calculated according to the NCI guidelines as follows:
    - If T (mean Abs of test) $\geq$ CN (mean Abs of negative control) : Cell growth is not inhibited. GI% = 0 or use formula for stimulation.
    - If T_0 (mean Abs at time zero) $\leq T <$ CN: GI% = $100 \times [(T - T_0)/(CN - T_0)]$. This represents net growth inhibition.
    - If $T < T_0$: GI% = $100 \times [(T - T_0)/(T_0)]$. This represents net cell kill (cytotoxicity).
19. Dose–response analysis: Plot GI% against the logarithm of compound concentration. Use software (e.g., Origin 6.0, GraphPad Prism) to determine the GI_{50} value (concentration

causing 50% growth inhibition) via non-linear regression (four-parameter logistic curve).

20. Selectivity index (SI): Perform the SRB assay identically on normal VERO cells. Calculate the SI as:

$$SI = \frac{GI_{50}\ (\text{VERO cells})}{GI_{50}\ (\text{Tumor cell line})}$$

An SI ≥2 is typically considered indicative of selective antiproliferative activity against the cancer cell line.

3.4 Preparation of Nuclear Extract from HT-29 Cells (for Topoisomerase Source)

1. Cell harvest: Grow HT-29 cells in a T150 flask to 80%–90% confluence. Wash twice with 10 mL of ice-cold PBS.
2. Scraping: Add 5 mL of fresh, ice-cold PBS. Gently scrape the cells using a sterile cell scraper. Transfer the cell suspension to a pre-chilled 15 mL conical tube.
3. Pellet cells: Centrifuge at 150 × *g* for 10 min at 4°C. Aspirate the supernatant completely.
4. Hypotonic lysis: Resuspend the cell pellet in 1 mL of ice-cold TEMP buffer (containing protease inhibitors: 0.5 mM PMSF, 0.5 mM DTT added fresh). Homogenize gently by pipetting up and down 20 times with a 1 mL pipette tip. Do not vortex.
5. Incubation: Place the tube on ice for 10 min, gently swirling every 2–3 min.
6. Low-speed spin: Centrifuge at 1500 × *g* for 10 min at 4°C. This step pellets the nuclei.
7. Nuclear wash: Carefully discard the supernatant (cytoplasmic fraction). Resuspend the crude nuclear pellet in 1 mL of TEMP buffer by gentle pipetting. Centrifuge again at 1500 × *g* for 10 min at 4°C.
8. High-salt extraction: Resuspend the washed nuclear pellet in 4× its volume of TEP buffer. While vortexing at a low speed, slowly add an equal volume of TEP buffer containing 2 M NaCl (final NaCl concentration = 1 M). This step extracts nuclear proteins such as topoisomerases.
9. Vigorous extraction: Vortex the mixture at high speed for 15 s. Place on ice for 30–60 min, vortexing briefly every 10 min.
10. Ultracentrifugation: Transfer the mixture to pre-chilled ultracentrifuge tubes. Centrifuge at 100,000 × *g* for 1 h at 4°C. Alternatively, a high-speed microcentrifuge can be used: centrifuge at 15,000 × *g* for 30 min at 4°C.

11. Collection: Carefully collect the clear supernatant (the nuclear extract containing topoisomerases) without disturbing the pellet. Aliquot into small volumes.
12. Storage: Flash-freeze aliquots in liquid nitrogen and store at −80°C. Determine protein concentration using the Bradford or Lowry assay before use in enzymatic assays.

3.5 Topoisomerase Inhibition Assays

General Notes:

- Use purified human topoisomerase I/IIα or a characterized nuclear extract as the enzyme source.
- Include controls: Substrate DNA only, DNA + enzyme (shows relaxation/decatenation), DNA + enzyme + known inhibitor (camptothecin for Topo I, etoposide for Topo IIα).

3.5.1 Topoisomerase I Inhibition Assay (DNA Relaxation Assay)

1. Reaction setup (20 μL final volume):
   - Test reaction: 0.152 μg (or 100 ng) of supercoiled pBR322 DNA, 5 μL of nuclear extract (or 4 U of purified Topo I), 1× Topoisomerase I reaction buffer, and test compound at desired final concentration (e.g., 50–200 μM). Adjust volume with nuclease-free water.
   - Set up all controls.
2. Incubation: Mix gently by pipetting. Incubate the reaction mixtures at 37°C for 30 min in a thermal cycler or water bath.
3. Reaction termination: Add 4 μL of SDS stop solution to each tube and mix well. The SDS denatures the enzyme.
4. Gel electrophoresis:
   a. Prepare a 1% agarose gel in 1× TBE buffer.
   b. Load the entire 24 μL of each reaction mixture into the wells.
   c. Run the gel at 80–100 V for 45–60 min in 1× TBE buffer until the dye front has migrated sufficiently.
5. Visualization: Stain the gel in a GelRed solution (1× in water or TBE) for 20–30 min with gentle agitation. Destain in water for 10 min if background is high. Visualize under a UV transilluminator.
6. Interpretation: Supercoiled DNA (Form I) migrates fastest. Topo I relaxation converts it to nicked/open circular (Form II) and relaxed circular forms. Inhibition is indicated by the persistence of supercoiled DNA in test samples compared to the fully relaxed DNA in the "DNA + enzyme" control.

3.5.2 Topoisomerase IIα Inhibition Assay (kDNA Decatenation Assay)

1. Reaction setup (20 μL final volume):
   - Test reaction: 0.164 μg (or 200 ng) of catenated kinetoplast DNA (kDNA), 5 μL of nuclear extract (or 2 U of purified Topo IIα), 1× Topoisomerase II reaction buffer (including 1 mM ATP), and test compound. Adjust the volume with water.
   - Set up controls.
2. Incubation: Mix gently. Incubate at 37°C for 60 min.
3. Reaction Termination: Add 4 μL of Sarkosyl stop solution to each tube and mix.
4. Gel electrophoresis:
   a. Prepare a 1% agarose gel in 1X TBE.
   b. Load samples. Include a lane with marker DNA.
   c. Run at 80 V for 45–60 min.
5. Visualization: Stain with GelRed as above.
6. Interpretation: Intact kDNA remains in the well or migrates as a high-molecular-weight smear. Active Topo IIα decatenates it, releasing minicircle DNA products that migrate as a distinct, fast-moving band. Inhibition is indicated by the absence or reduction of these minicircle bands and the persistence of kDNA near the well.

References

1. Dignam JD, Lebovitz RM, Roeder RG (1983) Accurate transcription initiation by RNA polymerase II in a soluble extract from isolated mammalian nuclei. Nucleic Acids Res 11(5):1475–1489
2. Trask DK, Muller MT (1983) Biochemical characterization of topoisomerase I purified from avian erythrocytes. Nucleic Acids Res 11(9):2779–2800
3. Liu LF, Rowe TC, Yang L, Tewey KM, Chen GL (1983) Cleavage of DNA by mammalian DNA topoisomerase II. J Biol Chem 258(24):15365–15370
4. Vichai V, Kirtikara K (2006) Sulforhodamine B colorimetric assay for cytotoxicity screening. Nat Protoc 1(3):1112–1116
5. Skehan P, Storeng R, Scudiero D, Monks A, McMahon J, Vistica D et al (1990) New colorimetric cytotoxicity assay for anticancer-drug screening. J Natl Cancer Inst 82(13):1107–1112

Chapter 6

Evaluation of Cytotoxic Selectivity and Gene Expression Modulation by Novel Antitumor Compounds

Abstract

This protocol provides a comprehensive experimental framework for evaluating the selective cytotoxicity of novel synthetic compounds against human tumor cell lines compared to normal peripheral blood mononuclear cells (PBMCs), coupled with molecular analysis of gene expression modulation. The methodology encompasses PBMC isolation from healthy donors using Ficoll-Paque density gradient centrifugation, followed by MTT-based cytotoxicity assessment across multiple cancer cell lines, including HL-60, CCRF-CEM, MCF-7, and Jurkat cells. The calculation of selectivity indices (SI) enables quantitative assessment of tumor-specific cytotoxicity. For mechanistic investigations, the protocol details TRIzol-based RNA extraction from HL-60 cells, DNase treatment to eliminate genomic DNA contamination, cDNA synthesis using high-capacity reverse transcription kits, and quantitative real-time PCR (qPCR) employing TaqMan gene expression assays. Target genes include those involved in apoptosis (BID, RIP-3), cell cycle regulation (p21), stress responses (GADD153/CHOP), and nuclear receptor signaling (PPARγ), with 18S rRNA serving as the endogenous reference. Relative quantification using the $2^{-\Delta\Delta Ct}$ method enables determination of compound-induced transcriptional changes. Statistical analysis guidelines ensure rigorous data interpretation, establishing this protocol as a robust tool for both primary cytotoxicity screening and mechanistic gene expression studies in anticancer drug discovery.

Keywords PBMC isolation, Selective cytotoxicity, MTT assay, Gene expression, qPCR

1 Introduction

Novel anticancer compounds must demonstrate selective cytotoxicity toward tumor cells while sparing normal cells to minimize adverse effects. Peripheral blood mononuclear cells (PBMCs) from healthy donors serve as a model for non-cancerous human cells in selectivity assays. The cytotoxic potential of candidate molecules is commonly assessed using the MTT assay across various tumor cell lines [1]. Furthermore, to investigate the molecular mechanisms of action, quantitative real-time PCR (qPCR) is employed to evaluate the expression of genes involved in apoptosis, cell cycle regulation, and stress responses.

Karuppusamy Arunachalam et al., *Advanced Protocols in Cancer Research*, Springer Protocols Handbooks,
https://doi.org/10.1007/978-1-0716-5348-7_6,

2 Aim

To assess the selective cytotoxicity of new synthetic compounds against tumor cell lines compared to normal PBMCs, and to determine their effects on gene expression in HL-60 cells.

3 Materials

3.1 Reagents and Chemicals

- Ficoll-Paque PLUS (GE Healthcare).
- RPMI-1640 medium (GIBCO).
- Fetal bovine serum (FBS), heat-inactivated.
- Dimethyl sulfoxide (DMSO).
- MTT (Sigma-Aldrich).
- SDS 20% solution.
- TRIzol® Reagent (Invitrogen).
- Chloroform, Isopropanol, 75% ethanol.
- DNase I (Promega).
- Sodium acetate, pH 4.0–4.6.
- RNase/DNase-free water.
- High-Capacity cDNA Reverse Transcription Kit (Applied Biosystems).
- RNaseOUT (Invitrogen).
- TaqMan Gene Expression Assays (Applied Biosystems).

3.2 Cell Lines

- HL-60, HL-60/MX1, CCRF-CEM, NG97, T47D, Raji, Jurkat.

3.3 Equipment

- 96- and 6-well culture plates.
- CO_2 incubator (37°C, 5% CO_2).
- Neubauer chamber.
- Plate reader (e.g., EL808, BioTek).
- Real-time PCR system (ABI Prism 7900HT).
- Microcentrifuge.
- Vortex mixer.
- Spectrophotometer (BioPhotometer Plus, Eppendorf).

4 Experimental Procedure

4.1 Blood Collection and PBMC Isolation (Ficoll-Paque® Method)

Day 0–1:

1. **Blood Collection:**
   - Collect 20–30 mL of venous blood from healthy, non-smoking donors into sterile EDTA or heparin vacutainer tubes.
   - Process within 2 h of collection.
2. **PBMC Isolation:**
   - Dilute blood 1:1 with sterile PBS (e.g., 10 mL blood + 10 mL PBS).
   - Using a serological pipette, slowly layer 15 mL of diluted blood over 15 mL of Ficoll-Paque® PLUS (room temperature) in a 50 mL conical tube at a 45° angle to preserve the interface.
   - Centrifuge at 400 × *g* for 30–35 min at 18–20°C with no brake during deceleration.
   - Using a sterile transfer pipette, carefully collect the buffy coat layer (opaque interface containing PBMCs) into a fresh 50 mL tube.
   - Wash PBMCs by adding 30 mL of PBS, centrifuge at 300 × *g* for 10 min at 4°C.
   - Discard supernatant, resuspend pellet in 10 mL RBC lysis buffer (155 mM NH_4Cl, 12 mM $NaHCO_3$, 0.1 mM EDTA, pH 7.2–7.4), incubate for 10 min at 4°C.
   - Add 30 mL PBS, centrifuge at 300 × *g* for 10 min at 4°C.
   - Repeat wash with PBS once more.
3. **Cell Counting and Viability Assessment:**
   - Resuspend PBMC pellet in 5 mL complete RPMI-1640 (10% FBS, 1% Pen-Strep).
   - Mix 10 μL cell suspension with 10 μL 0.4% trypan blue.
   - Count using a Neubauer hemocytometer:
     - Viable cells appear bright/clear.
     - Non-viable cells stain blue.
     - Viability (%) = [Viable cells/(Viable + Non-viable)] × 100.
   - Acceptance criterion: Viability >98% before proceeding.
4. **PBMC Culture and Treatment:**
   - Adjust cell concentration to 2×10^6 cells/mL in complete RPMI-1640 + 20 ng/mL IL-2 (to maintain viability).
   - Seed 100 μL/well (2×10^5 cells) in 96-well flat-bottom tissue culture plates.

- Incubate for 24 h at 37°C, 5% CO_2.
- Prepare compound solutions in complete medium (from DMSO stocks, final DMSO ≤0.2%).
- Add 100 µL of medium containing 2× final concentrations (50, 100, 150 µM) for final concentrations of 25, 50, 75 µM.
- Include controls: untreated (medium only), vehicle control (0.2% DMSO), positive control (2 µM staurosporine).
- Incubate for 48 h before MTT assay.

4.2 Tumor Cell Culture and Cytotoxicity Assessment

4.2.1 Cell Line Maintenance and Plating

Day −1:

1. **Cell Culture:**
   - Maintain tumor cell lines (e.g., HL-60, MCF-7, etc.) in appropriate media (RPMI-1640 or DMEM + 10% FBS + 1% Pen-Strep).
   - Harvest cells in logarithmic growth phase (70%–80% confluency for adherent lines).
2. **Cell Seeding for Assay:**
   - Prepare single-cell suspensions, count, and adjust concentration:
     - **Adherent lines:** 2×10^4 cells/mL in complete medium.
     - **Suspension lines (HL-60):** 2×10^5 cells/mL.
   - Seed 100 µL/well in 96-well plates:
     - **Adherent:** 2000 cells/well.
     - **Suspension:** 20,000 cells/well.
   - Incubate 24 h at 37°C, 5% CO_2 for adherence/equilibration.

4.2.2 Compound Treatment and MTT Assay

Day 0–3:

1. **Compound Preparation:**
   - Prepare 50 mM stock solutions in DMSO, aliquot and store at −20°C.
   - On the day of treatment, prepare serial dilutions in complete medium to achieve 2× final concentrations.
   - Final concentrations typically: 1, 10, 25, 50, 75 µM (adjust based on preliminary screening).

- **Include controls:** medium only (blank), vehicle control (0.2% DMSO), positive control (10 μM cisplatin).

2. **Treatment:**
   - Remove 50 μL medium from each well.
   - Add 50 μL of 2× compound solution (or control medium).
   - Final well volume: 100 μL.
   - Incubate for 72 h at 37°C, 5% CO_2.
3. **MTT Assay Protocol:**
   - After 72 h, prepare 5 mg/mL MTT solution in PBS, filter-sterilize (0.22 μm).
   - Add 10 μL MTT solution per well (final 0.5 mg/mL).
   - Incubate for 3–4 h at 37°C, 5% CO_2 in the dark.
   - Do not remove medium. Add 85 μL of solubilization solution (20% SDS in 0.02 N HCl).
   - Cover plate with foil, incubate overnight at 37°C to dissolve formazan crystals completely.
   - Next day, gently mix plate on orbital shaker for 5 min.
   - Measure absorbance at 570 nm with reference at 630–690 nm.

4.3 Data Analysis and IC_{50} Determination [2]

4.3.1 Calculation of Cell Viability and Inhibition

1. **Corrected Absorbance Values:**
   - Subtract blank (medium + MTT + SDS, no cells) from all readings.
2. **Percentage Viability:**

$$\text{Viability}(\%) = \left[\frac{\text{Abs}_{\text{sample}} - \text{Abs}_{\text{blank}}}{\text{Abs}_{\text{vehicle control}} - \text{Abs}_{\text{blank}}}\right] \times 100$$

3. **Percentage Inhibition:**

$$\text{Inhibition } (\%) = 100 - \text{Viability } (\%)$$

4.3.2 IC_{50} Determination (GraphPad Prism v9.0+)

1. **Dose–Response Curve Fitting:**
   - Enter $\log_{10}$(concentration) vs. inhibition (%) data.

- Use nonlinear regression (curve fit) → [Agonist] vs. response—variable slope (four parameters).

2. **Four-Parameter Logistic Model:**

$$\Upsilon = \text{Bottom} + \frac{\text{Top} - \text{Bottom}}{1 + 10^{(\log IC_{50} - X)\times \text{HillSlope}}}$$

Where:

- Υ = Response (% Inhibition),
- $X = \log[\text{Compound}]$,
- Top/Bottom = plateaus,
- HillSlope = steepness.

3. **Quality Parameters:**
   - $R^2 > 0.90$.
   - 95% confidence interval for IC_{50}.
   - Hill slope between −5 and −0.5 (typically −1.0 to −3.0).

4. **Selectivity Index (SI):**

$$SI = \frac{IC_{50}(\text{PBMC})}{IC_{50}(\text{Tumor cell line})}$$

Interpretation: SI >3 indicates selective cytotoxicity toward tumor cells.

4.4 RNA Extraction, DNase Treatment, and cDNA Synthesis [3]

4.4.1 Total RNA Extraction (TRIzol® Method)

1. **Cell Treatment and Harvest:**
   - SeedHL-60 cells at 2×10^6 cells/well in six-wellplates (2 mL/well).
   - Treat with: test compounds (25 μM), amsacrine (100 nM), rosiglitazone (25 μM), vehicle control.
   - Incubate for 10 h at 37°C, 5% CO_2.
   - Transfer cells to 2 mL microcentrifuge tubes, centrifuge at 500 × *g* for 5 min at 4°C.
   - Wash pellet with 1 mL ice-cold PBS, centrifuge again.

2. **RNA Extraction:**
   - Add 800 μL TRIzol® Reagent, vortex vigorously for 15 s, incubate for 5 min at 25°C.

- Add 160 μL chloroform (0.2 volumes), shake vigorously for 15 s, incubate for 3 min at 25°C.
- Centrifuge at 12,000 × *g* for 15 min at 4°C.
- Transfer ~400 μL of the upper aqueous phase to a new tube.
- Add 500 μL isopropanol (0.5 volumes) + 1 μL GlycoBlue™ coprecipitant, mix by inversion.
- Incubate for 10 min at 25°C, then centrifuge at 12,000 × *g* for 15 min at 4°C.
- Wash pellet with 1 mL 75% ethanol (in DEPC-treated water), centrifuge at 7500 × *g* for 5 min at 4°C.
- Air-dry pellet for 5–7 min (do not over-dry).
- Dissolve in 20–30 μL RNase-free water, incubate for 10 min at 55–60°C with gentle mixing.

3. **Quantification and Quality Control:**
   - Measure absorbance at 260 nm and 280 nm using a spectrophotometer.
   - **Purity:** A260/A280 ratio of 1.9–2.1
   - **Concentration (μg/μL):** (A260 × 40 × dilution factor)/1000
   - Check RNA integrity by agarose gel electrophoresis (28S:18S ≈ 2:1) or Bioanalyzer (RIN >8.0).

4.4.2 DNase I Treatment

1. **Reaction Setup:**
   - For 4 μg total RNA in ≤8 μL volume:

Component	Volume
RNA (4 μg)	X μL
10× DNase I Buffer	2.0 μL
DNase I, RNase-free (1 U/μL)	2.0 μL
RNaseOUT™ (40 U/μL)	0.5 μL

2. **Incubation:**
   - Incubate for 30–60 min at 37°C.
   - Add 2 μL 50 mM EDTA, incubate for 10 min at 65°C to inactivate DNase I.

3. **RNA Precipitation:**
   - Add 2.2 μL 3 M sodium acetate (pH 5.2) + 66 μL 100% ethanol.
   - Mix, store overnight at −80°C or 2 h at −20°C.

- Centrifuge at 20,000×*g* for 30 min at 4°C.
- Wash with 200 μL 75% ethanol, centrifuge again at 20,000×*g* for 15 min at 4°C.
- Resuspend pellet in 20 μL RNase-free water.

4.4.3 cDNA Synthesis (High-Capacity cDNA Kit)

1. **Reaction Setup (20 μL total):**

Component	Volume
DNase-treated RNA (up to 2 μg)	X μL
10 × RT Buffer	2.0 μL
25 × dNTP Mix (100 mM)	0.8 μL
10 × RT Random Primers	2.0 μL

2. **Thermal Cycling:**
   - 25°C for 10 min (primer annealing).
   - 37°C for 120 min (reverse transcription).
   - 85°C for 5 min (enzyme inactivation).
   - Hold at **4°C.**
3. **Dilution and Storage:**
   - Dilute cDNA 1:5-1:10 with nuclease-free water.
   - Store at −20°C for short-term, −80°C for long-term.

4.5 Quantitative Real-Time PCR (qPCR) [4]

4.5.1 TaqMan® qPCR Setup

1. **Reaction Components (10 μL Total Volume):**

Reaction Component	Volume(μL)
TaqMan™Fast Advanced Master Mix (2×)	5.0
TaqMan™ Gene Expression Assay (20×)	0.5
cDNA template (diluted)	2.0
Nuclease-free water	2.5

2. **Assay Information:**
   - **Target genes:** PPARγ (Hs01115513_m1), p21 (Hs00355782_m1), BID (Hs00609632_m1), GADD153/CHOP (Hs00358796_g1), RIP-3 (Hs00819388_m1).
   - **Reference gene:** 18S rRNA (Hs03928990_g1).
   - **Include:** no-template control (NTC), no-reverse transcription control (NRT).

3. **qPCR Cycling Parameters (ABI Prism 7900HT):**
   - **Step 1:** 50°C for 2 min (UDG incubation).
   - **Step 2:** 95°C for 20 s (polymerase activation).
   - **Step 3 (40 cycles):** 95°C for 1 s → 60°C for 20 s.
   - **Dissociation curve:** 95°C for 15 s → 60°C for 1 min → 95°C for 15 s.

4.5.2 Data Analysis ($2^{-\Delta\Delta Ct}$ Method)

1. **Calculate ΔCt:**

$$\Delta Ct_{\text{sample}} = Ct_{\text{target gene}} - Ct_{\text{18S rRNA}}$$

2. **Calculate ΔΔCt:**

$$\Delta\Delta Ct = \Delta Ct_{\text{treated}} - \Delta Ct_{\text{vehicle control}}$$

3. **Calculate Fold Change:**

$$\text{Fold Change} = 2^{-\Delta\Delta Ct}$$

4. **Normalization:**
   - Vehicle control set to 1.0.
   - **Upregulation:** Fold change >1.5.
   - **Downregulation:** Fold change <0.67.

4.6 Statistical Analysis

4.6.1 Data Presentation and Analysis

1. **Data Format:**
   - All data presented as mean ± SEM of ≥3 independent biological replicates.
   - Each biological replicate = separate experiment on different days.
2. **Statistical Tests** [5]**:**
   - **Two-group comparisons:** Unpaired Student's *t*-test (two-tailed).
   - **Multiple group comparisons:** One-way ANOVA) followed by Bonferroni's post-hoc test.
   - **Dose–response data:** Nonlinear regression for IC_{50}.
   - **qPCR data:** One-way ANOVA on ΔCt values.

3. **Software and Settings:**
   - GraphPad Prism v9.0+ or Origin Pro 8.5+.
   - Significance level: $\alpha = 0.05$.
   - ***p*-value notation:** $*p < 0.05$, $**p < 0.01$, $***p < 0.001$, $****p < 0.0001$.
4. **Power Analysis:**
   - For animal studies: n = 8 per group ($\alpha = 0.05$, power = 80%).
   - For cell studies: n = 3–6 biological replicates.

4.6.2 Quality Control Parameters

Acceptance Criteria:

- MTT assay: CV between replicates <15%.
- RNA quality: A260/A280 = 1.9–2.1, RIN > 8.0.
- qPCR: Amplification efficiency = 90%–110%, $R^2 > 0.98$.
- cDNA synthesis: No amplification in NRT controls.
- Statistical power: ≥80% for main comparisons.

4.7 Safety and Compliance

4.7.1 Biosafety

- Perform all cell culture in Class II biosafety cabinet.
- Decontaminate waste with 10% bleach or autoclave.
- Use appropriate PPE: lab coat, gloves, safety glasses.

4.7.2 Ethical Compliance

- Human PBMC collection: Informed consent + IRB approval.
- Animal studies: IACUC approval following ARRIVE guidelines.
- Data management: FAIR principles (Findable, Accessible, Interoperable, Reusable).

4.7.3 Data Recording

- Electronic lab notebook for all procedures.
- Raw data files backed up in institutional repository.
- Metadata: Date, operator, reagent lot numbers, instrument calibrations.

References

1. Boyum A (1968) Isolation of mononuclear cells and granulocytes from human blood. Scand J Clin Lab Invest 21(97):77–89
2. Mosmann T (1983) Rapid colorimetric assay for cellular growth and survival. J Immunol Methods 65(1-2):55–63
3. Chomczynski P, Sacchi N (2006) Single-step method of RNA isolation. Nat Protoc 1(2):581–585
4. Livak KJ, Schmittgen TD (2001) Analysis of relative gene expression data using real-time quantitative PCR. Methods 25(4):402–408
5. Motulsky HJ (2014) Intuitive biostatistics, 4th edn. Oxford University Press

Chapter 7

Evaluation of the Cytotoxic and Antiproliferative Effects of Phytocompound on Human Glioblastoma Cell Lines

Abstract

This protocol outlines a comprehensive experimental approach for evaluating the in vitro anticancer potential of a phytocompound against human glioblastoma multiforme (GBM) cell lines U87-MG and U373-MG, with complementary molecular docking studies to predict potential protein targets. The methodology integrates multiple functional assays to characterize cytotoxic and antiproliferative effects, beginning with an MTT-based viability assessment to determine half-maximal inhibitory concentrations (IC_{50}) and calculate selectivity indices against non-tumoral HEK-293 cells. Mechanistic investigations include acridine orange/propidium iodide (AO/PI) dual staining coupled with confocal microscopy to discriminate between apoptotic and necrotic cell death morphologies, colony formation assays to evaluate clonogenic survival following compound exposure, and three-dimensional (3D) spheroid migration assays using the hanging drop method to assess inhibition of tumor cell invasiveness. The protocol further incorporates molecular docking simulations using Molegro Virtual Docker to predict binding interactions between the phytocompound and key oncogenic kinases implicated in GBM pathogenesis, including ERK1/2 (PDB: 5LCJ), JNK-1 (PDB: 2G01), and PKB/Akt (PDB: 1GZN). This integrated workflow combines phenotypic cellular assays with computational target prediction, providing a robust platform for both efficacy evaluation and mechanistic hypothesis generation in glioblastoma drug discovery.

Keywords Glioblastoma, Phytocompound, Cytotoxicity, Spheroid migration, Molecular docking

1 Introduction

Glioblastoma multiforme (GBM) is the most aggressive and common primary malignant brain tumor in adults, characterized by rapid proliferation, diffuse infiltration, and high resistance to conventional therapies [1]. The identification of novel compounds with selective cytotoxicity against glioma cells remains a critical area of oncology research. A newly synthesized or isolated chemical entity is of interest for its potential anticancer properties. This protocol outlines a comprehensive in vitro assessment of compound effects on glioma cell viability, proliferation, death mechanisms, and migration, using both two-dimensional (2D) and three-dimensional (3D) culture models. Complementary moleculardocking studies are included to predict potential protein targets involved in its mechanism of action.

Karuppusamy Arunachalam et al., *Advanced Protocols in Cancer Research*, Springer Protocols Handbooks, https://doi.org/10.1007/978-1-0716-5348-7_7,

2 Aim

To evaluate the in vitro anticancer potential of the compound against human glioblastomacell lines (U87-MG and U373-MG), assessing its cytotoxicity, selectivity, induction of cell death, inhibition of colony formation and migration, and to predict its interaction with key oncogenic kinases via molecular docking simulation.

3 Materials

3.1 Reagents and Consumables

- **Cell culture:** Dulbecco's modified Eagle's medium (DMEM), high glucose (Sigma-Aldrich®); fetal bovine serum (FBS) (GIBCO®); L-glutamine (Nutricell®); penicillin–streptomycin solution (10,000 U/mL and 10 mg/mL) (Sigma-Aldrich®); 0.25% trypsin–EDTA solution (GIBCO®); phosphate-buffered saline (PBS), pH 7.4 (Sigma-Aldrich®).
- **Test compound:** Synthesized (dissolved in DMSO to create a stock solution and stored at −20°C). Note: Final DMSO concentration in all assays must not exceed 0.5% (v/v).
- **Controls:** Demecolcine (positive control for cytotoxicity); Triton X-100 (1% v/v, positive control for cell lysis in MTT); DMSO (vehicle control).
- **Assay reagents:** Trypan blue solution (0.4%) (Sigma-Aldrich®); MTT reagent (3-(4,5-dimethylthiazol-2-yl)-2,5-diphenyltetrazolium bromide) (Sigma-Aldrich®); dimethyl sulfoxide (DMSO) (Dinâmica®); acridine orange (AO) (1 mg/mL); propidium iodide (PI) (1 mg/mL) (Thermo Fisher®); gentian violet solution; Annexin V-FITC Apoptosis Detection Kit (optional, for flow cytometry validation) (Thermo Fisher®); pharmacological blockers (as required for mechanistic studies).
- **Molecular docking:** software: Marvin Sketch (ChemAxon), Spartan'14 (Wavefunction), Molegro Virtual Docker 6.0.1 (Molexus). Protein Data Bank (PDB) IDs: 5LCJ (ERK1/2), 2G01 (JNK-1), 1GZN (PKB/Akt).

3.2 Cell Lines

- U87-MG (human glioblastoma, Grade IV; ATCC® HTB-14™).
- U373-MG (human glioblastoma, Grade III; ECACC 08061901).
- HEK-293 (human embryonic kidney; non-tumoral control; ATCC® CRL-1573™).

3.3 Equipment

- **Cell culture:** Class II biological safety cabinet (Telstar®); CO_2 incubator (37°C, 5% CO_2, humidified) (Panasonic®); inverted phase-contrast microscope (Olympus®).

- **General laboratory:** Refrigerated centrifuge (Hettich®); microplate reader (BioTek®); confocal laser scanning microscope (Leica®); electronic analytical balance (Shimadzu®); water bath (LAUDA®); digital shaker (IKA®).
- **Analysis:** Software: GraphPad Prism 8.0 (statistical analysis), ImageJ (colony and migration analysis).

4 Laboratory Working Protocol (Fig. 1)

4.1 *Cell Culture Maintenance*

1. Culture all cell lines in T-25 or T-75 flasks with complete growth medium: DMEM (high glucose) supplemented with 10% (v/v) FBS, 1% (v/v) L-glutamine, and 1% (v/v) penicillin–streptomycin.
2. Maintain cultures at 37°C in a humidified incubator with 5% CO_2.
3. Monitor cell confluence daily. Subculture cells when they reach 80%–90% confluence using 0.25% trypsin–EDTA.
4. For subculture: Aspirate medium, rinse with PBS, add trypsin, incubate at 37°C for ~3–5 min, neutralize with complete medium, centrifuge at 1400 rpm for 4 min, and resuspend pellet in fresh medium.
5. Determine cell count and viability using a Neubauer chamber and trypan blue exclusion (0.4%). Use only suspensions with > 95% viability for experiments.

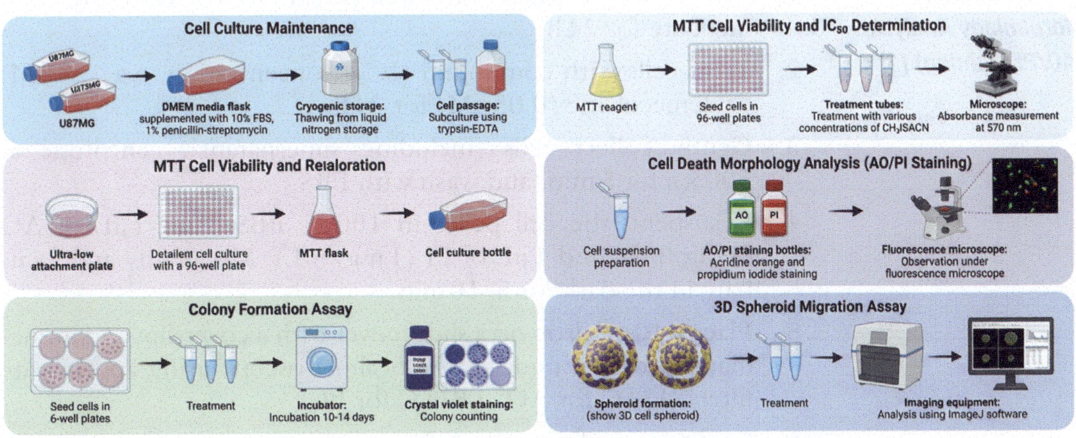

Fig. 1 Flowchart for evaluation of the cytotoxic and antiproliferative effects of phytocompound on human glioblastomacell lines

4.2 MTT Cell Viability and IC_{50} Determination [2]

1. Seed cells in 96-well plates at a density of 1×10^4 cells/well in 100 µL of complete medium. Include blank wells (medium only). Incubate for 24 h to allow adherence.
2. Prepare serial dilutions of compound and demecolcine in complete medium. Critical: Ensure final DMSO concentration is $\leq 0.5\%$.
3. Aspirate medium from the plate and add 100 µL of each drug concentration to the test wells. Include controls: negative control (complete medium + 0.5% DMSO), positive control (1% Triton X-100).
4. Incubate the plate for 24 h.
5. Add 10 µL of MTT stock solution (5 mg/mL in PBS) to each well. Incubate for 4 h at 37°C, protected from light.
6. Carefully remove the supernatant and add 100 µL of DMSO to each well to solubilize the formazan crystals. Shake gently for 10 min.
7. Measure the absorbance at 570 nm (reference 630 nm) using a microplate reader.
8. Calculate cell viability: % Viability = [(Abs Sample − Abs Blank)/(Abs Negative Control − Abs Blank)] × 100.
9. Determine the IC_{50} (concentration that inhibits 50% of cell viability) using non-linear regression analysis (e.g., log(inhibitor) vs. response in GraphPad Prism).
10. Calculate the selectivity index (SI): SI = IC_{50}(HEK-293)/IC_{50}(glioma cell line).

4.3 Cell Death Morphology Analysis (AO/PI Staining) [3]

1. Seed U87-MG cells in 24-well plates (1×10^4 cells/mL) and incubate for 24 h.
2. Treat cells with compound (IC_{50} concentration, e.g., 24 µM) or demecolcine (0.05 µM) for 24 h.
3. Gently collect cells (including supernatant), centrifuge at 500 × *g* for 5 min, and wash with PBS.
4. Resuspend the cell pellet in 100 µL PBS. Add 1 µL of AO (1 mg/mL) and 1 µL of PI (1 mg/mL). Mix gently and incubate in the dark for 5–10 min.
5. Place a 10 µL drop on a slide, cover with a coverslip, and immediately observe under a confocalmicroscope using appropriate filters (FITC for AO, TRITC for PI).
6. Categorize cells based on fluorescence:

   - **Viable:** Uniform green nucleus, intact structure.
   - **Early apoptotic:** Bright green nucleus with condensed or fragmented chromatin.

- **Late apoptotic:** Orange/red nucleus (AO+PI) with condensed chromatin.
- **Necrotic:** Uniform red nucleus (PI only), structure may be swollen.

4.4 Colony Formation Assay (Clonogenic Survival) [4]

1. Seed U87-MG cells at a low density (~200–500 cells/well) in 24-well plates in complete medium. Allow cells to attach for 6–8 h.
2. Treat cells with compound (e.g., 12 and 24 μM) or demecolcine. Include a vehicle control (0.2% DMSO). Incubate for 7–10 days, replacing the medium/treatment every 2–3 days.
3. Post-incubation, aspirate medium, wash wells gently with PBS.
4. Fix colonies with 100% methanol for 15 min at room temperature.
5. Stain with 0.5% gentian violet solution for 30 min.
6. Rinse thoroughly with tap water and air-dry the plate.
7. Image wells under a stereomicroscope. Count colonies (defined as aggregates of >50 cells) manually or using ImageJ software. Express results as % colony formation relative to the control.

4.5 3D Spheroid Migration Assay [5]

1. **Spheroid formation:** Using the "hanging drop" method, pipette 25 μL drops of a U87-MG cell suspension (4×10^4 cells/mL) onto the inner lid of a sterile Petri dish. Invert the lid over the dish filled with PBS to maintain humidity. Incubate for 72 h to form compact spheroids.
2. **Treatment:** Carefully transfer one spheroid per well to a 48-well ultra-low attachment plate. Allow to settle for 30 min. Add 1 mL of treatment per well: control medium, compound (12 and 24 μM), or demecolcine (0.05 μM).
3. **Imaging and analysis:** Capture bright-field images of each spheroid at the equatorial plane at time points: 0, 3, 6, 18, and 24 h post-treatment.
4. Using ImageJ, measure the total area covered by migrating cells at each time point.
5. Calculate the percentage of migration relative to the control group at $T = 0$ h. Perform statistical analysis using two-way ANOVA with Tukey's post-hoc test.

4.6 Molecular Docking Protocol [6]

1. **Protein preparation:** Download target proteinstructures(PDB: 5LCJ, 2G01, 1GZN) from the RCSB PDB. Remove water molecules and co-crystallized ligands (except for defining the active site) using MVD software. Add hydrogen atoms and assign charges.
2. **Ligand preparation:** Draw the 2D structure of compound and MK2206 (control) in Marvin Sketch. Optimize their 3D

geometry and minimize energy using the AM1 method in Spartan'14. Save in .mol2 format.

3. **Active site definition:** For proteins with co-crystallized inhibitors (5LCJ, 2G01), use the ligand's position to define the binding cavity. For 1GZN, use cavity detection tools based on known active site residues.
4. **Docking simulation:** Load the prepared protein and ligands into MVD 6.0. Set docking parameters: MolDock SE algorithm, grid resolution of 0.30 Å, search radius of 15 Å, ten runs per ligand.
5. **Analysis:** Evaluate the best pose for each ligand based on the MolDock score (kcal/mol) and rerank score. Analyze key hydrogen bonds, hydrophobic, and electrostatic interactions with amino acid residues in the active site.
6. **Validation:** Re-dock the native co-crystallized ligand and calculate the RMSD between the docked and original pose. An RMSD <2.0 Å indicates a reliable docking protocol.

4.7 Statistical Analysis

- Perform all experiments in at least three independent replicates ($n = 3$), each with technical triplicates.
- Express data as mean ± standard error of the mean (SEM).
- Use GraphPad Prism 8.0 for analysis. Compare multiple groups using one-way or two-way ANOVA, followed by Tukey's post-hoc test.
- A p-value <0.05 is considered statistically significant.

References

1. Franken NA, Rodermond HM, Stap J, Haveman J, van Bree C (2006) Clonogenic assay of cells in vitro. Nat Protoc 1(5):2315–2319
2. Gao W et al (2020) The application of acridine orange staining in the assessment of apoptosis. Methods Mol Biol 2115:195–200.
3. Mosmann T (1983) Rapid colorimetric assay for cellular growth and survival: application to proliferation and cytotoxicity assays. J Immunol Methods 65(1-2):55–63
4. Robbins E, Marcus PI (1963) Dynamics of acridine orange-cell interaction. J Cell Biol 18(2):237–250
5. Sousa F et al (2023) Confocal microscopy for apoptosis detection in glioma cells. STAR Protoc 4(1):102039
6. Thomsen R, Christensen MH (2006) MolDock: a new technique for high-accuracy molecular docking. J Med Chem 49(11):3315–3321

Chapter 8

Hemolytic Activity Assay

Abstract

This protocol describes a standardized hemolytic activity assay for evaluating the membrane-disrupting potential of test compounds using mouse erythrocytes as a model system. The method is based on spectrophotometric quantification of hemoglobin release following exposure of red blood cells to increasing concentrations of test substances, providing a direct measure of membrane damage that correlates with general cytotoxicity. Blood collected from Swiss mice via orbital plexus is processed to obtain a washed 2% erythrocyte suspension, which is then incubated with serial dilutions of test compounds (ranging from 3.9 to 200 μg/mL) in 96-well microplates for 1 h at room temperature. Following incubation and centrifugation, the supernatant absorbance is measured at 540 nm, with 1% Triton X-100 serving as the positive control for 100% hemolysis and saline as the negative control for spontaneous hemoglobin release. The percentage of hemolysis is calculated using a standardized formula, and results are expressed as mean ± SEM from independent experiments, with statistical significance determined by one-way ANOVA followed by the Student–Newman–Keuls post-hoc test. This assay provides essential preliminary data on the membrane-toxic potential of candidate compounds, serving as a crucial biocompatibility screen prior to advanced preclinical evaluation.

Keywords Hemolysis, Erythrocytes, Membrane disruption, Cytotoxicity, Biocompatibility

1 Introduction

The hemolytic assay is a well-established in vitro method used to assess the potential of chemical substances to disrupt cell membranes, particularly red blood cells (RBCs). This assay provides insight into the membrane-damaging activity of test compounds, which may indicate general cytotoxicity [1]. When erythrocytes are exposed to harmful agents, hemoglobin is released into the surrounding medium and can be quantified spectrophotometrically.

2 Aim

To evaluate the hemolytic potential of test compounds by measuring their ability to cause membrane disruption in mouse erythrocytes.

Karuppusamy Arunachalam et al., *Advanced Protocols in Cancer Research*, Springer Protocols Handbooks,
https://doi.org/10.1007/978-1-0716-5348-7_8,

3 Materials

- **Biological material**: Blood from Swiss *Mus musculus* mice (three animals).
- **Reagents**:
  - Saline solution (0.85% NaCl + 10 mM $CaCl_2$).
  - Test compounds (dissolved in DMSO; stock: 2000 μg/mL).
  - Triton X-100 (1% solution as positive control).
- **Equipment:**
  - 96-well flat-bottom microplates.
  - Micropipettes and sterile tips.
  - Centrifuge (capable of 1500 and 5000 rpm).
  - Spectrophotometer or microplate reader (540 nm).
  - Orbital shaker or gentle rocker.
- **Others:**
  - Anesthetic for animal handling (per ethical protocol).
  - Ice, tubes, gloves, lab coat.

4 Step-by-Step Laboratory Protocol [2, 3]

4.1 Blood Collection and Erythrocyte Preparation

1. Anesthetize three Swiss mice and collect blood via the orbital plexus.
2. Immediately dilute the pooled blood in 30 volumes of cold saline solution (0.85% NaCl + 10 mM $CaCl_2$).
3. Centrifuge at 1500 rpm for 3 min.
4. Discard the supernatant and repeat the wash twice.
5. Resuspend the washed erythrocytes in saline to obtain a 2% suspension.

4.2 Sample Preparation and Plate Setup

1. Prepare test sample stock solutions in DMSO (2000 μg/mL).
2. Set up a 96-well plate with the following layout:
   - Row 1: 100 μL of saline (blank control).
   - Row 2: 50 μL saline + 50 μL 10% DMSO (vehicle control).
   - Row 3: 100 μL saline + 100 μL test compound (starting conc.).
   - Rows 4–11: Serial 1:2 dilutions from Row 3 to create a concentration range of 3.9–200 μg/mL.
   - Row 12: 80 μL saline + 20 μL Triton X-100 (positive control).

3. Add 100 μL of 2% erythrocyte suspension to all wells.

4.3 Incubation and Hemolysis Detection

1. Incubate the plate at room temperature (26 ± 2°C) for 1 h on an orbital shaker or with gentle agitation.
2. Centrifuge the plate at 5000 rpm for 3 min.
3. Transfer 100 μL of supernatant from each well to a new microplate.
4. Read absorbance at 540 nm using a microplate reader.

4.4 Data Analysis

4.4.1 Calculation of Hemolysis Percentage

The percentage of hemolysis for each test sample was calculated using the following formula:

$$\text{Hemolysis }(\%) = \frac{A_{\text{sample}} - A_{\text{PBS}}}{A_{\text{Triton X}-100} - A_{\text{PBS}}} \times 100$$

Where:

- A_{sample} = Absorbance of the test sample (compound + erythrocytes).
- A_{PBS} = Absorbance of the negative control (PBS + erythrocytes), representing spontaneous hemolysis (0%).
- $A_{\text{Triton X}-100}$ = Absorbance of the positive control (1% Triton X-100 + erythrocytes), representing 100% hemolysis.

4.4.2 Data Presentation

Results for each experimental condition are presented as the mean ± standard error of the mean (SEM) from *n* independent experiments.

4.4.3 Statistical Analysis

Statistical significance was determined using one-way analysis of variance (ANOVA). When ANOVA indicated a significant difference ($p < 0.05$), post-hoc comparisons between groups were performed using the Student–Newman–Keuls (SNK) test. A *p*-value of less than 0.05 was considered statistically significant.

References

1. Adhikari A, Mondal S, Biswas P, Paul P, Bhattacharya S, Pal U, Bhattacharyya M (2019) Hemocompatible cationic polymers: a rationale for the molecular design. J Mater Chem B 7(43):6752–6765. https://doi.org/10.1039/C9TB01658H
2. Fotakis G, Timbrell JA (2006) In vitro cytotoxicity assays: comparison of LDH, neutral red, MTT and protein assay in hepatoma cell lines following exposure to cadmium chloride. Toxicol Lett 160(2):171–177. https://doi.org/10.1016/j.toxlet.2005.07.001
3. Mohan P, Rapoport N (2010) Doxorubicin as a molecular nanotheranostic agent: effect of doxorubicin encapsulation in micelles or nanoemulsions on the ultrasound-mediated intracellular delivery and nuclear trafficking. Mol Pharm 7(6):1959–1973. https://doi.org/10.1021/mp100269f

Part II

Mechanistic and Molecular Pharmacology

Check for updates

Chapter 9

Evaluation of DNA Intercalation and Oxidative Cleavage by Bioactive Compounds

Abstract

This protocol describes a comprehensive experimental approach for evaluating the DNA intercalation and oxidative cleavage potential of naphthoquinone compounds, combined with in vitro biological assays to assess their cytotoxic and genotoxic effects on MCF-7 breast adenocarcinoma cells. The methodology integrates biophysical and cell-based techniques to elucidate mechanisms of DNA interaction and cellular responses. DNA intercalation is assessed using the ethidium bromide displacement assay, where test compounds compete with intercalated ethidium bromide for binding sites on calf thymus DNA (CT-DNA), resulting in fluorescence quenching measured at 492/620 nm. Oxidative DNA cleavage is evaluated by quantifying thiobarbituric acid (TBA)-reactive species following compound exposure, with absorbance measured at 532 nm to detect propenal–TBA complex formation indicative of ROS-mediated DNA degradation. Complementary cell-based assays include MTT viability testing to determine half-maximal inhibitory concentrations (IC_{50}), intracellular ROS measurement using the DCFH-DA fluorescent probe, comet assay for direct visualization of DNA fragmentation, colony formation assays to assess long-term antiproliferative effects, and Western blotting to detect apoptosis-related proteins, including cleaved caspase-3, PARP, p53, Bcl-2, Bax, cyclin D1, and p21. All assays are performed with and without sodium ascorbate co-treatment to investigate redox-dependent mechanisms, providing an integrated workflow for characterizing the DNA-targeting and anticancer properties of naphthoquinones.

Keywords DNA intercalation, Oxidative cleavage, Naphthoquinones, MCF-7 cells, Comet assay

1 Introduction

Naphthoquinones are bioactive quinonoid compounds known for their redox properties, which allow them to interact with cellular macromolecules such as DNA. Their ability to intercalate into DNA and induce oxidative cleavage is linked to their cytotoxic and therapeutic potential, particularly in cancer research. Understanding these interactions is essential for assessing the genotoxic or chemotherapeutic properties of such compounds [1].

Karuppusamy Arunachalam et al., *Advanced Protocols in Cancer Research*, Springer Protocols Handbooks, https://doi.org/10.1007/978-1-0716-5348-7_9,

2 Aim

To investigate the DNA intercalation and oxidative cleavage potential of naphthoquinones in vitro using calf thymus DNA (CT-DNA) and standard spectroscopic assays [2].

3 Materials: Chemical Reagents and Antibodies (Sect. 4.1)

- **Cell Culture Reagents**: Dulbecco's modified Eagle's medium (DMEM), fetal bovine serum (FBS), and antibiotics (Gibco, USA).
- **Chemical Reagents** (Sigma-Aldrich, USA):
  - Juglone, sodium ascorbate, CT-DNA, agarose, DMSO.
  - DCFH-DA, DTNB, BSA, ethidium bromide, TBA.
  - Protease inhibitor cocktail, catalase (CAT), glutathione reductase.
  - NADPH, doxorubicin.
- **Other Reagents:**
  - 80-phosphate inhibitor cocktail (Calbiochem, Merck Biosciences).
  - Chemiluminescent kit for HRP-based protein detection (Millipore, USA).
- All other reagents were of ACS-grade purity.

4 Experimental Procedures

4.1 Evaluation of DNA Intercalation Using Ethidium Bromide Displacement Assay

1. **Objective**
   To assess the ability of naphthoquinones to intercalate into calf thymus DNA (CT-DNA) using fluorescence displacement of ethidium bromide (EtdBr) as an indicator.
2. **Materials Required**
   - CT-DNA (calf thymus DNA).
   - Ethidium bromide (EtdBr).
   - Naphthoquinones (test compounds).
   - Sodium ascorbate.
   - Doxorubicin (positive control).
   - 50 mM phosphate buffer (pH 7.4) containing 0.1 M NaCl.
   - Distilled water.
   - TECAN Infinite M200 microplate reader.

- 96-well black flat-bottom microplates.
- Micropipettes and tips.
- Vortex mixer.

3. **Preparation of Solutions**
   1. CT-DNA Stock: Dissolve CT-DNA in 50 mM phosphate buffer containing 0.1 M NaCl to make a 12.17 mM stock solution. Store at 4°C.
   2. Working DNA Solution: Dilute CT-DNA to 10 µM in the same buffer before use.
   3. Ethidium Bromide: Prepare a 1 mM stock solution in distilled water. Protect from light.
   4. Naphthoquinone Solutions: Prepare 10 mM stock solutions in DMSO and dilute to final concentrations of 0–50 µM with buffer.
   5. Ascorbate: Prepare a 100 mM stock in distilled water. Dilute to 1 mM as required.
   6. Doxorubicin Control: Prepare 10 mM stock in water or DMSO and dilute to 0–50 µM.

4. **Procedure**
   1. **Fluorescence Binding Assay Setup:**
      - In each well of a 96-well black microplate, add:
        - 100 µL of 10 µM CT-DNA solution.
        - 1 µM Ethidium bromide.
      - Incubate for 10 min at room temperature to ensure binding.
   2. **Determining Saturation Concentration:**
      - To determine DNA saturation with EtdBr, vary CT-DNA concentrations (1–100 µM) and measure fluorescence to determine optimal binding (saturation typically occurs at 3 µM DNA).
   3. **Intercalation Assay:**
      - Add increasing concentrations of naphthoquinones (0, 1, 5, 10, 20, 30, 40, and 50 µM) to separate wells containing the DNA–EtdBr complex.
      - Set up additional wells with 1 mM sodium ascorbate to assess redox-dependent intercalation.
      - Mix gently and incubate for 10 min at room temperature in the dark.

4. **Fluorescence Measurement:**
   - Measure fluorescence using the TECAN Infinite M200 reader with:
     - **Excitation wavelength:** 492 nm.
     - **Emission wavelength:** 620 nm.
5. **Positive Control:**
   - Include wells with doxorubicin (0–50 μM) as a standard intercalating compound.
6. **Data Analysis:**
   - A decrease in fluorescence intensity compared to the DNA–EtdBr control indicates displacement due to intercalation by the test compound.

4.2 Evaluation of Oxidative Cleavage of DNA by Naphthoquinones

1. **Objective**
   To evaluate the ability of naphthoquinones to induce oxidative cleavage of CT-DNA through the generation of reactive oxygen species (ROS), using thiobarbituric acid (TBA) reaction as an indicator of DNA degradation [3].
2. **Materials Required**
   - CT-DNA (0.5 mM working concentration).
   - Naphthoquinones (10 μM).
   - Sodium ascorbate (1 mM).
   - Thiobarbituric acid (TBA) 1% in 50 mM NaOH.
   - Glacial acetic acid.
   - Positive control: $[Fe(EDTA)]^{2-}$ (100 μM) + H_2O_2 (10 mM).
   - 50 mM phosphate buffer (pH 7.2).
   - Eppendorf tubes (1.5 mL).
   - Water bath or dry heating block (100°C).
   - Ice bath or refrigerator.
   - Spectrophotometer or TECAN Infinite M200 reader.
   - Micropipettes and tips.
3. **Preparation of Solutions**
   1. CT-DNA: Prepare a 0.5 mM solution in 50 mM phosphate buffer (pH 7.2).
   2. Naphthoquinones: Prepare 10 mM stock in DMSO; dilute to 10 μM.
   3. Ascorbate: Prepare 100 mM stock; dilute to 1 mM.

4. TBA Solution: Dissolve 1% TBA in 50 mM NaOH freshly.
5. Acetic Acid: Use glacial acetic acid as provided.

4. **Procedure**

1. **Sample Setup:**
   - In 1.5 mL microcentrifuge tubes, add:
     - 100 μL of 0.5 mM CT-DNA.
     - 10 μM naphthoquinones (test compound).
     - 1 mM sodium ascorbate (optional).
     - Make up the volume to 500 μL with phosphate buffer.
   - Prepare the following groups:
     - Test (naphthoquinones ± ascorbate).
     - Negative control (no naphthoquinones or ascorbate).
     - Positive control ($[Fe(EDTA)]^{2-}$ + H_2O_2).
2. **Incubation:**
   - Incubate all tubes at 37°C for 2 h.
3. **Reaction with TBA:**
   - After incubation, add:
     - 500 μL of 1% TBA in NaOH.
     - 500 μL glacial acetic acid.
     - Final ratio = 1:1:1 (sample:TBA:acetic acid).
   - Mix gently and incubate at 100 °C for 30 min using a heating block or water bath.
4. **Cooling:**
   - Immediately transfer the tubes to ice to stop the reaction.
5. **Measurement:**
   - Measure the absorbance at 532 nm using a spectrophotometer or microplate reader.
6. **Data Interpretation:**
   - An increase in absorbance at 532 nm indicates formation of the propenal–TBA complex, suggesting oxidative DNA cleavage.

- Compare the absorbance values of test samples to controls to assess the oxidative potential of the test compounds.

4.3 In Vitro Biological Assays

4.3.1 MCF-7 Cell Culture

1. **Objective**
   To culture and maintain human breast adenocarcinoma cells (MCF-7) under optimal conditions for experimental assays.
2. **Materials**
   - MCF-7 cell line (Cell Bank of Rio de Janeiro, Brazil).
   - Dulbecco's modified Eagle's medium (DMEM, Gibco).
   - Fetal bovine serum (FBS), heat-inactivated.
   - Penicillin (100 U/mL).
   - Streptomycin (100 μg/mL).
   - Trypsin–EDTA (0.25%).
   - Phosphate-buffered saline (PBS, pH 7.4).
   - T-25 or T-75 tissue culture flasks.
   - CO_2 incubator (37°C, 5% CO_2, 95% humidity).
   - Biosafety cabinet.
   - Inverted phase contrast microscope.
3. **Procedure**
   1. **Thawing Cells**
      - Quickly thaw frozen MCF-7 vial in a 37°C water bath (~1–2 min).
      - Transfer contents to a 15 mL tube containing 10 mL warm DMEM.
      - Centrifuge at 200 × *g* for 5 min; discard supernatant.
      - Resuspend the pellet in 5 mL complete DMEM (DMEM + 10% FBS + antibiotics).
      - Transfer to a T-25 flask and incubate at 37°C, 5% CO_2.
   2. **Routine Maintenance**
      - Replace medium every 48–72 h.
      - When confluency reaches ~80%–90%, passage the cells.
   3. **Passaging Cells**
      - Aspirate old medium, wash once with sterile PBS.
      - Add trypsin–EDTA and incubate at 37°C for 3–5 min.

- Add fresh medium to neutralize trypsin.
- Centrifuge and resuspend cells for counting and reseeding.

4.3.2 Cell Viability Assay (MTT Assay)

1. **Objective**
   To evaluate the cytotoxic effects of naphthoquinones on MCF-7 cells by measuring mitochondrial dehydrogenase activity via the MTT reduction assay.
2. **Materials**
   - Cultured MCF-7 cells.
   - Naphthoquinones (diluted in DMSO).
   - Sodium ascorbate (1 mM).
   - MTT reagent (3-(4,5-dimethylthiazol-2-yl)-2,5-diphenyl tetrazolium bromide), 5 mg/mL in PBS.
   - DMSO (for formazan solubilization).
   - DMEM complete medium.
   - 96-well culture plates.
   - Multichannel pipette.
   - Microplate reader (TECAN Infinite M200 or equivalent).
   - Sterile 0.22 μm filter.
3. **Procedure**
   1. **Seeding Cells**
      - Plate 1×10^4 MCF-7 cells per well in a 96-well plate.
      - Incubate for 24 h to allow cell attachment.
   2. **Treatment**
      - Remove medium and add 200 μL of fresh medium containing:
        - Naphthoquinones (0–80 μM), with or without 1 mM ascorbate.
        - Control wells with 1% DMSO as vehicle control.
      - Incubate for 24 h.
   3. **MTT Incubation**
      - Add 20 μL of MTT solution (5 mg/mL) to each well.
      - Incubate for 4 h at 37°C in the dark.
   4. **Formazan Solubilization**
      - Remove medium carefully.
      - Add 100 μL of DMSO per well.
      - Shake gently for 10 min to dissolve formazan crystals.

5. **Measurement**
   - Measure absorbance at 540 nm using a microplate reader.
6. **Data Analysis**
   - Perform all treatments in triplicate.
   - Calculate percent viability relative to control and determine IC_{50} using GraphPad Prism software.

4.3.3 Intracellular ROS Measurement (DCFH-DA Assay)

1. **Objective**
   To measure the level of intracellular reactive oxygen species (ROS) in MCF-7 cells following treatment, using DCFH-DA as a fluorescent probe.
2. **Materials**
   - MCF-7 cells.
   - DCFH-DA (10 μM working concentration).
   - Hank's Balanced Salt Solution (HBSS)
   - Naphthoquinones (2.5, 5, 10, 20 μM).
   - Sodium ascorbate (1 mM).
   - 96-well black plates with clear bottoms.
   - TECAN Infinite M200 plate reader.
3. **Procedure**
   1. **Seeding Cells**
      - Seed 15,000 cells per well in a black 96-well plate.
      - Incubate for 24 h for attachment.
   2. **Loading with DCFH-DA**
      - Remove medium and wash cells with HBSS.
      - Add 100 μL of 10 μM DCFH-DA in HBSS per well.
      - Incubate at 37°C for 30 min, protected from light.
   3. **Treatment**
      - Remove excess dye and wash once with HBSS.
      - Add 100 μL of treatment medium containing naphthoquinones ± ascorbate.
      - Incubate for 2 h at 37°C.
   4. **Post-treatment Wash**
      - Wash twice with HBSS.
      - Add 100 μL HBSS for fluorescence reading.

5. **Measurement**
   - Measure fluorescence at:
     - Excitation: 485 nm.
     - Emission: 530 nm.
6. **Data Analysis**
   - Calculate ROS increase using the formula:
     $\Delta F = (F - F_0)/F_0$,
     where F = post-treatment fluorescence, F_0 = baseline fluorescence.

4.3.4 DNA Fragmentation Assay (Comet Assay)

1. **Objective**
   To evaluate the extent of DNA fragmentation in MCF-7 cells after treatment using the alkaline comet assay.
2. **Materials**
   - MCF-7 cells.
   - Naphthoquinones (25, 50, 75 μM).
   - Sodium ascorbate (1 mM).
   - Doxorubicin (positive control).
   - Trypsin–EDTA.
   - PBS (pH 7.4).
   - Normal melting agarose (1%).
   - Low-melting-point agarose (0.5%).
   - Microscope slides.
   - Coverslips.
   - Lysis solution (2.5 M NaCl, 100 mM EDTA, 10 mM Tris, 1% Triton X-100, 10% DMSO, pH 10).
   - Electrophoresis buffer (300 mM NaOH, 1 mM EDTA, pH 13).
   - Electrophoresis unit (horizontal tank).
   - Fluorescent DNA dye (e.g., ethidium bromide or SYBR Green).
   - Fluorescencemicroscope with imaging software.
3. **Procedure**
   1. **Cell Seeding and Treatment**
      - Plate 5×10^4 MCF-7 cells per well in a 24-well plate.
      - After 24 h, treat with test compounds for an additional 24 h.
   2. **Harvesting Cells**

- Wash with PBS, trypsinize, and neutralize with complete medium.
- Centrifuge at 1000 × *g* for 10 min. Discard supernatant.

3. **Embedding Cells**
   - Resuspend pellet in 100 μL of 0.5% low-melting agarose (42°C).
   - Drop onto pre-coated slides (1% normal agarose).
   - Place coverslip and cool at 4°C for 5 min to solidify.
4. **Lysis**
   - Remove coverslip and immerse slides in cold lysis solution at 4°C for 2 h.
5. **DNA Unwinding**
   - Place slides in alkaline buffer for 20 min at 4°C to unwind DNA.
6. **Electrophoresis**
   - Perform electrophoresis at 25 V and 300 mA for 20 min at 4°C.
7. **Neutralization and Staining**
   - Neutralize with PBS or Tris buffer (pH 7.5), stain with DNA dye.
   - Store slides in a humid chamber protected from light until analysis.
8. **Microscopy**
   - Analyze comets using fluorescencemicroscopy.
   - Quantify DNA damage (e.g., tail length, tail moment) using image analysis software.

4.3.5 Colony Formation Assay

1. **Objective**
   To assess the long-term antiproliferative effect of naphthoquinones (ascorbate) on MCF-7 cells by evaluating their ability to form colonies after treatment.
2. **Scientific Principle**
   The colony formation(clonogenic) assay measures the ability of a single cell to grow into a colony over time. A reduction in the number or size of colonies after treatment indicates cytostatic or cytotoxic effects of the tested compound.
3. **Materials**
   - MCF-7 cells.
   - Naphthoquinones (2.5, 5, 10, 20 μM).
   - Sodium ascorbate (1 mM).
   - Dimethyl sulfoxide (DMSO, 1%).

- Dulbecco's modified Eagle's medium (DMEM) + 10% FBS.
- Six-well tissue culture plates.
- PBS (pH 7.4).
- Crystal violet solution (0.2% in methanol).
- Methanol (fixative).
- Sterile pipettes and tips.
- Cell culture incubator (37°C, 5% CO_2).
- Biosafety cabinet.
- Inverted microscope.
- Image analysis software (optional).

4. **Procedure**
   1. **Seeding Cells**
      - Seed 500 MCF-7 cells per well in a six-well plate with 2 mL complete DMEM.
      - Incubate for 24 h at 37°C to allow cell adhesion.
   2. **Treatment**
      - Replace medium with fresh medium containing:
        - Naphthoquinones at 2.5, 5, 10, or 20 μM, alone or with 1 mM sodium ascorbate.
        - Ascorbate-only control (1 mM).
        - Negative control: culture medium + 1% DMSO (vehicle).
      - Incubate for 24 h.
   3. **Post-Treatment and Long-Term Growth**
      - After 24 h, remove treatment medium and wash cells three times with pre-warmed PBS (37°C).
      - Add 2 mL of fresh complete medium to each well.
      - Incubate cells for 10–15 days, or until visible colonies (≥50 cells) form.
      - Change medium every 3–4 days to maintain optimal growth.
   4. **Fixation and Staining**
      - Remove medium and wash cells with PBS.
      - Fix cells with 1 mL of methanol for 15 min at room temperature.
      - Discard methanol and stain with 0.2% crystal violet solution for 30 min.

- Wash gently with distilled water to remove excess stain and air-dry.

5. **Colony Counting**

   - Count colonies manually using a stereomicroscope or analyze using image analysis software.
   - Express results as number of colonies per well or percentage relative to control.

4.3.6 Immunoelectrophoresis Assays (Western Blotting)

1. **Objective**
   To detect and quantify specific intracellular proteins in MCF-7 cells following treatment with naphthoquinones (±ascorbate) via SDS-PAGE and Western blotting.
2. **Scientific Principle**
   Western blotting allows for the detection of specific proteins using antibody-based recognition after protein separation by molecular weight via SDS-PAGE and electrotransfer to a nitrocellulose membrane.
3. **Materials**
   - MCF-7 cells.
   - Naphthoquinones (20 μM).
   - Sodium ascorbate (1 mM).
   - PBS (pH 7.4).
   - RIPA buffer: 25 mM Tris-HCl (pH 7.4), 150 mM NaCl, 1% NP-40, 0.25% sodium deoxycholate.
   - Protease inhibitor cocktail (1%).
   - Phosphatase inhibitor cocktail (3%).
   - Laemmli sample buffer: 60 mM Tris-HCl (pH 6.8), 2% SDS, 10% glycerol, 5% β-mercaptoethanol, 0.01% bromophenol blue.
   - Bradford protein assay kit (BioRad).
   - SDS-PAGE gel (10%–12%).
   - Nitrocellulose membrane.
   - Transfer buffer (25 mM Tris, 192 mM glycine, 20% methanol).
   - Blocking solution: 5% non-fat dry milk in TBST (TBS + 0.1% Tween-20).
   - Primary antibodies (as per Table 1).
   - HRP-conjugated secondary antibodies.
   - ECL chemiluminescence substrate.
   - ChemiDoc MP Imaging System (BioRad).
   - Microcentrifuge tubes, pipettes, ice, rocker.

Table 1
List of primary antibodies used in Western blot analysis

Target protein	Host species	Dilution	Supplier	Catalog number	Molecular weight (kDa)
β-actin (Loading control)	Mouse	1:5000	Sigma-Aldrich	A5316	~42
Caspase-3 (cleaved)	Rabbit	1:1000	Cell Signaling Technology	#9661	~17, ~19 (cleaved forms)
PARP (cleaved)	Rabbit	1:1000	Cell Signaling Technology	#9541	~89
p53	Mouse	1:1000	Santa Cruz Biotechnology	sc-126	~53
Bcl-2	Rabbit	1:1000	Abcam	ab32124	~26
Bax	Rabbit	1:1000	Abcam	ab32503	~21
Cyclin D1	Rabbit	1:1000	Cell Signaling Technology	#2978	~36
p21	Rabbit	1:1000	Cell Signaling Technology	#2947	~21

4. **Procedure**

   1. **Cell Treatment and Lysis**
      1. Seed 4×10^5 MCF-7 cells/well in a 12-well plate.
      2. Incubate for 24 h to allow attachment.
      3. Treat cells for 2 h with:
         - Naphthoquinone (20 μM).
         - Naphthoquinone + 1 mM ascorbate.
         - Untreated control.
      4. After treatment, wash wells three times with ice-cold PBS.
      5. Add RIPA lysis buffer (200 μL) supplemented with:
         - 1% protease inhibitor cocktail.
         - 3% phosphatase inhibitor cocktail.
      6. Scrape cells and transfer lysates to microcentrifuge tubes.
      7. Incubate on ice for 30 min, vortexing every 10 min.
   8. Centrifuge at $12{,}000 \times g$ for 15 min at 4°C.
   9. Transfer clear supernatant (protein lysate) to fresh tubes and store on ice or at −80°C.

2. **Protein Quantification**
    1. Determine protein concentration using the Bradford assay.
    2. Prepare a standard curve using BSA.
    3. Measure absorbance at 595 nm.
3. **SDS-PAGE and Protein Transfer**
    1. Mix 25 μg of total protein with Laemmli buffer, heat at 95°C for 5 min.
    2. Load samples into SDS-PAGE wells and run at 100 V until dye front reaches bottom.
    3. Transfer proteins to a nitrocellulose membrane using a wet/tank transfer system (100 V for 1 h at 4°C).
4. **Membrane Blocking and Antibody Incubation**
    1. Block membrane in 5% milk/TBST for 1 h at room temperature.
    2. Incubate overnight at 4°C with primary antibody diluted in 1% milk/TBST, following manufacturer's instructions.
    3. Wash membrane three times for 5 min each in TBST.
    4. Incubate with HRP-conjugated secondary antibody for 1 h at room temperature.
    5. Wash membrane as above.
5. **Detection and Analysis**
    1. Apply ECL detection substrate to membrane.
    2. Capture images using the ChemiDoc MP system.
    3. Quantify band intensities using Image Lab software.
    4. Normalize expression levels to β-actin (loading control).

5 Notes and Tips

- Always include proper controls (untreated, vehicle, and positive controls).
- For accurate colony counting, define colony size threshold (e.g., ≥50 cells).
- For immunoblotting, run molecular weight markers in parallel for protein size estimation.
- Ensure all antibodies are validated for human proteins and optimized for dilution.
- Minimize light exposure during ECL detection.

6 Notes on Antibodies

- All antibodies were diluted in 1% non-fat dry milk in TBST unless otherwise specified.
- Secondary antibodies (goat anti-rabbit or goat anti-mouse HRP-conjugated) were used at 1:5000 dilution and matched to the host species of the primary antibodies.
- Incubation with primary antibodies was performed overnight at 4°C, and with secondary antibodies for 1 h at room temperature.

References

1. Zheng H, Zeng Y, Huang X, Zhang H, Pu F, Cheng H, Hu A (2023) Synthesis, reaction mechanism, DNA cleavage and antitumor properties of naphthoquinone-based enediynes. Asian J Org Chem 12(8):e202300306
2. Ourique F, Kviecinski MR, Felipe KB, Correia JFG, Farias MS, Castro LS, Pedrosa RC (2015) DNA damage and inhibition of Akt pathway in MCF-7 cells and Ehrlich tumor in mice treated with 1, 4-naphthoquinones in combination with ascorbate. Oxid Med Cell Longev 2015(1):495305
3. Vukic MD, Vukovic NL, Obradovic A, Matic M, Djukic M, Avdovic E (2020) Redox status, DNA and HSA binding study of naturally occurring naphthoquinone derivatives. EXCLI J 19:48

Check for updates

Chapter 10

Comprehensive Analysis of Oxidative Stress Markers in Tumor Ascitic Exudate from a Murine Model

Abstract

This protocol describes a comprehensive panel of spectrophotometric assays for evaluating oxidative stress markers and antioxidant defense system status in tumor ascitic exudate (TAE) from a murine tumor model. The methodology encompasses sample preparation through homogenization in phosphate buffer and protein normalization using the Lowry method to ensure standardized comparisons across samples. Oxidative damage to macromolecules is assessed via lipid peroxidation measured as thiobarbituric acid-reactive substances (TBARS) at 540 nm, and protein carbonylation quantified by reaction with 2,4-dinitrophenylhydrazine (DNPH) with absorbance read at 360 nm. Non-enzymatic antioxidant capacity is evaluated through reduced glutathione (GSH) content using the DTNB (Ellman's) reagent at 412 nm. A complete panel of enzymatic antioxidant activities is measured using kinetic spectrophotometric assays: superoxide dismutase (SOD) via inhibition of adrenaline autoxidation at 480 nm, catalase (CAT) through direct decomposition of hydrogen peroxide monitored at 240 nm, and the glutathione-dependent enzymes including glutathione peroxidase (GPx), glutathione reductase (GR), and glutathione S-transferase (GST), all coupled to NADPH oxidation or conjugate formation measured at 340 nm. All results are normalized to sample protein content, enabling quantitative comparison of oxidative stress status and antioxidant capacity between experimental groups. This integrated workflow provides a robust tool for investigating the role of oxidative stress in tumor biology and evaluating the antioxidant or pro-oxidant effects of therapeutic interventions.

Keywords Oxidative stress, Lipid peroxidation, Antioxidant enzymes, Glutathione, Tumor ascitic exudate

1 Introduction

Oxidative stress, resulting from an imbalance between reactive oxygen species (ROS) production and the cellular antioxidant capacity, plays a significant role in cancer progression and therapy response. Tumor microenvironments often exhibit elevated ROS, leading to macromolecular damage such as lipid peroxidation and protein carbonylation. Concurrently, the activity of enzymatic antioxidants is frequently altered. This protocol details a standardized panel of spectrophotometric assays to evaluate these critical parameters in a biological fluid (TAE) from a murine tumor model. Accurate assessment requires

Karuppusamy Arunachalam et al., *Advanced Protocols in Cancer Research*, Springer Protocols Handbooks, https://doi.org/10.1007/978-1-0716-5348-7_10,

initial sample homogenization and protein normalization to ensure comparable results across samples [1].

2 Aim

To quantitatively assess the level of oxidative stress and the status of the antioxidant defense system in tumor-bearing mice by measuring specific biomarkers—lipid peroxidation, protein carbonylation, reduced glutathione (GSH) content, and the activity of key antioxidant enzymes(SOD, CAT, GPx, GR, GST)—in tumor ascitic exudate (TAE) samples.

3 Materials

1. **Biological Sample:** Tumor ascitic exudate (TAE) from tumor-bearing mice.
2. **Chemicals and Reagents:**
   - Potassium phosphate buffer (20 mM, pH 7.4, with 150 mM NaCl, 0.1% Triton X-100).
   - Trichloroacetic acid (TCA), 12% and 20% (w/v).
   - Thiobarbituric acid (TBA), 0.73% (w/v) in 60 mM Tris-HCl (pH 7.4).
   - 2,4-Dinitrophenylhydrazine (DNPH), 10 mM in 2 N HCl.
   - Ethanol: ethyl acetate (1:1 v/v).
   - Guanidine hydrochloride, 6 M in 20 mM KH_2PO_4 (pH 2.3).
   - 5,5′-Dithio-bis-(2-nitrobenzoic acid) (DTNB), 2.5 mM in 1% sodium citrate.
   - Adrenaline (epinephrine), 60 mM (freshly prepared in 0.1 N HCl).
   - Hydrogen peroxide (H_2O_2), 30 mM in 50 mM phosphate buffer (pH 7.0).
   - Reduced glutathione (GSH), oxidized glutathione (GSSG).
   - β-Nicotinamide adenine dinucleotide phosphate (NADPH).
   - tert-Butyl hydroperoxide (t-BuOOH).
   - 1-Chloro-2,4-dinitrobenzene (CDNB).
   - Diethylenetriaminepentaacetic acid (DPTA).
   - Glutathione reductase (GR, from yeast).

- Glycine buffer (50 mM, pH 10.2).
- All other salts and buffers as specified.

3. **Equipment:**

- Refrigerated microcentrifuge.
- Spectrophotometric microplate reader (capable of kinetic readings at 240, 340, 360, 412, 480, and 540 nm).
- Heating block or water bath (95–100°C).
- Vortex mixer.
- Analytical balance.
- Micropipettes (1–1000 μL range).
- 96-well clear flat-bottom microplates.
- 1.5 mL and 2.0 mL microcentrifuge tubes.
- Ice bucket.

4 Methods

4.1 Sample Preparation and Protein Quantification

1. **TAE Homogenate Preparation:**
   a. Thaw TAE samples on ice if frozen.
   b. For each sample, prepare a 1:4 (v/v) homogenate by adding 400 μL of TAE to 1600 μL of ice-cold potassium phosphate buffer (20 mM, pH 7.4, containing 150 mM NaCl and 0.1% Triton X-100).
   c. Homogenize thoroughly by vortexing for 30 s.
   d. Centrifuge the homogenate at 5000 × *g* for 5 min at 4°C.
   e. Carefully collect the clear supernatant into a fresh, labeled tube placed on ice. This supernatant (S1) will be used for all subsequent assays.
2. **Total Protein Determination (Lowry Method):**
   a. Determine the total protein concentration of each S1 sample using the standardized Lowry method (or a compatible kit such as the DC Protein Assay).
   b. Prepare a standard curve using bovine serum albumin (BSA, 0–100 μg/mL).
   c. Normalize all subsequent oxidative stress marker measurements to the protein content (per mg protein) to account for variations in sample cellularity [2].

4.2 Oxidative Damage Marker Assays

4.2.1 Lipid Peroxidation (TBARS Assay)

1. In a 1.5 mL heat-resistant microcentrifuge tube, add 100 µL of S1.
2. Add sequentially with mixing:
   - 1.0 mL of 12% (w/v) trichloroacetic acid (TCA).
   - 900 µL of 0.73% (w/v) thiobarbituric acid (TBA) prepared in 60 mM Tris-HCl buffer (pH 7.4).
3. Cap the tubes tightly, vortex, and incubate in a heating block at 95°C for 60 min.
4. Cool the tubes to room temperature in an ice bath or cold water for 10 min.
5. Centrifuge at 10,000 × *g* for 5 min to remove precipitate.
6. Transfer 200 µL of the clear pink supernatant in duplicate to a 96-well plate.
7. Measure the absorbance at 540 nm using a microplate reader.
8. **Calculation:** Determine MDA concentration using an extinction coefficient (ε) of 156 mM^{-1} cm^{-1}. Express results as nmol of MDA per mg of protein [3].

4.2.2 Protein Carbonylation (DNPH Assay)

1. For each sample, prepare two tubes: one for the DNPH reaction and one as an HCl control.
2. To the sample tube, add 100 µL of S1 + 600 µL of 10 mM DNPH in 2 N HCl.
3. To the control tube, add 100µL of S1 + 600µL of 2 N HCl (without DNPH).
4. Incubate both tubes in the dark at room temperature for 60 min, vortexing every 15 min.
5. Precipitate proteins by adding 700 µL of ice-cold 20% (w/v) TCA to each tube. Mix and incubate on ice for 10 min.
6. Centrifuge at 10,000 × *g* for 5 min at 4°C. Discard the supernatant.
7. Wash the protein pellet three times with 1 mL of ethanol:ethyl acetate mixture (1:1 v/v). Centrifuge and discard the supernatant after each wash.
8. Dissolve the final pellet in 900 µL of 6 M guanidine hydrochloride (in 20 mM KH_2PO_4, pH adjusted to 2.3 with HCl).
9. Incubate at 37°C for 60 min with occasional vortexing to ensure complete solubilization.
10. Transfer 200 µL in duplicate to a 96-well plate.

11. Read the absorbance at 360 nm. Subtract the absorbance of the HCl control from the DNPH sample absorbance.
12. **Calculation:** Use an extinction coefficient (ε) of 22,000 $M^{-1}cm^{-1}$ for protein hydrazones. Express results as nmol of carbonyl groups per mg of protein [4].

4.3 Non-Enzymatic Antioxidant Assay

4.3.1 Reduced Glutathione (GSH) Content (DTNB Assay)

1. Prepare an acid extract separately from S1 to preserve GSH. Mix 200 μL of TAE with 800 μL of 12% (w/v) TCA in a fresh tube.
2. Vortex vigorously and centrifuge at 10,000 × *g* for 10 min at 4°C.
3. Collect the clear supernatant (acid extract, AE).
4. In a 96-well plate, prepare the reaction mix per well:
   - 190 μL of 0.2 M phosphate buffer (pH 8.0).
   - 10 μL of AE (from step 3).
   - 20 μL of 2.5 mM DTNB reagent (in 1% sodium citrate).
5. Mix gently and incubate at room temperature for exactly 3 min.
6. Measure the absorbance at 412 nm.
7. Calculation: Determine GSH concentration from a standard curve of pure GSH (0–50 μM). Express results as μmol of GSH per mg of protein [5].

4.4 Enzymatic Antioxidant Activity Assays

*(For all enzyme assays, use S1. Adjust supernatant volume based on preliminary activity range-finding. Perform kinetic readings.)

4.4.1 Superoxide Dismutase (SOD) Activity (Adrenaline Autoxidation Inhibition)

1. Prepare fresh adrenaline solution (60 mM in 0.1 N HCl, kept on ice in the dark).
2. In a 96-well plate, add 5–60 μL of S1 (depending on activity) and bring the volume to 200 μL with 50 mM glycine buffer (pH 10.2).
3. Initiate the reaction by rapidly adding 5 μL of the fresh adrenaline solution to each well.
4. Immediately start reading the increase in absorbance at 480 nm every 30 s for 10 min.
5. **Calculation:** One unit (U) of SOD activity is defined as the amount of enzyme that causes 50% inhibition of adrenaline autoxidation to adrenochrome under the assay conditions. Calculate the percentage inhibition and interpolate the volume

giving 50% inhibition. Express activity as units of SOD per mg of protein (U SOD/mg protein) [6].

4.4.2 Catalase (CAT) Activity (H_2O_2 Degradation)

1. In a 96-well plate, add 200 μL of 30 mM H_2O_2 solution prepared in 50 mM phosphate buffer (pH 7.0).
2. Initiate the reaction by adding 5 μL of S1 to the well. Mix immediately by pipetting.
3. Immediately start the kinetic measurement of the decrease in absorbance at 240 nm every 15 ss for 5 min.
4. Calculation: Use the molar extinction coefficient of H_2O_2 ($\varepsilon = 43.6\ M^{-1}cm^{-1}$). Calculate the rate of H_2O_2 decomposition. Express activity asnmol of H_2O_2 consumed per minute per mg of protein (nmol min^{-1} mg^{-1} protein) [7].

4.4.3 Glutathione Peroxidase (GPx) Activity (Coupled Assay with t-BuOOH)

1. Prepare the reaction mixture (per well) on ice:
   - 0.1 M phosphate buffer (pH 7.0).
   - 1 mM GSH.
   - 0.24 U/mL glutathione reductase (GR).
   - 0.1 mM NADPH.
   - 0.5 mM DPTA.
2. In a 96-well plate, add 200 μL of the reaction mixture and 5 μ L of S1. Pre-incubate for 3 min at 25°C.
3. Initiate the reaction by adding 5 μL of 3.75 mM *tert*-butyl hydroperoxide (t-BuOOH).
4. Immediately start reading the decrease in absorbance at 340 nm every 30 s for 3 min.
5. **Calculation:** Use the extinction coefficient of NADPH ($\varepsilon = 6.22\ mM^{-1}cm^{-1}$). Express activity as nmol of NADPH oxidized per minute per mg of protein (nmol min^{-1} mg^{-1} protein) [8].

4.4.4 Glutathione Reductase (GR) Activity

1. Prepare the reaction mixture (per well):
   - 0.1 M phosphate buffer (pH 7.0).
   - 1 mM oxidized glutathione (GSSG).
   - 0.1 mM NADPH.
   - 0.5 mM DPTA.
2. In a 96-well plate, add 200 μL of reaction mixture and 5 μL of S1. Mix gently.
3. Immediately start reading the decrease in absorbance at 340 nm every 30 s for 3 min.
4. **Calculation:** Use the extinction coefficient of NADPH ($\varepsilon = 6.22\ mM^{-1}\ cm^{-1}$). Express activity as nmol of NADPH

oxidized per minute per mg of protein (nmol min^{-1} mg^{-1} protein) [9].

4.4.5 Glutathione S-Transferase (GST) Activity (CDNB Conjugation)

1. In a 96-well plate, add sequentially:
   - 250 μL of 0.1 M phosphate buffer (pH 7.0).
   - 5 μL of S1.
   - 5 μL of 20 mM reduced glutathione (GSH).
2. Initiate the reaction by adding 5 μL of 20 mM 1-chloro-2,4-dinitrobenzene (CDNB) in ethanol.
3. Immediately start reading the increase in absorbance at 340 nm every 30 s for 3 min.
4. **Calculation:** Use the extinction coefficient of the CDNB–GSH conjugate ($\varepsilon = 9.6\,mM^{-1}cm^{-1}$). Express activity as nmol of conjugate formed per minute per mg of protein (nmol min^{-1} mg^{-1} protein) [10].

References

1. Dogra S, Adhikari L, Benbrook DM, Bohn JA, Burgett A, Chandra V, Dockery L, Singh A, McNally L, Rai R, Isingizwe ZR (2025) Harnessing ovarian cancer ascites for translational science: models, biomarkers, and therapeutics. Mol Cancer 24(1):257
2. Lowry OH, Rosebrough NJ, Farr AL, Randall RJ (1951) Protein measurement with the Folin phenol reagent. J Biol Chem 193(1):265–275
3. Ohkawa H, Ohishi W, Yagi K (1979) Assay for lipid peroxides in animal tissues by thiobarbituric acid reaction. Anal Biochem 95(2):351–358
4. Levine RL, Williams JA, Stadtman ER, Shacter E (1994) Carbonyl assays for determination of oxidatively modified proteins. Methods Enzymol 233:346–357
5. Ellman GL (1959) Tissue sulfhydryl groups. Arch Biochem Biophys 82(1):70–77
6. Misra HP, Fridovich I (1972) The role of superoxide anion in the autoxidation of epinephrine and a simple assay for superoxide dismutase. J Biol Chem 247(10):3170–3175
7. Aebi H (1984) Catalase in vitro. Methods Enzymol 105:121–126
8. Flohé L, Günzler WA (1984) Assays of glutathione peroxidase. Methods Enzymol 105:114–121
9. Carlberg I, Mannervik B (1985) Glutathione reductase. Methods Enzymol 113:484–490
10. Habig WH, Pabst MJ, Jakoby WB (1974) Glutathione S-transferases. The first enzymatic step in mercapturic acid formation. J Biol Chem 249(22):7130–7139

Chapter 11

Evaluation of Oxidative Stress Markers: Experimental Procedure

Abstract

This protocol provides a detailed experimental procedure for the comprehensive evaluation of oxidative stress markers in tumor ascitic exudate (TAE) samples from murine models. The methodology encompasses a complete panel of spectrophotometric assays to assess both oxidative damage to macromolecules and the status of enzymatic and non-enzymatic antioxidant defense systems. Following standardized sample preparation through homogenization in phosphate buffer and protein normalization by the Lowry method, lipid peroxidation is quantified via the thiobarbituric acid-reactive substances (TBARS) assay, measuring malondialdehyde (MDA) at 540 nm, while protein oxidative damage is assessed by carbonyl content determination using 2,4-dinitrophenylhydrazine (DNPH) with absorbance read at 360 nm. Reduced glutathione (GSH) levels are measured through reaction with DTNB (Ellman's reagent) at 412 nm. The enzymatic antioxidant profile is comprehensively evaluated through kinetic assays: superoxide dismutase (SOD) activity via inhibition of adrenaline autoxidation monitored at 480 nm, catalase (CAT) through direct decomposition of hydrogen peroxide at 240 nm, and the glutathione-dependent enzymes including glutathione peroxidase (GPx), glutathione reductase (GR), and glutathione S-transferase (GST) through NADPH oxidation or conjugate formation measured at 340 nm. All results are normalized to sample protein content, enabling quantitative comparison of oxidative stress status and antioxidant capacity between experimental groups. This integrated workflow serves as a robust tool for investigating the role of oxidative stress in tumor biology and evaluating the effects of therapeutic interventions on redox homeostasis.

Keywords Oxidative stress, Lipid peroxidation, Protein carbonylation, AntiOxidant enzymes, Glutathione

1 Introduction

To assess oxidative stress parameters in tumor ascitic exudate (TAE) samples, various biochemical assays were performed targeting lipid peroxidation, protein oxidation, antioxidant enzyme activity, and glutathione status [1]. All procedures were performed using homogenates prepared in a 1:4 ratio with phosphate buffer (20 mM, 150 mM NaCl, 0.1% Triton, pH 7.4), followed by centrifugation at 5000 ×*g* for 5 min unless stated otherwise. Protein concentrations were determined by the Lowry method prior to all assays.

Karuppusamy Arunachalam et al., *Advanced Protocols in Cancer Research*, Springer Protocols Handbooks,
https://doi.org/10.1007/978-1-0716-5348-7_11,

2 Lipid Peroxidation Assay (TBARS Method)

Objective: To quantify malondialdehyde (MDA) levels as an index of lipid peroxidation [2].

Method:

1. Prepare TAE homogenate in a 1:4 (v/v) ratio with phosphate buffer.
2. Centrifuge at 5000 × *g* for 5 min.
3. In a microcentrifuge tube, add:
   - 100 μL sample supernatant.
   - 1 mL of 12% trichloroacetic acid (TCA).
   - 900 μL of 60 mM Tris-HCl buffer (pH 7.4).
   - 0.73% thiobarbituric acid (TBA).
4. Incubate samples in a boiling water bath for 1 h.
5. Cool samples in an ice bath for 10 min.
6. Centrifuge at 5000 × *g* for 5 min.
7. Transfer 200 μL of each supernatant into a 96-well plate.
8. Measure absorbance at 540 nm using a microplate reader.

   Expression of Results: nmol MDA/mg protein.

3 Protein Carbonylation Assay

Objective: To assess oxidative damage to proteins by quantifying carbonyl content [3].

Method:

1. Prepare and centrifuge TAE homogenate as above.
2. Add 100 μL of supernatant to 600 μL of 10 mM DNPH in 2 N HCl.
3. Incubate for 1 h at room temperature in the dark with continuous mixing.
4. Add 600 μL of 20% TCA and incubate in an ice bath for 10 min.
5. Centrifuge at 10,000 × *g* for 5 min. Discard supernatant.
6. Wash the pellet three times using 1:1 ethanol:ethyl acetate.
7. After the final wash, remove solvent using a cotton swab.
8. Add 900 μL of 6 M guanidine in 20 mM KH_2PO_4 and incubate at 37°C for 1 h.
9. Transfer 200 μL into a 96-well plate and read absorbance at 360 nm.

   Expression of Results: nmol carbonyl/mg protein.

4 Reduced Glutathione (GSH) Assay

Objective: To determine intracellular levels of reduced GSH [4].

Method:

1. Prepare an acid extract (200 µL TAE + 800 µL of 12% TCA).
2. Centrifuge at 5000 × g for 5 min.
3. In a 96-well plate, add:
   - 10 µL sample supernatant.
   - 190 µL of 0.2 M phosphate buffer (pH 8.0).
   - 20 µL of 2.5 mM DTNB in 1% sodium citrate.
4. After 3 min, read absorbance at 412 nm.

Expression of Results: µmol GSH/mg protein.

5 Superoxide Dismutase (SOD) Activity Assay

Objective: To assess antioxidant enzyme activity against superoxide radicals [5].

Method:

1. Prepare and centrifuge homogenate.
2. In a 96-well plate, mix 5–60 µL of sample supernatant with glycine buffer to 200 µL total volume.
3. Add 5 µL of 60 mM adrenaline solution (prepared fresh, pH ~2.0).
4. Read absorbance kinetically at 480 nm for 10 min.

Expression of Results: USOD/mg protein (1 unit = 50% inhibition of adrenochrome formation).

6 Catalase (CAT) Activity Assay

Objective: To determine catalase activity by H_2O_2 degradation [6].

Method:

1. Prepare and centrifuge homogenate.
2. In a 96-well plate, add:
   - 5 µL of sample supernatant.
   - 200 µL of 30% H_2O_2 prepared in 50 mM phosphate buffer (pH 7.0).
3. Immediately perform kinetic reading at 240 nm for 5 min.

Expression of Results: nmol H_2O_2 degraded/(min·mg protein).

7 Glutathione Peroxidase (GPx) Activity Assay

Objective: To measure GPx activity based on NADPH consumption [7].

Method:

1. Prepare and centrifuge homogenate.
2. Prepare reaction medium containing:
   - 25 mL of 0.1 M phosphate buffer (pH 7.0).
   - 8.6 mg NADPH.
   - 10 mL of 5 mM DPTA.
   - 15 mL distilled water.
   - 24 mg GSH.
   - 5 U GR.
3. In a 96-well plate, add:
   - 5 μL sample.
   - 200 μL reaction medium.
   - 5 μL t-BuOOH.
4. Read absorbance at 340 nm for 3 min.

Expression of Results: μmol NADPH oxidized/(min·mg protein).

8 Glutathione Reductase (GR) Activity Assay

Objective: To evaluate GR activity based on NADPH oxidation [8].

Method:

1. Prepare and centrifuge homogenate.
2. Prepare reaction mix containing:
   - 0.1 M phosphate buffer (pH 7.0).
   - 8.6 mg NADPH.
   - 30.6 mg oxidized glutathione (GSSG).
   - 5 mM DPTA.
3. In a 96-well plate, add:
   - 5 μL sample supernatant.
   - 200 μL reaction mix.
4. Measure absorbance at 340 nm for 3 min.

Expression of Results: μmol NADPH oxidized/(min·mg protein).

9 Glutathione S-Transferase (GST) Activity Assay

Objective: To assess GST-mediated conjugation of GSH to CDNB [9].

Method:

1. Prepare and centrifuge homogenate.
2. Prepare fresh solutions of 0.1 M CDNB (in ethanol) and 0.1 M GSH (in phosphate buffer pH 7.0).
3. In a 96-well plate, combine:
   - 5 μL sample.
   - 250 μL 0.1 M phosphate buffer (pH 7.0).
   - 5 μL CDNB.
   - 5 μL GSH.
4. Read absorbance at 340 nm for 3 min.

Expression of Results: μmol conjugated product formed/(min·mg protein).

References

1. Halliwell B, Whiteman M (2004) Measuring reactive species and oxidative damage in vivo and in cell culture: how should you do it and what do the results mean?. Br J Pharmacol 142(2):231–255. https://doi.org/10.1038/sj.bjp.0705776
2. Ohkawa H, Ohishi N, Yagi K (1979) Assay for lipid peroxides in animal tissues by thiobarbituric acid reaction. Anal Biochem 95(2):351–358. https://doi.org/10.1016/0003-2697(79)90738-3
3. Levine RL, Williams JA, Stadtman ER, Shacter E (1994) Carbonyl assays for determination of oxidatively modified proteins. Methods Enzymol 233:346–357. https://doi.org/10.1016/S0076-6879(94)33040-9
4. Ellman GL (1959) Tissue sulfhydryl groups. Arch Biochem Biophys 82(1):70–77. https://doi.org/10.1016/0003-9861(59)90090-6
5. Misra HP, Fridovich I (1972) The role of superoxide anion in the autoxidation of epinephrine and a simple assay for superoxide dismutase. J Biol Chem 247(10):3170–3175. https://doi.org/10.1016/S0021-9258(19)45228-9
6. Aebi H (1984) Catalase in vitro. Methods Enzymol 105:121–126. https://doi.org/10.1016/S0076-6879(84)05016-3
7. Flohe L, Günzler WA (1984) Assays of glutathione peroxidase. Methods Enzymol 105:114–121. https://doi.org/10.1016/S0076-6879(84)05015-1
8. Carlberg I, Mannervik B (1985) Glutathione reductase. Methods Enzymol 113:484–490. https://doi.org/10.1016/S0076-6879(85)13062-4
9. Habig WH, Pabst MJ, Jakoby WB (1974) Glutathione S-transferases. The first enzymatic step in mercapturic acid formation. J Biol Chem 249(22):7130–7139. https://doi.org/10.1016/S0021-9258(19)42083-8

Chapter 12

In Vitro Evaluation of Cytotoxicity (Dark and Phototoxic), Cell Death Mechanism, and Confocal Imaging in NIH-3T3 and B16-F10 Cells

Abstract

This protocol describes a comprehensive experimental approach for evaluating the in vitro cytotoxic activity and elucidating the mechanisms of action of synthetic metal-based compounds, including copper(II) and platinum(II) complexes, against a panel of human cancer cell lines representing both solid tumors (H460, A549, MDA-MB-231, PC3) and hematologic malignancies (U937, MOLT-4, THP-1). The methodology integrates initial cytotoxicity screening using the MTT colorimetric assay to determine half-maximal inhibitory concentrations (IC_{50}) following 48-h compound exposure, followed by a suite of flow cytometry-based mechanistic assays to characterize cell death pathways. Cell cycle analysis with propidium iodide (PI) staining enables quantification of the Sub-G_1 apoptotic population, while mitochondrial membrane potential ($\Delta\Psi m$) disruption is assessed using JC-1 dye, where loss of red fluorescence indicates mitochondrial depolarization associated with early apoptosis. Reactive oxygen species (ROS) generation is measured using the DCFH-DA fluorescent probe, with parallel experiments incorporating the antioxidant N-acetylcysteine (NAC) to confirm oxidative stress involvement. All flow cytometry data are acquired using a BD FACSCalibur™ instrument with FL1 (JC-1 monomers, DCF) and FL2 (PI, JC-1 aggregates) channel detection, and analyzed using WinMDI software. This integrated workflow enables comprehensive characterization of compound-induced cytotoxicity from initial potency determination through detailed mechanistic investigation of apoptosis induction, mitochondrial dysfunction, and oxidative stress.

Keywords Metal-based compounds, Cytotoxicity, Apoptosis, Mitochondrial membrane potential, Reactive oxygen species

1 Introduction

Naturally occurring anthraquinone derivative with potential antitumor activity. To enhance its bioavailability and selective delivery, it can be encapsulated in nanostructured systems. This study aims to assess the in vitro behavior of nanoparticles in murine fibroblast (NIH-3T3) and melanoma (B16-F10) cell lines. This includes evaluating cellular internalization, dark and phototoxic cytotoxicity, cell death pathways, and intracellular localization using flow cytometry and confocalmicroscopy [1].

Karuppusamy Arunachalam et al., *Advanced Protocols in Cancer Research*, Springer Protocols Handbooks,
https://doi.org/10.1007/978-1-0716-5348-7_12,

2 Aim

To evaluate the cellular uptake, cytotoxic potential under dark and photodynamic conditions, and the mode of cell death induced by nanoparticles in NIH-3T3 and B16-F10 cells.

3 Materials

3.1 Cell Lines and Culture Supplies

- NIH-3T3 (ATCC® CRL-1658™).
- B16-F10 (ATCC® CRL-6475™).
- DMEM and RPMI-1640 media (Sigma-Aldrich or Gibco).
- Fetal bovine serum (FBS).
- Streptomycin/penicillin (1%).
- Amphotericin B (0.5%).
- Amino acids (1%) for NIH-3T3.
- 75 cm^2 culture flasks and 96-/24-well plates (Corning).
- Trypsin–EDTA solution (0.05%, Corning).
- Cryogenic vials, Mr. Frosty™ Freezing Container.

3.2 Assays and Reagents

- MTT reagent (5 mg/mL, Sigma).
- DCFH-DA (ROS assay).
- JC-1 dye (Mitochondrial potential).
- Guava Nexin® kit (Merck Millipore).
- Paraformaldehyde (PFA, 2% and 4%).
- Triton X-100 (0.1%).
- Glycine (100 mM).
- PBS (1×, sterile).
- Isopropanol (analytical grade).
- Alexa Fluor® 488 (Life Technologies).
- ProLong® Diamond Antifade Mountant with DAPI.

3.3 Instruments

- CO_2 incubator (37°C, 5%).
- Cytation 5 Multi-Mode Reader (BioTek).
- Flow cytometer (Guava EasyCyte 8HT).
- Confocalmicroscope.
- LED light source (450 ± 20 nm, MMO Dental LEC-Plus).
- Plate shaker (IKA KS 260).
- Centrifuge.

4 Experimental Procedures

4.1 Cell Culture and Expansion

1. Thaw cryopreserved NIH-3T3 and B16-F10 cells rapidly in a 37°C water bath.
2. Transfer cells into 75 cm^2 flasks containing:
   - NIH-3T3: 10 mL DMEM + 10% FBS + 1% streptomycin/penicillin + 0.5% amphotericin + 1% amino acids.
   - B16-F10: 10 mL RPMI-1640 + 10% FBS + 1% streptomycin/penicillin + 0.5% amphotericin.
3. Incubate at 37°C in 5% CO_2 until 80%–90% confluence.
4. Subculture using 2 mL of 0.05% trypsin for 5 min, neutralize with complete medium.
5. For cryopreservation: Suspend 1–1.5 × 10^6 cells/mL in freezing medium (90% FBS + 10% DMSO), place in Mr. Frosty container at −80°C overnight, then transfer to liquid nitrogen.

4.2 Cellular Internalization of QZ-NPs

1. Seed 1.5 × 10^4 cells/well in black 96-well plates.
2. Incubate for 24 h to allow adhesion.
3. Add QZ-NPs at concentrations ranging from 8 to 268 μg/mL. Include empty NP controls.
4. Incubate for 3 h at 37°C.
5. Wash cells three times with sterile PBS.
6. Add 100 μL RPMI (phenol red-free) to each well.
7. Read fluorescence using Cytation 5:
   - Excitation: 470 nm.
   - Emission: 500–700 nm.
8. Subtract empty NP fluorescence from synthesized NP values.

4.3 Cytotoxicity Under Dark Conditions (MTT Assay)

1. Plate 1.5 × 10^4 cells/well in 96-well plates.
2. After 24 h, treat with synthesized NPs (8 to 268 μg/mL) and empty NPs for 3 h.
3. Wash 3× with PBS.
4. Incubate for 24 h in fresh medium.
5. Add 200 μL of 5 mg/mL MTT to each well.
6. Incubate for 4 h at 37°C.
7. Remove MTT solution; add 200 μL isopropanol.
8. Shake plate for 10 min; measure absorbance at 560 and 690 nm.
9. Calculate % cell viability relative to control.

4.4 Phototoxicity Assay

1. Seed 4×10^4 cells/well in 24-well plates.
2. After 24 h, treat with synthesized NPs at 111 and 222 μg/mL for 3 h.
3. Wash with PBS; add fresh medium.
4. Irradiate using 450 nm LED light at fluences 1–25 J/cm^2.
5. Incubate 24 h post-irradiation.
6. Perform MTT assay as above.
7. Analyze data with ANOVA and Tukey's post-hoc test.

4.5 Cell Death Pathway by Flow Cytometry

1. Seed cells in 24-well plates and treat as above.
2. Detach cells using 200 μL trypsin–acutase (1:1).
3. Collect in labeled tubes and centrifuge (1000 rpm, 5 min, 4°C).
4. Discard supernatant; resuspend in 200 μL Guava Nexin® reagent.
5. Incubate 20 min in the dark.
6. Transfer to 96-well U-bottom plates and analyze with Guava EasyCyte 8HT.
7. Quantify viable, apoptotic, and necrotic cells using CytoSoft software.

4.6 Confocal Microscopy

1. Seed 3×10^4 cells/well on coverslips in 24-well plates.
2. After 24 h, treat with synthesized NPs and empty NPs for 3 h.
3. Wash 3× with PBS.
4. Fix with 2% PFA for 20 min.
5. Wash 5× with PBS + 100 mM glycine.
6. Permeabilize with 0.1% Triton X-100 for 10 min.
7. Wash 2× with PBS.
8. Incubate with Alexa Fluor 488 (1:20) for 15 min.
9. Wash 3× with PBS and mount with ProLong® Diamond + DAPI.
10. Observe under confocalmicroscope (63× or 100× oil immersion lens).

Reference

1. Mosmann T (1983) Rapid colorimetric assay for cellular growth and survival: application to proliferation and cytotoxicity assays. J Immunol Methods 65(1–2):55–63

Chapter 13

Evaluation of Antiproliferative, Pro-Apoptotic, and Immunomodulatory Effects of Test Compounds on Human Leukemic Cell Lines and Primary Peripheral Blood Mononuclear Cells (PBMCs)

Abstract

This protocol provides a comprehensive experimental framework for evaluating the antiproliferative, pro-apoptotic, and immunomodulatory effects of test compounds against human leukemic cell lines (HL60 for acute myeloid leukemia and K562 for chronic myeloid leukemia) and primary peripheral blood mononuclear cells (PBMCs) isolated from leukemia patients and healthy donors. The methodology integrates multiple complementary assays to characterize compound activity across cellular and molecular levels. Initial cytotoxicity screening employs the MTT colorimetric assay across 24–72 h treatment periods to determine half-maximal inhibitory concentrations (IC_{50}). Long-term antiproliferative effects are assessed through colony formation assays in methylcellulose-based semi-solid medium, enabling quantification of clonogenic potential following compound exposure at IC_{50} and 2× IC_{50} concentrations. Cell cycle analysis by flow cytometry with propidium iodide (PI) staining reveals compound-induced perturbations in G_1, S, and G_2/M phase distribution. Mechanistic immunomodulatory studies include evaluation of cyclooxygenase (COX-1 and COX-2) inhibitory activity in LPS-stimulated HL60 cell lysates using a colorimetric substrate-based assay, and quantification of cytokine secretion profiles (IL-4, IL-6, IL-10, IL-12, IFN-γ, TNF-α) in PBMC culture supernatants by enzyme-linked immunosorbent assay (ELISA). Statistical analyses are performed using GraphPad Prism with appropriate tests (ANOVA, *t*-test, Mann–Whitney, Chi-square) and significance set at $p < 0.05$. This integrated approach enables comprehensive characterization of compound bioactivity from initial cytotoxicity through detailed investigation of cell cycle effects and immunomodulatory mechanisms in leukemic models.

Keywords Leukemia, Cytotoxicity, Colony formation, Cell cycle, Immunomodulation

1 Introduction

Acute and chronic myeloid leukemias (AML, CML) represent aggressive hematological malignancies with a need for novel therapeutic strategies. In vitro models using established cell lines (e.g., HL60 for AML, K562 for CML) and primary patient-derived peripheral blood mononuclear cells (PBMCs) are crucial for screening the biological activity of new compounds [1]. Key mechanisms of interest for anticancer agents include the inhibition of cell proliferation, induction of

Karuppusamy Arunachalam et al., *Advanced Protocols in Cancer Research*, Springer Protocols Handbooks,
https://doi.org/10.1007/978-1-0716-5348-7_13,

cell cycle arrest, reduction of clonogenic potential, and modulation of inflammatory pathways, including cyclooxygenase (COX) enzyme activity and cytokine secretion. This protocol details a comprehensive in vitro assessment to evaluate these mechanisms.

2 Aim

To assess the cytotoxic, anti-clonogenic, cell cycle-disturbing, and immunomodulatory effects of test compounds on human leukemic cell lines (HL60, K562) and primary PBMCs isolated from leukemia patients and healthy donors.

3 Materials and Methods

3.1 Cell Culture and Maintenance

Cell Lines: HL60 (AML), K562 cells (CML), and Vero (non-cancerous control) cell lines were used.

- **Culture Media:**
  - **HL60, K562, PBMCs:** RPMI 1640 medium supplemented with 10% heat-inactivated fetal bovine serum (FBS), 100 μg/mL penicillin, and 100 μg/mL streptomycin.
  - **Vero cells:** Dulbecco's modified Eagle's medium (DMEM) supplemented with 10% FBS and 100 μg/mL streptomycin.
- **Culture Conditions:** All cells were maintained at 37°C in a humidified atmosphere of 5% CO_2.

3.2 Isolation of Human Peripheral Blood Mononuclear Cells (PBMCs)

PBMCs were isolated from heparinized peripheral blood samples of leukemia patients and healthy donors using density gradient centrifugation with Ficoll-Hypaque. Isolated PBMCs were washed thrice with RPMI 1640 before culture.

3.3 Cell Viability Assay (MTT Assay)

Cell viability was determined using the MTT assay as described by Oliveira et al. (2020). Cells (1×10^5 cells/well for lines; 5×10^5 cells/well for PBMCs) were seeded in 96-well plates, treated with compounds (3–100 μg/mL), and incubated for 24, 48, and 72 h. MTT (5 mg/mL) was added, followed by incubation and solubilization with acidic isopropanol. Absorbance was measured at 570 nm. Viability was calculated as: (A_{570} treated/A_{570} untreated) × 100. The half-maximal inhibitory concentration (IC_{50}) was determined via nonlinear regression.

3.4 Colony Formation Assay

The clonogenic potential of HL60 and K562 cells was assessed. Briefly, 0.5×10^3 cells were seeded in methylcellulose-based semi-solid medium (MethoCult 4230) containing IC_{50} or 2× IC_{50} of the compounds in 12-well plates. Colonies were counted microscopically after 8–10 days. MTT (1 mg/mL) was added to stain colonies, and quantification was performed using ImageJ software.

3.5 Cell Cycle Analysis by Flow Cytometry

HL60 and K562 cells treated with IC_{50} or 2× IC_{50} concentrations for 24 h were fixed in 70% ethanol, treated with RNase A, and stained with propidium iodide (PI). DNA content was analyzed using a BD FACS Calibur flow cytometer. Cell cycle distribution (G1, S, G2/M phases) was determined using FlowJo software.

3.6 Cyclooxygenase (COX-1 and COX-2) Inhibitory Activity Assay

COX inhibitory activity was evaluated using a commercial inhibitor screening kit. HL60 cells ($>1 \times 10^8$) were stimulated with LPS (10 μ g/mL) for 6 h, then treated with the IC_{50} concentration of the compound for 24 h. Cell lysates were incubated with assay buffer, heme, colorimetric substrate, and arachidonic acid. Absorbance was read at 590 nm to determine COX activity.

3.7 Cytokine Measurement by ELISA

PBMCs (5×10^5 cells/well) were treated with IC_{50} or 2× IC_{50} concentrations for 24 h. Culture supernatants were collected, and levels of IL-4, IL-6, IL-10, IL-12, IFN-γ, and TNF-α were quantified using commercial ELISA kits according to the manufacturer's instructions.

3.8 Statistical Analysis

Data are presented as mean ± standard deviation. Statistical analyses were performed using GraphPad Prism v8.0. Tests included ANOVA, Student's *t*-test, Mann–Whitney test, Chi-square, or Fisher's exact test as appropriate. A p-value < 0.05 was considered statistically significant.

4 Step-by-Step Laboratory Working Protocol [1, 2]

4.1 Cell Culture and Treatment 1

1. Maintain HL60, K562, and PBMCs in complete RPMI 1640 medium. Maintain Vero cells in complete DMEM.
2. Incubate all cultures at 37°C, 5% CO_2.
3. For experiments, harvest cells in the logarithmic growth phase. Count using a hemocytometer or automated cell counter.
4. Seed cells at specified densities in appropriate multi-well plates.
5. Prepare stock solutions of test compounds in a suitable solvent (e.g., DMSO). Ensure final solvent concentration is ≤0.5% (v/v) in all wells, including vehicle controls.
6. Add treatment compounds to wells at desired final concentrations (e.g., 3–100 μg/mL for MTT; IC_{50}/2× IC_{50} for other assays). Include untreated (medium only) and vehicle control wells.
7. Return plates to the incubator for the designated treatment period (24, 48, 72 h).

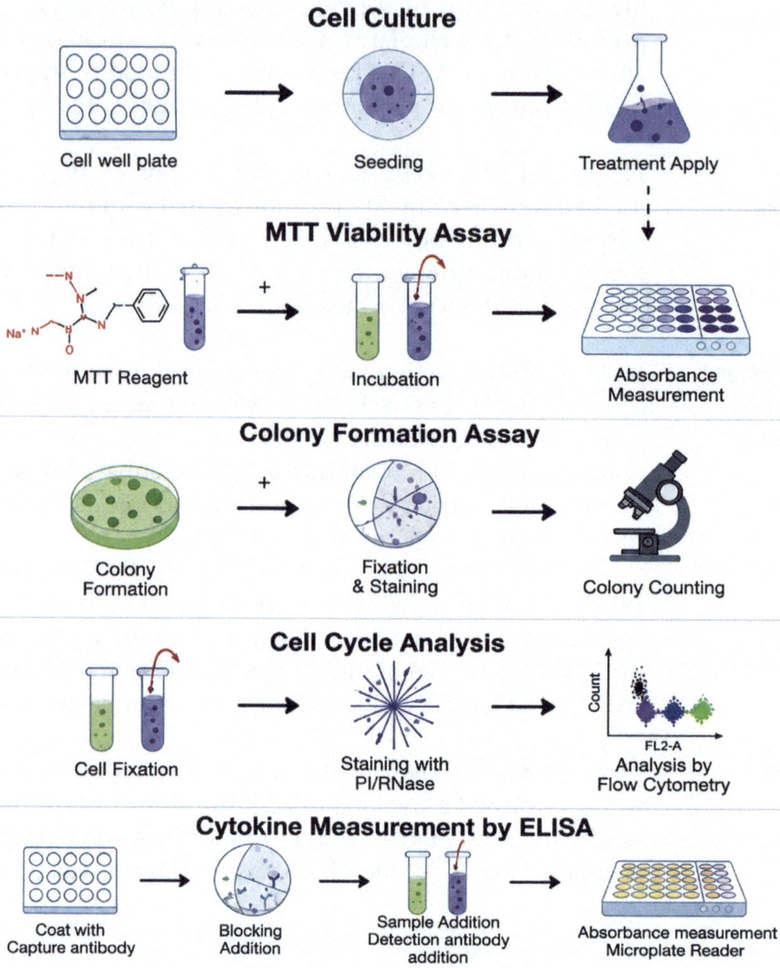

Fig. 1 Schematic representation of antiproliferative, pro-apoptotic, and immunomodulatory effects of tests

4.2 MTT Cell Viability Assay [1]

1. After treatment incubation, add 10 μL of MTT solution (5 mg/mL in PBS) directly to each well of the 96-well plate.
2. Incubate the plate at 37°C for 4 h.
3. Carefully remove the medium without disturbing the formed formazan crystals.
4. Add 100 μL of 0.1 N HCl in anhydrous isopropanol to each well to solubilize the crystals.

5. Gently shake the plate on an orbital shaker for 10–15 min until all crystals are dissolved.
6. Measure the absorbance of each well at 570 nm using a microplate reader.
7. Calculate the percentage viability relative to the untreated control.

4.3 Colony Formation Assay

1. Prepare working concentrations of compounds in complete culture medium.
2. Mix 0.5×10^3 cells with 1.5 mL of semi-solid methylcellulose medium (MethoCult 4230) containing the appropriate compound concentration (IC_{50} or 2× IC_{50}) in a tube.
3. Vortex thoroughly and then pipette 1 mL of the cell–methylcellulose mixture into each well of a 12-well plate in duplicate/triplicate.
4. Incubate plates undisturbed for 8–10 days at 37°C, 5% CO_2.
5. After incubation, add 100 μL of MTT solution (1 mg/mL) to each well and incubate for 4–6 h at 37°C to stain colonies.
6. Image wells and count colonies using ImageJ software.

4.4 Cell Cycle Analysis Protocol

1. Treat cells in six-well plates (e.g., 2×10^5 cells/well) for 24 h.
2. Harvest cells by centrifugation (300 × *g*, 5 min). Wash once with cold PBS.
3. Gently resuspend the cell pellet in 300 μL of PBS.
4. While vortexing gently, add 700 μL of ice-cold 70% ethanol dropwise to fix cells. Fix at 4°C for at least 2 h or overnight.
5. Pellet fixed cells (500 × *g*, 5 min) and wash twice with PBS.
6. Resuspend cell pellet in 500 μL of PBS containing 100 μg/mL RNase A and 40 μg/mL Propidium Iodide (PI).
7. Incubate in the dark at 37°C for 30 min.
8. Analyze samples on a flow cytometer using a 488 nm laser for excitation and detecting PI fluorescence in the FL2 or FL3 channel (e.g., 585/42 nm bandpass filter). Acquire at least 10,000 events per sample.
9. Analyze data using doublet discrimination and fit cell cycle phases using software (e.g., FlowJo'sDean–Jett–Fox model).

4.5 COX Activity Assay (Kit-Based)

Note: Perform all steps per manufacturer's (Cayman Chemical) instructions.

1. Stimulate HL60 cells with LPS (10 μg/mL) for 6 h in a 24-well plate.
2. Treat cells with compound at IC_{50} for 24 h.

3. Lyse cells on ice with cold lysis buffer (0.1 M Tris-HCl, pH 7.8, 1 mM EDTA). Centrifuge at 10,000 × *g* for 15 min at 4°C.
4. Collect supernatant. Determine protein concentration.
5. In a 96-well plate, combine 150 μL assay buffer, 10 μL heme, 10 μL sample or inhibitor control, and 20 μL colorimetric substrate.
6. Initiate reaction by adding 20 μL of arachidonic acid solution.
7. Incubate at room temperature for 5 min.
8. Read absorbance immediately at 590 nm.

4.6 Cytokine Measurement by ELISA

1. Culture PBMCs (5×10^5/well) in a 96-well plate with treatments for 24 h.
2. Centrifuge plate at 300 × *g* for 5 min. Carefully collect 100 μL of supernatant from each well without disturbing the cell pellet.
3. Store supernatants at −80°C until analysis.
4. Thaw samples on ice. Perform ELISA for target cytokines (IL-4, IL-6, IL-10, IL-12, IFN-γ, TNF-α) strictly according to the kit manufacturer's (ImunoTools) protocol.
5. Read absorbance at the specified wavelength (typically 450 nm with a reference filter).
6. Calculate cytokine concentration (pg/mL) from the standard curve.

References

1. Oliveira ACR, De Oliveira FS, Braz AF, Oliveira JS, Lima-Santos J, Dias AA (2024) Unveiling the anticancer potential of the ethanolic extract from Trichoderma asperelloides. Front Pharmacol 15:1398135
2. Plaimee P, Khamphio M, Weerapreeyakul N, Barusrux S, Johns NP (2014) Immunomodulatory effect of melatonin in SK-LU-1 human lung adenocarcinoma cells co-cultured with peripheral blood mononuclear cells. Cell Prolif 47(5):406–415

Part III

Advanced Culture Models: 3D, Co-Culture, and Bioengineering

Check for updates

Chapter 14

Advanced 2D and 3D Co-Culture Systems for Studying Breast Cancer Cell Interactions and GLS Inhibition

Abstract

This protocol describes advanced two-dimensional (2D) and three-dimensional (3D) co-culture systems for investigating the effects of glutaminase (GLS) inhibition on breast cancer cell behavior and tumor-immune interactions, with a focus on triple-negative breast cancer (TNBC) models. The methodology employs a panel of genetically modified human and murine breast cancer cell lines, including Hs578T variants (parental, mKO2, shGFP, shGLS), MDA-MB-231, MCF-7, and 4T1 (Mock and GAB), to explore GLS dependency. Three-dimensional culture models are established using multiple approaches: magnetized spheroids generated via NanoShuttle® nanoparticle-mediated aggregation on magnetic drives, gravity-induced spheroids in ultra-low attachment (ULA) plates, and mammospheres cultured in MammoCult™ medium over 7–11 days. Viability assessment of 3D structures employs Calcein AM, propidium iodide (PI), and Hoechst 33342 staining coupled with high-content imaging on the Operetta® system and quantitative analysis using Columbus® software for spheroid metrics (diameter, area, volume) and viability calculations. Tumor-immune interactions are investigated through co-culture of 4T1 spheroids with primary murine bone marrow-derived macrophages (BMDMs), established via M-CSF-driven differentiation, using either co-seeding or macrophage addition to pre-formed spheroids. Downstream analyses include RNA extraction from pooled spheroids using TRI Reagent, cDNA synthesis with GoScript™ Reverse Transcriptase, and quantitative real-time PCR (qPCR) with EvaGreen® dye for gene expression profiling normalized to Hprt housekeeping gene. Immunofluorescence staining of cryosectioned spheroids enables spatial localization of macrophage markers (F4/80, CD68, CD206) and GLS2 expression using confocal microscopy. This integrated workflow provides a physiologically relevant platform for studying metabolic dependencies and immune cell dynamics in breast cancer.

Keywords 3D co-culture, Spheroids, Mammospheres, Glutaminase inhibition, Tumor-associated macrophages

1 Introduction

Breast cancer comprises various molecular subtypes with distinct biological behaviors and treatment responses. Triple-negative breast cancer (TNBC) is particularly aggressive and lacks targeted therapeutic options. In vitro 3D culture models, such as spheroids and mammospheres, more accurately replicate the tumor microenvironment compared to traditional 2D models. In this study, a panel of genetically modified breast cancer cell lines, including knockdown

Karuppusamy Arunachalam et al., *Advanced Protocols in Cancer Research*, Springer Protocols Handbooks,
https://doi.org/10.1007/978-1-0716-5348-7_14,

and overexpression variants, is employed to explore glutaminase (GLS) dependency and immune-tumor interactions. Co-culture systems with primary murine macrophages provide insight into tumor-immune dynamics, particularly in the context of glutamine metabolism inhibition using CB-839, a GLS inhibitor. Downstream analysis involves high-content imaging, RNA expression profiling, and immunofluorescencemicroscopy [1].

2 Aim

To investigate the impact of GLS inhibition on breast cancer cell growth, spheroid/mammosphere formation, and immune cell interactions using2D/3D cultures, macrophage co-cultures, and molecular characterization techniques.

3 Materials

3.1 Cell Lines & Culture Media

- Hs578T (parental, mKO2, shGFP, shGLS).
- MDA-MB-231 (TNBC), MCF-7 (ER+, PR+).
- 4T1 Mock and 4T1 GAB (murine TNBC).
- RPMI-1640 medium, supplemented with:
  - 10% Fetal Bovine Serum (FBS).
  - 1% Penicillin-Streptomycin.
  - Optional: 1× non-essential amino acids, sodium pyruvate, vitamin solution.

3.2 Reagents & Kits

- NanoShuttle® (Greiner).
- CB-839 (GLS inhibitor).
- Calcein AM, Hoechst 33342, Propidium Iodide.
- Mammocult™ Human Medium Kit (STEMCELL Technologies).
- TRI Reagent (Sigma).
- GoScript™ Reverse Transcriptase Kit (Promega).
- HOT FIREPol® EvaGreen® qPCR Mix Plus (Solis BioDyne).

3.3 Plates & Labware

- ULA 96-well plates (Corning/Greiner).
- CellCarrier Spheroid ULA 384-well plates.
- 24-well plates.
- Poly-HEMA treated U-bottom plates.
- Cryomolds, TissueTek® O.C.T.
- Microscope slides pre-coated with HistoGrip (Sigma).

3.4 Antibodies

- Primary: anti-F4/80, anti-CD68, anti-CD206, anti-GLS2.
- Secondary: Alexa Fluor® 647-rat, 488-mouse, 546-rabbit.

3.5 Equipment

- Operetta®High Content Imaging System (Perkin Elmer).
- Columbus® Image Analysis Software.
- Leica TCS SP8 X® confocal microscope.
- Standard tissue culture equipment and cryostat.

4 Methods: Detailed Procedures [2]

4.1 Cell Culture Maintenance & Preparation for Experiments

- **Procedure:**

1. **Thawing:** Rapidly thaw frozen vials of cell lines (Hs578T variants, MDA-MB-231, MCF-7, 4T1 Mock, 4T1 GAB) in a 37°C water bath. Immediately transfer cells to 9 mL of pre-warmed complete RPMI-1640 medium (RPMI + 10% FBS + 1% Pen-Strep) in a 15 mL conical tube.
2. **Centrifugation & Seeding:** Centrifuge at $300\times g$ for 5 min. Aspirate supernatant, gently resuspend cell pellet in 5 mL fresh complete medium, and seed into a T-75 culture flask. Incubate at 37°C, 5% CO_2.
3. **Maintenance:** Monitor daily. Replace medium every 2–3 days. For genetically modified lines, maintain appropriate selection antibiotics (e.g., puromycin for shRNA lines) as per validation protocols.
4. **Passaging:** At 70%–80% confluency, aspirate medium, wash with 5 mL PBS, and add 2 mL of 0.25% Trypsin-EDTA. Incubate at 37°C for 3–5 min. Neutralize with 8 mL complete medium. Centrifuge, resuspend, and split at desired ratios (typically 1:5 to 1:10) into new flasks.
5. **Experimental Preparation:** For all assays, harvest cells in the logarithmic growth phase. Perform a viable cell count using trypan blue exclusion on a hemocytometer or automated counter. Adjust cell concentration for specific assays as follows.

4.2 Formation of Magnetized Spheroids (NanoShuttle® Method)

- **Procedure:**

1. Prepare a single-cell suspension of Hs578T cellsNano-Shuttle® as in Sect. 1.5. Adjust concentration to 5×10^5 cells/mL.
2. To 1 mL of cell suspension (~5×10^5 cells), add 5 μL of NanoShuttle®Spheroid models stock solution (1 μL per 1×10^4 cells). Mix gently by pipetting.

3. Incubate the cell-nanoparticle mixture for 30 min at 37°C, 5% CO_2, with gentle shaking every 10 min.
4. Transfer the mixture to a 15 mL tube. Wash three times to remove unbound nanoparticles: Add 10 mL fresh medium, centrifuge at 300 × *g* for 5 min, and carefully aspirate the supernatant. Repeat twice.
5. Resuspend the final pellet in complete medium to a concentration of 1.25×10^5 cells/mL.
6. Seed 200 μL of this suspension (containing 25,000 cells) into each well of a 96-well, ultra-low attachment (ULA), cell-repellent plate.
7. Immediately place the plate on a magnetic drive (e.g., Spheroid Drive) for 24 h to aggregate cells.
8. After 24 h, carefully remove the magnet. Compact, spherical aggregates should be visible. Allow spheroids to mature for an additional 24 h before initiating treatments.

4.3 Formation of Non-Magnetized Spheroids (Gravity-Induced)

- **Procedure:**

1. Prepare single-cell suspensions of desired cell lines (Hs578T variants, 4T1 lines). Adjust concentration to 1.5×10^4 cells/mL for 384-well plates or as optimized.
2. Using a multichannel pipette, seed 50 μL of cell suspension (~750 cells) into each well of a CellCarrier SpheroidULA 384-well plate. Ensure even distribution.
3. **Centrifuge:** The plate at 300 × *g* for 3 min to gently pellet cells at the bottom of the U-bottom well, promoting aggregation.
4. Incubate plate undisturbed at 37°C, 5% CO_2 for 48–72 h to allow spheroid self-assembly. Monitor formation using a brightfield microscope.
5. **Treatment:** After spheroid formation (Day 2–3), prepare 2× concentrated drug solutions of CB-839 in fresh medium. Carefully add 50 μL of the 2× drug solution directly to each well containing the existing 50 μL medium and spheroid, resulting in a final 1× drug concentration (e.g., 1 μM) and 100 μL total volume. For vehicle control, add medium with equivalent DMSO (final conc. ≤0.1%).

4.4 Mammosphere Formation Assay

- **Procedure:**

1. Prepare MammoCult™ Human Medium according to kit instructions (add hydrocortisone, heparin, and fresh antibiotics). Pre-warm medium.
2. Harvest MCF-7, MDA-MB-231, or Hs578T cells. Perform a viable count and resuspend cells in MammoCult™ medium at a density of 1000 cells/mL.

3. Seed 200 µL of cell suspension (200 cells/well) into each well of a 96-well ULA plate. For treatment at seeding, add CB-839 directly to the cell suspension medium to the desired final concentration (e.g., 1 µM) before seeding.
4. Incubate plates for 7–11 days at 37°C, 5% CO_2. Do not disturb. Refuel cultures on Day 4 by carefully adding 20 µL of fresh MammoCult™ medium (± drug) per well.
5. **For treatment of pre-formed mammospheres:** On Day 7, gently collect mammospheres by centrifugation (300 × *g*, 5 min) in a conical tube. Aspirate old medium, gently resuspend mammospheres in fresh MammoCult™ medium containing CB-839 or vehicle, and re-seed into a new ULA plate. Incubate for an additional 3–4 days.

4.5 Viability Staining and High-Content Imaging of 3D Structures

- **Procedure:**

1. Prepare a master staining solution in phenol-free, serum-free medium (e.g., FluoroBrite DMEM): 2 µM Calcein AM (live cells), 4 µg/mL Propidium Iodide (PI) (dead cells), 10 µg/mL Hoechst 33342 (nuclei).
2. For each well of a 96- or 384-well plate containing spheroids/mammospheres, carefully aspirate 100 µL of old medium.
3. Add 100 µL of the pre-warmed staining solution per well.
4. Incubate plate at 37°C, 5% CO_2 for 2 h.
5. Image Acquisition (Operetta® CLS):
   - Use a 5× or 10× objective suitable for 3D imaging.
   - Set up a Z-stack to encompass the entire spheroid volume (e.g., 150 µm total, 20 µm steps).
   - Configure channels: Hoechst (Ex 355-385, Em 430-500), Calcein (Ex 460-490, Em 500-550), PI (Ex 530-560, Em 570-650).
   - Acquire images for all experimental wells using an automated scan pattern.
6. **Analysis (Columbus®):**
   - Use the "Find Spheroids" building blockColumbus® software based on the Hoechst channel to identify objects.
   - Apply a size filter to exclude debris.
   - Measure spheroid metrics: diameter (µm), cross-sectional area (μm^2), and volume (calculated from radius).
   - Calculate viability: (Total Calcein+ area / Total Hoechst+ area) × 100 for each spheroid.

4.6 Primary Bone Marrow-Derived Macrophage (BMDM) Generation

- **Procedure:**
  1. Euthanize 8–12 week old female BALB/c mice using CO_2 asphyxiation followed by cervical dislocation.
  2. Sterilize hind legs with 70% ethanol. Dissect out femurs and tibias under aseptic conditions, removing all muscle tissue.
  3. Place bones in a sterile petri dish with cold PBS. Cut both ends of the bones to expose the marrow cavity.
  4. Flush marrow from each bone using a 3 mL syringe fitted with a 26G needle and 5 mL of cold, sterile PBS into a 50 mL conical tube.
  5. Dissociate cell clumps by gently pipetting up and down 10–15 times. Pass the cell suspension through a 70 μm cell strainer.
  6. Centrifuge at 300 × *g* for 5 min at 4°C. Aspirate supernatant.
  7. Lyse RBCs: Resuspend pellet in 3 mL of RBC Lysis Buffer (155 mM NH_4Cl, 12 mM $NaHCO_3$, 0.1 mM EDTA, pH 7.3). Incubate at room temperature for 2 min. Immediately quench with 10 mL of cold PBS.
  8. Centrifuge (300 × *g*, 5 min, 4°C). Resuspend pellet in BMDM Culture Medium: RPMI-1640 + 10% FBS + 1% Pen-Strep + 1× NEAA + 1 mM Sodium Pyruvate + 10 mM HEPES + 20 ng/mL recombinant murine M-CSF.
  9. Count viable cells. Seed 1×10^6 cells per well in a 6-well tissue culture plate in 3 mL of BMDM medium.
  10. Incubate at 37°C, 5% CO_2. On Day 3, add an additional 1 mL of fresh BMDM medium per well. On Day 5 or 6, macrophages (adherent, elongated) are ready. Gently scrape with a cell scraper for co-culture experiments.

4.7 3D Tumor-Macrophage Co-Culture Setup

- **Procedure:**
  1. **Option A: Co-seeding**
     - Prepare a single-cell suspension of 4T1 Mock or GAB cells and freshly harvested BMDMs.
     - Mix cells at desired ratios (e.g., 1:0.5 tumor:macrophage = 25,000:12,500 cells/well) in complete medium.
     - Seed the mixed suspension in 200 μL volume into wells of a poly-HEMA coated, U-bottom 96-well plate.
     - Centrifuge at 300 × *g* for 3 min to initiate contact.
     - Incubate for 7 days, with a 50% medium change (careful aspiration) on Day 3 or 4.

2. **Option B: Adding Macrophages to Pre-formed Spheroids**

   - Generate 4T1 spheroids (25,000 cells/well) in ULA plates for 48 h as in Sect. 2 or 3.
   - On the day of co-culture, gently harvest BMDMs by scraping. Wash, count, and resuspend.
   - Using a wide-bore pipette tip, carefully aspirate 100 μL of medium from the spheroid well.
   - Gently add 100 μL of macrophage suspension (containing the desired number of cells) to the well. Swirl plate gently to distribute.
   - Incubate co-cultures for an additional 3–5 days before analysis.

4.8 RNA Extraction and qPCR from 3D Co-Cultures

- **Procedure:**

1. Pool 10–15 spheroids/co-culture wells per condition into a 1.5 mL microcentrifuge tube. Let spheroids settle or centrifuge briefly (100 × *g*, 2 min).
2. Aspirate medium completely. Add 500 μL of TRI Reagent to the pellet. Vortex vigorously for 1 min to lyse spheroids.
3. Incubate 5 min at RT. Add 100 μL of chloroform. Shake tube vigorously for 15 s. Incubate 3 min at RT.
4. Centrifuge at 12,000 × *g* for 15 min at 4°C. Transfer the upper, clear aqueous phase (~250 μL) to a new tube.
5. Add 250 μL of isopropanol, mix by inversion. Incubate at −20°C for 1 h or overnight to precipitate RNA.
6. Centrifuge at 12,000 × *g* for 15 min at 4°C. Wash pellet with 500 μL of 75% ethanol (in DEPC-water). Centrifuge 5 min.
7. Air-dry pellet for 5–10 min. Dissolve in 20 μL of RNase-free water. Quantify RNA using a Nanodrop (Fig. 1).
8. **cDNA synthesis**: For each sample, combine 1 μg of total RNA, 4 μL of GoScript 5× Reaction Buffer, 1 μL of Random Primers (0.5 μg), 2 μL of $MgCl_2$ (25 mM), 1 μL of dNTP Mix (10 mM each), 1 μL of GoScript Reverse Transcriptase, and Nuclease-Free Water to 20 μL total. Run in a thermocycler: 25°C for 5 min, 42°C for 60 min, 70°C for 15 min, 4°C hold.
9. **qPCR:** Prepare a master mix per reaction: 10 μL EvaGreen qPCR Mix (2×), 0.6 μL forward primer (10 μM), 0.6 μL reverse primer (10 μM), 6.8 μL Nuclease-Free Water, and 2 μL of diluted cDNA (1:10). Run in triplicate. Use cycling: 95°C for 10 min, then 40 cycles of (95°C for 15 s, 60°C for 60 s), followed by a melt curve. Analyze via the $2^{-\Delta\Delta Ct}$ method using *Hprt* as housekeeper.

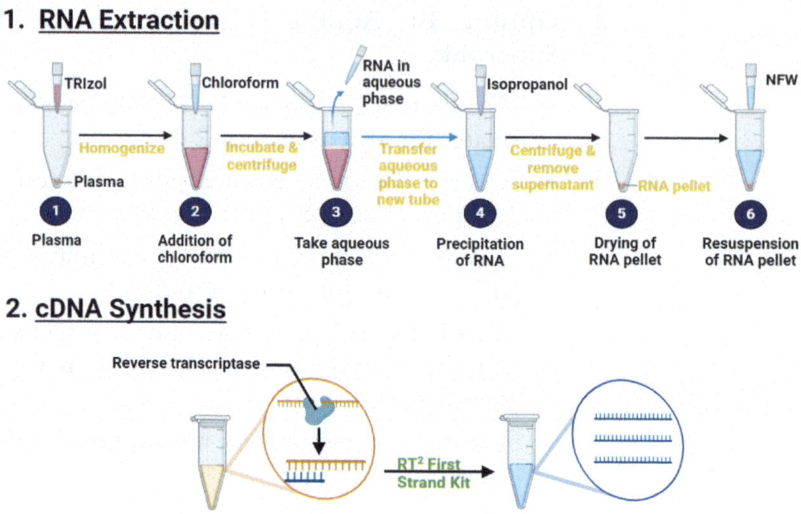

Fig. 1 Experimental procedure of RNA extraction and cDNA synthesis

4.9 Immuno-fluorescence Staining of Cryosectioned Spheroids

- **Procedure:**

1. **Embedding:** Pool and wash spheroids in PBS. Carefully aspirate PBS and resuspend in a small volume of TissueTek® O.C.T. compound. Pipette into a cryomold, orienting spheroids. Slowly lower into liquid nitrogen-chilled isopentane and freeze. Store at −80°C.
2. **Sectioning:** Equilibrate block to −20°C in cryostat. Cut 10 μm sections and mount on HistoGrip-coated microscope slides. Air-dry sections for 30 min at RT.
3. **Fixation & Permeabilization:** Immerse slides in 4% Paraformaldehyde (PFA) in PBS for 15 min at RT. Wash 3×5 min with PBS. Permeabilize with 0.2% Triton X-100 in PBS for 10 min. Wash 3×5 min with PBS.
4. **Blocking:** Apply Image-iT FX Signal Enhancer for 30 min at RT. Wash with PBS. Then, apply blocking buffer (1% BSA + 5% normal serum from secondary antibody host species in PBS) for 1 h at RT in a humidified chamber.
5. **Primary Antibody Incubation:** Prepare primary antibody cocktail in blocking buffer (e.g., rat anti-F4/80 1:200, rabbit anti-CD206 1:100, mouse anti-GLS2 1:150). Apply to sections, ensuring full coverage. Incubate overnight at 4°C in a humidified chamber.
6. **Secondary Antibody & Counterstain:** Wash slides 3× 10 min with PBS-T (0.1% Tween-20). Apply appropriate Alexa Fluor-conjugated secondary antibodies (e.g., AF647-anti-rat, AF546-anti-rabbit, AF488-anti-mouse)

diluted 1:500 in blocking buffer. Incubate for 1 h at RT in the dark.

7. Wash 3×1 0 min in PBS-T in the dark. Apply DAPI (0.25 μ g/mL) for 5 min at RT. Wash 2×5 min with PBS.

8. **Mounting:** Apply a drop of anti-fade mounting medium (e.g., ProLong Diamond) and carefully lower a coverslip, avoiding bubbles. Seal edges with clear nail polish. Store slides at 4°C in the dark.

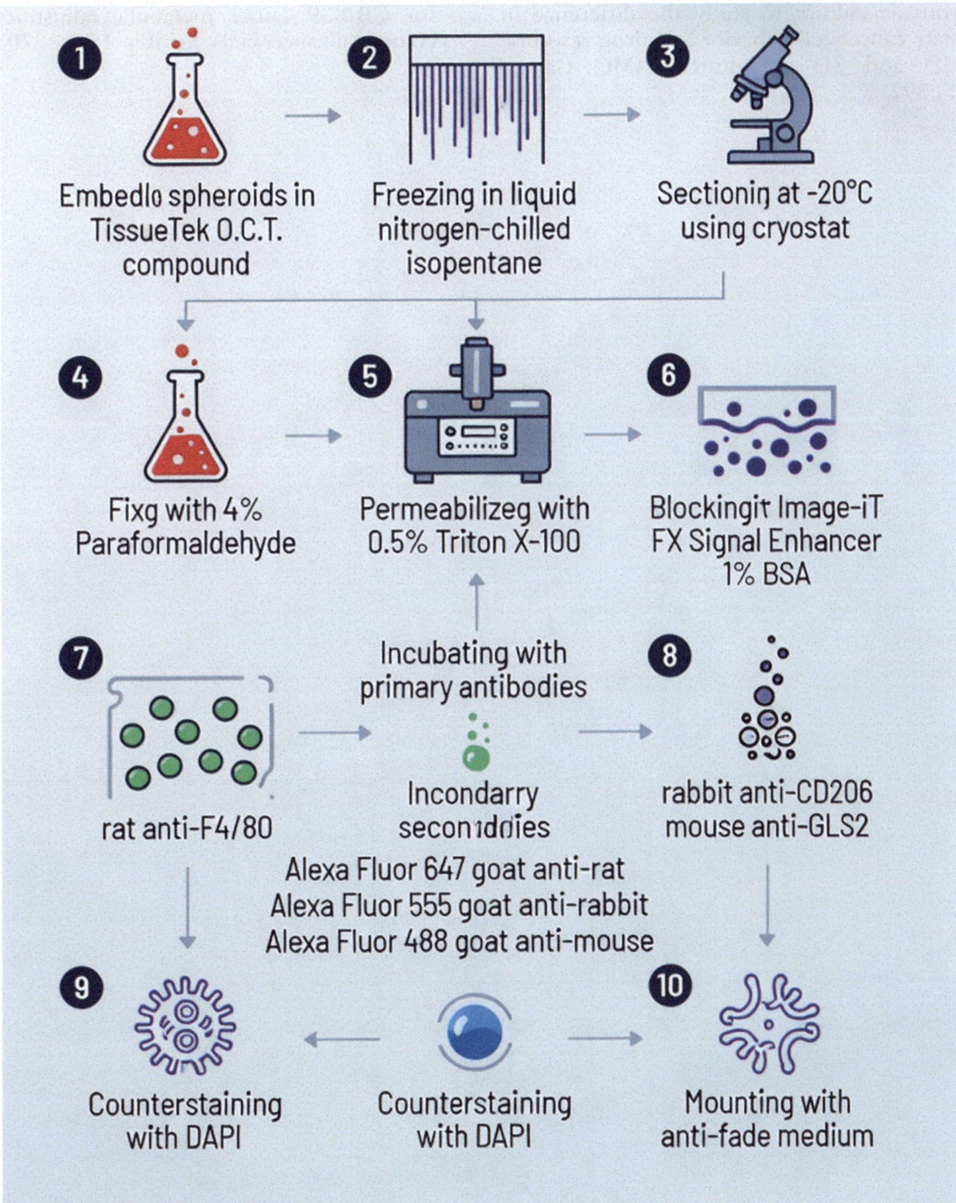

Fig. 2 Experimental design of immunofluorescence staining of cryosectioned spheroids

9. **Imaging:** Acquire high-resolution Z-stacks using a Leica SP8 confocal microscope with a 40× oil immersion objective. Use sequential scanning to avoid channel cross-talk. Analyze fluorescence intensity and localization using LAS X or Fiji/ImageJ software (Fig. 2).

References

1. Mosaad E, Chambers K, Futrega K, Clements J, Doran MR (2018) Using high throughput microtissue culture to study the difference in prostate cancer cell behavior and drug response in 2D and 3D co-cultures. BMC Cancer 18(1):592
2. Spada M, Piras C, Leoni VP, Casula M, Simbula G, Noto A et al (2025) Glutaminase inhibitor CB-839 causes metabolic adjustments in colorectal cancer cells. Sci Rep 15(1):37028

Chapter 15

In Vitro Breast and Cervical Cancer 2D and 3D Co-Culture Models

Abstract

This protocol provides a comprehensive methodology for establishing, optimizing, and characterizing two-dimensional (2D) and three-dimensional (3D) co-culture models of breast and cervical cancer using MCF-7 (human breast adenocarcinoma), HeLa (human cervical adenocarcinoma), and primary human dermal fibroblasts (hFIB) to recapitulate tumor-stroma interactions. The experimental workflow encompasses cell culture maintenance, ratio-based co-culture seeding (cancer:fibroblast ratios of 1:0, 3:1, 1:1, 1:3, 0:1), and multi-parametric analysis of cellular behavior. Metabolic activity in 2D co-cultures is quantitatively assessed using the resazurin reduction assay (excitation 560 nm/emission 590 nm) across 24–96 h. Three-dimensional heterotypic spheroids are generated via the liquid-overlay technique on 1% agarose-coated plates, with seeding densities optimized at 5×10^3, 1×10^4, and 1.5×10^4 cells per well, and cultured under gentle agitation (60–80 rpm) to promote symmetric aggregation. Structural characterization employs bright-field microscopy for growth kinetics (projected area, diameter, circularity), scanning electron microscopy (SEM) with critical point drying and gold/palladium sputter-coating for surface ultrastructure visualization, and confocal laser scanning microscopy (CLSM) using WGA-Alexa Fluor™ 594 membrane staining for 3D architectural reconstruction. For nanoparticle uptake studies, CellLight™ Actin-GFP-labeled MCF-7 cells are co-cultured with unlabeled hFIB in Collagen IV-coated Ibidi µ-Slides, exposed to CH-H-R/RITC-pDNA nanoparticles, and analyzed by CLSM with orthogonal projections and flow cytometry to quantify cell-type-specific uptake based on GFP (FL-1) and RITC (FL-2) fluorescence. This integrated platform enables detailed investigation of tumor-stroma interactions, nanoparticle targeting, and therapeutic response in physiologically relevant co-culture systems.

Keywords Co-culture, Spheroids, Tumor–stroma interaction, Nanoparticle uptake, Confocal microscopy

1 Introduction

The tumor microenvironment plays a pivotal role in cancer progression, therapeutic response, and metastasis. Co-culture models that incorporate both cancer cells and stromal cells, such as fibroblasts, more accurately recapitulate the in vivo conditions. This lab manual outlines standardized procedures for the development and analysis of 2D and 3D co-culture models using MCF-7 (human breast cancer), HeLa (human cervical cancer), and primary human dermal fibroblasts (hFIB). These models are employed for evaluating cell viability,

Karuppusamy Arunachalam et al., *Advanced Protocols in Cancer Research*, Springer Protocols Handbooks,
https://doi.org/10.1007/978-1-0716-5348-7_15,

morphology, and nanoparticle uptake using advanced imaging and analytical methods [1].

2 Aim

To establish, optimize, and characterize 2D and 3D co-culture in vitro models of breast and cervical cancer for studying cellular interactions, morphology, viability, and nanoparticle uptake.

3 Materials

- Cell lines: MCF-7, HeLa (ATCC), hFIB (Promocell).
- Culture media: DMEM-F12, DMEM-High Glucose.
- Supplements: FBS, streptomycin, gentamycin.
- Reagents: Trypsin-EDTA (0.18%, 5 mM), resazurin (0.1%), agarose, PBS.
- Labeling dyes: Hoechst 33342, CellLight Actin-GFP BacMam 2.0, WGA-Alexa 594.
- Plates and flasks: T-75 flasks, 6-well plates, 96-well plates, 24-well plates, Ibidi µ-Slides.
- Nanoparticles: CH-H-R/RITC-pDNA.
- Equipment: Inverted microscope, CLSM (Zeiss LSM 710), SEM (Hitachi S-2700), flow cytometer (BD FACSCalibur), microplate reader (Gemini XS), microplate shaker (Grant-bio PMS-1000).

4 Procedures [2, 3]

4.1 Thawing and Initial Culture

- Rapidly thaw cryovials containing MCF-7 (human breast adenocarcinoma) or hFIB (human foreskin fibroblasts) in a 37°C water bath for 60–90 s.
- Immediately transfer cell suspension to a 15 mL conical tube containing 9 mL of pre-warmed complete growth medium: DMEM/F-12 supplemented with 10% (v/v) Fetal Bovine Serum (FBS) and 1% (v/v) Penicillin-Streptomycin (e.g., 100 U/mL penicillin, 100 µg/mL streptomycin).
- Centrifuge at 300 × *g* for 5 min to pellet cells and remove residual cryoprotectant.

- Resuspend the pellet in 5 mL of complete medium and transfer to a T-25 culture flask. Incubate at 37°C in a humidified 5% CO_2 incubator.
- For HeLa (human cervical adenocarcinoma) cells, use DMEM-High Glucose supplemented with 10% FBS and 1% antibiotics.

4.2 Maintenance and Subculturing

- Monitor cells daily. Replace medium every 2–3 days or when color indicates acidification (yellow-orange).
- Subculture at 70%–80% confluence. Aspirate medium and wash the monolayer gently with 2–3 mL of Dulbecco's Phosphate-Buffered Saline (DPBS) without Ca^{2+}/Mg^{2+}.
- Add enough 0.18% Trypsin-EDTA solution to cover the monolayer (e.g., 1 mL for a T-25 flask). Incubate at 37°C for 3–5 min.
- Critical Note: Monitor detachment under an inverted microscope. Do not exceed 5 min for hFIBs. Neutralize trypsin by adding an equal volume of complete medium containing FBS.
- Transfer the cell suspension to a centrifuge tube, pellet at $300 \times g$ for 5 min, and resuspend in fresh complete medium.

4.3 Cell Counting and Viability Assessment

- Mix 10 μL of the cell suspension with 10 μL of 0.4% Trypan Blue solution. Load 10 μL onto a hemocytometer.
- Count live (unstained) and dead (blue-stained) cells in the four corner quadrants.
- Calculate cell concentration and viability:
  - Cells/mL = (Average count per quadrant × Dilution Factor (2) × 10^4).
  - % Viability = (Total live cells/Total cells) × 100. Only cultures with >95% viability should be used for co-culture experiments.

4.4 Establishment and Optimization of 2D Co-Culture Models

Principle: Direct 2D co-culture allows for heterotypic cell–cell contact and paracrine signaling, mimicking tumor-stroma interactions [3].

Detailed Procedures

1. Preparation of Single-Cell Suspensions: Harvest and count MCF-7, HeLa, and hFIB cells separately as in 5.1.
2. **Ratio-Based Seeding:**
   - Ratios, e.g., 1:0, 3:1, 1:1, 1:3, 0:1 cancer:hFIB, calculate the required number of each cell type for a final density of 2×10^4 total cells per well of a 6-well plate.
   - Example for a 1:1 ratio: Mix 1×10^4 MCF-7 cells with 1×10^4 hFIB cells in a 1.5 mL microcentrifuge tube.

3. **Co-culture Seeding:**
   - Pellet the mixed cell suspension at 300×*g* for 5 min. Resuspend in the appropriate complete medium (DMEM/F-12 for MCF-7:hFIB, DMEM-HG for HeLa:hFIB).
   - Seed the suspension evenly into the wells. Gently rock the plate side-to-side and front-to-back for even distribution.
   - Include monoculture controls for MCF-7, HeLa, and hFIB alone at the same total seeding density.
4. **Incubation:** Place plates in the 37°C, 5% CO_2 incubator. Monitor daily for attachment, morphology, and confluence.

4.5 Microscopic Analysis of 2D Co-Cultures

Detailed Procedure:

1. At designated time points (24, 48, 72, 96 h), remove the plate from the incubator.
2. Using an inverted phase-contrast microscope, observe each well systematically. Note differences in morphology: epithelial cancer cells (MCF-7/HeLa) typically form cohesive islands, while fibroblasts (hFIB) are spindle-shaped and less densely packed.
3. Capture representative bright-field images at 10× objective (to assess overall distribution and cluster formation) and 40× objective (to examine individual cell morphology and cell-cell contacts). Ensure consistent focus and illumination across all samples and time points.

4.6 Metabolic Activity Assessment via Resazurin Assay (2D)

Principle: Viable cells reduce non-fluorescent resazurin (blue) to fluorescent resorufin (pink), providing a quantifiable measure of metabolic activity [4].

Detailed Procedures:

1. Seeding: Seed 1×10^4 total cells/well in a 96-well plate in quintuplicate (n=5) for each condition (co-culture ratios & monocultures). Include blank wells with medium only.
2. Assay Execution: After 24 h of incubation, carefully aspirate the old medium from each well and replace with 100 µL of fresh, pre-warmed medium.
3. Add 10 µL of 0.1% (w/v) filter-sterilized resazurin sodium salt solution directly to each well (final concentration ~0.01%).
4. Return the plate to the incubator and incubate for 4–6 h (or overnight for low-metabolism cultures).
5. Measurement: Using a fluorescence microplate reader, measure the fluorescence intensity with Excitation at 560 nm and Emission at 590 nm.

6. Data Analysis: Subtract the average fluorescence of blank wells from all sample readings. Normalize data to the initial time point (e.g., 24 h) or to control monocultures to determine fold-change in metabolic activity over time (48, 72, 96 h).

4.7 Development of 3D Heterotypic Spheroid Co-Cultures

Principle: The liquid-overlay technique on agarose-coated plates prevents cell attachment, promoting self-aggregation into spheroids that recapitulate 3D architecture and microenvironmental gradients [5].

Detailed Procedures:

1. Agarose Coating: Prepare a 1% (w/v) agarose solution in ultrapure water or serum-free medium. Autoclave or microwave to dissolve completely. While still warm (≈60°C), dispense 300 μL into each well of a 24-well plate to form a thin, non-adherent base. Allow to solidify completely at room temperature (≈20 min). Critical: Pre-warm plates with 500 μ L of medium in the incubator for 1 h before cell seeding to equilibrate.
2. Spheroid Formation: Harvest and count cells as before. Mix MCF-7 or HeLa with hFIB at the desired ratios.
3. Seed the mixed cell suspensions in 100–200 μL of complete medium at varying densities (e.g., 5×10^3, 1×10^4, and 1.5×10^4 cells/well) directly atop the agarose layer.
4. Carefully place the plates on a horizontal shaker inside the incubator (e.g., 60–80 rpm) to enhance nutrient exchange and promote symmetric spheroid formation.
5. Monitor spheroid formation daily under the microscope for up to 6 days. Compact, spherical aggregates typically form within 24–72 h.

4.8 Structural Analysis of 3D Spheroids

4.8.1 Optical Microscopy for Spheroid Growth Kinetics

- Image spheroids daily under bright-field illumination. Use image analysis software (e.g., ImageJ) to measure projected area, diameter, and circularity from the captured images to track growth and compaction over time.

4.8.2 Scanning Electron Microscopy (SEM) for Surface Ultrastructure

1. Fixation: Gently transfer spheroids to a microcentrifuge tube. Wash with 0.1 M sodium cacodylate buffer (pH 7.4) containing 1% sucrose for 1 h. Post-fix with 2.5% glutaraldehyde in the same buffer for 2 h at room temperature.
2. Dehydration: Perform a graded ethanol series (50%, 60%, 70%, 80%, 90%, 100%—15 min each step) to remove all water.

3. Drying and Coating: Subject spheroids to critical point drying (CPD) using liquid CO_2 to preserve delicate 3D structure. Mount on SEM stubs and sputter-coat with a 10–15 nm layer of gold/palladium.
4. Imaging: Analyze spheroid surface topography and cell–cell interactions using an SEM (e.g., Hitachi S-2700) at accelerating voltages of 5–15 kV.

4.9 Confocal Laser Scanning Microscopy (CLSM) for 3D Architecture

Detailed Procedure (Live/Deep Imaging):

1. Fixation and Staining: Fix spheroids in 4% Paraformaldehyde (PFA) for 1 h at 4°C. Wash 3× with PBS.
2. Membrane Staining: Incubate spheroids with Wheat Germ Agglutinin, Alexa Fluor™ 594 conjugate (WGA-AF594, 5 μg/mL in PBS) for 30–60 min at RT in the dark to label glycoproteins on the plasma membrane.
3. Mounting: Carefully transfer stained spheroids to an imaging-compatible dish (e.g., Ibidi μ-Slide). Use a spacer to prevent crushing.
4. Image Acquisition: Using a confocalmicroscope (e.g., Zeiss LSM 710) with a 20×/0.8 NA or 40×/1.2 NA water-immersion objective, acquire z-stack images through the entire spheroid depth (step size: 1–2 μm).
5. 3D Reconstruction: Process z-stacks using software (e.g., ZEN, Imaris) to generate 3D reconstructions, ortho-slices, and volume renderings to visualize internal architecture.

4.10 CLSM Analysis of Nanoparticle Uptake in 2D Co-Cultures

Principle: This protocol visualizes cell-type-specific uptake in a co-culture system using fluorescently labeled cells and nanoparticles [4].

Detailed Procedures:

1. **Cell Labeling and Seeding:** Pre-label MCF-7 cells with CellLight™ Actin-GFP, BacMam 2.0 according to the manufacturer's protocol (overnight incubation, followed by a recovery period) to fluorescently tag the actin cytoskeleton.
2. **Co-culture Setup:** Pre-coat Ibidi μ-Slide wells with Collagen IV (5 μg/cm^2) for 30 min at 37°C. Seed a co-culture of GFP-labeled MCF-7 and unlabeled hFIB at a 1:1 ratio (2×10^4 total cells/well).
3. **Nanoparticle Treatment:** After 24 h, treat cells with CH-H-R/RITC-pDNA nanoparticles (dose: 1 μg/cm^2, where RITC provides red fluorescence) for 4 h.

4. **Staining and Fixation:** Wash wells with PBS. Fix cells with 4% PFA for 15 min at RT. Permeabilize with 0.1% Triton X-100 (optional) and stain nuclei with Hoechst 33342 (2 µg/mL) for 15 min.
5. **Imaging:** Acquire high-resolution z-stacks (slice interval ~0.23 µm) using a 63× oil objective. Use sequential scanning to avoid channel crosstalk.
6. **Analysis:** Use orthogonal (XZ, YZ) projections and 3D rendering to determine if RITC (nanoparticle) fluorescence co-localizes preferentially with GFP (MCF-7 or unlabeled (hFIB) cells.

4.11 Flow Cytometric Quantification of Nanoparticle Uptake [6]

Principle: Flow cytometry provides quantitative, cell-by-cell analysis of nanoparticle association/uptake in mixed populations.

Detailed Procedures:

1. Experimental Setup: Seed monocultures of GFP+ MCF-7 and hFIB, as well as their co-culture (1:1 ratio), in 6-well plates at 2×10^5 cells/well.
2. Treatment: After 24 h, add CH-H-R/RITC-pDNA nanoparticles (1 µg/cm^2) for 4 h.
3. Cell Harvesting: Wash cells 3× with cold PBS. Harvest using 0.18% trypsin/5 mM EDTA (incubate at 37°C for no more than 3 min to minimize internalization artifacts). Neutralize with complete medium, centrifuge (300 × *g*, 5 min), and resuspend in 500 µL of ice-cold PBS containing 1% BSA. Pass suspension through a 35–40 µm cell strainer.
4. **Flow Cytometry Acquisition:**
   - Use untreated GFP+ MCF-7 and hFIB to set compensation and establish gating: FSC-A vs. SSC-A to gate on live cells, then GFP (FL-1, 530/30 nm) to distinguish MCF-7 (GFP+) from hFIB (GFP-).
   - For nanoparticle detection, use the RITC/PE channel (FL-2, 585/42 nm).
   - Acquire at least 8000 events per sample within the live cell gate.
5. **Data Analysis:** Using software (e.g., FCS Express v.4), analyze the median fluorescence intensity (MFI) of RITC in both the GFP+ (MCF-7) and GFP- (hFIB) populations. Compare MFI values to untreated controls to quantify cell-type-specific nanoparticle uptakenanoparticle uptake[6].

References

1. Capes-Davis A, Freshney RI (2021) Freshney's culture of animal cells: A manual of basic technique and specialized applications. John Wiley & Sons
2. Fennema E, Rivron N, Rouwkema J, Van Blitterswijk C, De Boer J (2013) Spheroid culture as a tool for creating 3D complex tissues. Trends Biotechnol 31(2):108–115
3. Freshney, RI (2015) Culture of animal cells: a manual of basic technique and specialized applications. John Wiley & Sons
4. O'brien J, Wilson I, Orton T, Pognan F (2000) Investigation of the Alamar Blue (resazurin) fluorescent dye for the assessment of mammalian cell cytotoxicity. Eur J Biochem 267(17):5421–5426
5. Zanoni M, Piccinini F, Arienti C, Zamagni A, Santi S, Polico R, Bevilacqua A, Tesei A (2016) 3D tumor spheroid models for in vitro therapeutic screening: a systematic approach to enhance the biological relevance of data obtained. Sci Rep 6(1):19103
6. Mason J, Öhlund D (2023) Key aspects for conception and construction of co-culture models of tumor-stroma interactions. Front Bioeng Biotechnol 11:1150764

Chapter 16

Development of 3D Breast Cancer Spheroid Models and Evaluation of Paclitaxel Cytotoxicity in Monolayer Versus Spheroid Cultures

Abstract

This protocol describes a standardized methodology for establishing and characterizing three-dimensional (3D) tumor spheroid models of breast cancer using MDA-MB-231 (triple-negative) and MCF-7 (luminal A) cell lines, and for comparing their chemosensitivity to Paclitaxel relative to conventional two-dimensional (2D) monolayer cultures. Spheroids are generated using two complementary approaches: the agarose-based liquid-overlay technique with concentrations of 1.0% and 1.5% (w/v) and cell seeding densities ranging from 1000 to 50,000 cells per well, and the Geltrex®-enhanced method incorporating 1.5% or 2.0% (v/v) extracellular matrix components to promote more physiologically relevant tumor architecture. Spheroid formation and growth kinetics are monitored by inverted microscopy on days 4 and 7, with diameter measurements quantified using ImageJ software, and surface ultrastructure is characterized by scanning electron microscopy (SEM) following glutaraldehyde fixation, osmium tetroxide post-fixation, graded ethanol dehydration, and gold sputter-coating. Cytotoxicity assessment is performed using the AlamarBlue® metabolic assay (excitation 560 nm/emission 590 nm) following 72-h exposure to a dose range of Paclitaxel (0.5% DMSO vehicle) in both culture models, enabling comparative determination of half-maximal inhibitory concentrations (IC_{50}) via non-linear regression in GraphPad Prism. Statistical analyses include two-way ANOVA with Bonferroni post hoc for spheroid size comparisons and Kruskal-Wallis with Dunn's post hoc for cytotoxicity data, with significance set at $p < 0.05$. This protocol provides a robust platform for investigating the differential drug sensitivity conferred by 3D tumor architecture versus conventional monolayer cultures.

Keywords 3D spheroids, Breast cancer, Paclitaxel, Cytotoxicity, Drug resistance

1 Introduction

Breast cancer remains a leading cause of cancer-related mortality worldwide. In vitro studies using two-dimensional (2D) monolayer cultures have limitations in mimicking the complex tumor microenvironment. Three-dimensional (3D) cell culture models, such as multicellular tumor spheroids, offer a more physiologically relevant system for studying cancer biology and drug response. This study focuses on establishing and characterizing 3D spheroid models of two distinct breast cancer cell lines—the highly aggressive, triple-negative

Karuppusamy Arunachalam et al., *Advanced Protocols in Cancer Research*, Springer Protocols Handbooks,
https://doi.org/10.1007/978-1-0716-5348-7_16,

MDA-MB-231 and the less aggressive, hormone receptor-positive MCF-7—using agarose-based and Geltrex®-based methods [1, 2].

2 Aim

To establish and standardize 3D tumor spheroid models of MDA-MB-231 and MCF-7 breast cancer cell lines using agarose and Geltrex® matrices, and to compare the cytotoxic effects of Paclitaxel on these cells cultured in 2D monolayers versus 3D spheroids.

3 Materials

- **Cell Lines**: MDA-MB-231 (triple-negative), MCF-7 (luminal A).
- **Culture Media**: RPMI 1640 (for MDA-MB-231), DMEM High Glucose (for MCF-7), supplemented with 10% FBS, 1% Penicillin-Streptomycin, and 0.5% Amphotericin B.
- **3D Culture Matrices**: Agarose powder, Geltrex® (reduced growth factors).
- **Consumables**: 75 cm^2 flasks, 96-well flat-bottom plates, serological pipettes, and conical tubes.
- **Reagents**: PBS, Trypsin-EDTA, Trypan blue, Paclitaxel (Ontax®), DMSO, AlamarBlue® reagent, glutaraldehyde, osmium tetroxide, ethanol.
- **Equipment**: CO_2 incubator, inverted light microscope, centrifuge, Neubauer chamber, microplate spectrophotometer (Synergy H1), scanning electron microscope (JSM6610LV).

4 Working Procedure (Step-by-Step) [3–6]

4.1 2D Monolayer Culture Maintenance (Fig. 1)

1. Culture MDA-MB-231 and MCF-7 cells in their respective supplemented media in 75 cm^2 flasks at 37°C and 5% CO_2.
2. Change media two to three times weekly. Monitor confluence and morphology using an inverted microscope.
3. At ~80% confluence, wash cells with PBS, detach with trypsin-EDTA, and inactivate with complete medium.
4. Count viable cells using Trypan blue and a Neubauer chamber. Seed cells at required densities for experiments or for passaging.

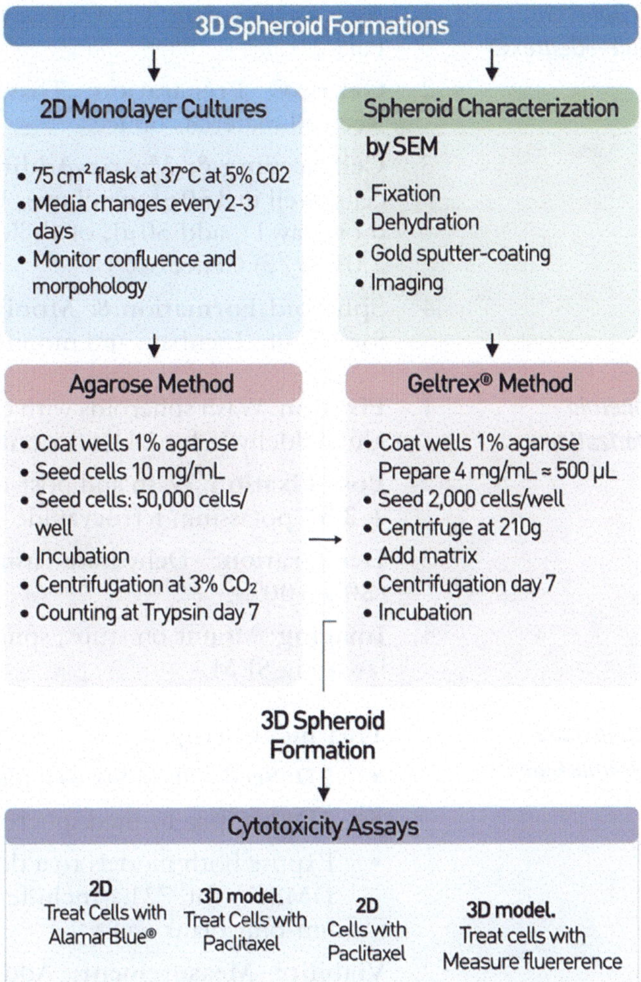

Fig. 1 The schematic representation of 3D tumor spheroid models of MDA-MB-231 and MCF-7 breast cancer cell lines using agarose and Geltrex® matrices

4.2 3D Spheroid Formation—Agarose Method

1. **Agarose Coating**: Dissolve agarose in distilled water, autoclave, and maintain at >60°C. Add 50 µL of 1.0% or 1.5% (w/v) agarose solution per well of a 96-well plate. UV-sterilize for 30 min.
2. **Cell Seeding**: Plate cells at densities ranging from 1000 to 50,000 cells/well in 200 µL of medium.
3. **Spheroid Formation**: Centrifuge plates at 1000 × *g* for 10 min. Incubate at 37°C, 5% CO_2.
4. **Monitoring**: Observe and image spheroids on days 4 and 7 using an inverted microscope. Measure spheroid diameters using ImageJ software.

4.3 3D Spheroid Formation—Geltrex® Method

1. **Agarose Coating:** Coat wells with 50 µL of 1.0% agarose as in Part 2.
2. **Geltrex® Preparation:** Thaw Geltrex®at 4°C overnight. Keep all materials on ice.
3. **Cell Seeding & Matrix Addition:** Plate cells (2000–10,000 cells/well in 150 µL medium). Immediately or 24 h later (Day 0 or Day 1), add 50 µL of chilled medium containing 1.5% or 2.0% (v/v) Geltrex®.
4. **Spheroid Formation & Monitoring:** Centrifuge at 1000 × *g* for 10 min. Incubate and monitor as in Part 2.

4.4 Spheroid Characterization (SEM)

1. **Fixation**: Wash spheroids with cacodylate buffer. Fix with 2.5% glutaraldehyde for 24 h at room temperature.
2. **Post-Fixation**: Wash and post-fix with 0.2% osmium tetroxide + 2.5% potassium ferrocyanide (1:1) for 1 h.
3. **Dehydration**: Dehydrate using a graded ethanol series (30%–100%).
4. **Imaging**: Mount on stubs, sputter-coat with gold, and visualize using SEM.

4.5 Cytotoxicity Assay (AlamarBlue®)

1. **Treatment Setup**:
   - **2D:** Seed cells in 96-well plates 24 h prior to treatment.
   - **3D:** Use pre-formed spheroids (~day 4, ~400 µm).
   - Expose both models to a dose range of Paclitaxel (in 0.5% DMSO) for 72 h. Include untreated control and medium-only blank wells.
2. **Viability Measurement**: Add AlamarBlue® reagent (10% v/v). Incubate for 4 h at 37°C.
3. **Readout**: Measure fluorescence (Ex: 560 nm/Em: 590 nm) using a microplate reader.
4. **Analysis**: Calculate % metabolic viability relative to control. Determine IC_{50} values using GraphPad Prism software.

4.6 Statistical Analysis

1. Test data for normality (Shapiro-Wilk) and homogeneity of variance (Levene's test).
2. Analyze spheroid size data using two-way ANOVA with Bonferroni post hoc.
3. Analyze cytotoxicity data using the Kruskal–Wallis test with Dunn's post hoc.
4. Consider $p < 0.05$ as statistically significant.

References

1. Cailleau R, Young R, Olive M, Reeves WJ Jr (1974) Breast tumor cell lines from pleural effusions. J Natl Cancer Inst 53(3):661–674
2. Comşa Ş, Cimpean AM, Raica M (2015) The story of MCF-7 breast cancer cell line: 40 years of experience in research. Anticancer Res 35(6):3147–3154
3. Friedrich J, Seidel C, Ebner R, Kunz-Schughart LA (2009) Spheroid-based drug screen: considerations and practical approach. Nat Protoc 4(3):309–324
4. Ivascu A, Kubbies M (2006) Rapid generation of single-tumor spheroids for high-throughput cell function and toxicity analysis. SLAS Discov 11(8):922–932
5. O'brien J, Wilson I, Orton T, Pognan F (2000) Investigation of the Alamar Blue (resazurin) fluorescent dye for the assessment of mammalian cell cytotoxicity. Eur J Biochem 267(17):5421–5426
6. Sadeghi-Oroumiyeh A, Valizadeh H, Zakeri-Milani P (2021) Determination of paclitaxel solubility and stability in the presence of injectable excipients. Pharm Chem J 55(9):983–987

Chapter 17

Evaluation of Doxorubicin Efficacy on 2D and 3D Cultures of Triple-Negative Breast Cancer Cells (MDA-MB-231)

Abstract

This protocol describes a comparative methodology for evaluating the cytotoxic and morphological effects of doxorubicin (DOX) on two-dimensional (2D) monolayer and three-dimensional (3D) spheroid cultures of MDA-MB-231 triple-negative breast cancer cells. The 3D spheroid model is established using the liquid-overlay technique on 1.5% (w/v) agarose-coated U-bottom 96-well plates, with cell seeding densities of 10,000–15,000 cells per well and centrifugation at 170 × *g* for 60 s to promote aggregation, followed by culture for up to 13 days with medium replacement every 3 days. Fully formed spheroids (day 7) and 2D monolayers are treated with doxorubicin (0.5–10.0 μg/mL) for 24 and 48 h, with spheroid cultures maintained on an orbital shaker at 90 rpm during treatment to enhance drug penetration. Cytotoxicity is assessed using the MTT assay (0.5 mg/mL, 2-h incubation, absorbance at 570 nm) following dissociation of spheroids into single-cell suspensions. Spheroid morphology and growth inhibition are monitored by bright-field microscopy, with two-dimensional area measurements (μm^2) quantified using ImageJ software. Histological analysis of spheroid architecture is performed by hematoxylin and eosin (H&E) staining following 4% paraformaldehyde fixation, paraffin embedding, and 4 μm sectioning. Statistical comparisons between treatment groups and time points are conducted using two-way ANOVA with Dunnett's multiple comparisons test in GraphPad Prism 8.3.0, with significance set at $p < 0.05$. This protocol enables direct comparison of drug efficacy between conventional 2D cultures and more physiologically relevant 3D tumor models.

Keywords Triple-negative breast cancer, 3D spheroids, Doxorubicin, MTT assay, Histology

1 Introduction

Triple-negative breast cancer (TNBC) is an aggressive subtype of breast cancer characterized by the absence of estrogen, progesterone, and HER2 receptors, which limits treatment options. In vitro models such as 2D monolayers and 3D spheroids offer valuable tools for studying drug responses and tumor biology. While 2D cultures are simple and widely used, 3D spheroids better mimic the tumor microenvironment, including gradients of oxygen, nutrients, and drug penetration [1]. This study aims to assess the cytotoxicity and morphological impact of doxorubicin (DOX) on both 2D and 3D models of MDA-MB-231 cells, providing comparative insights into drug efficacy in physiologically relevant conditions.

Karuppusamy Arunachalam et al., *Advanced Protocols in Cancer Research*, Springer Protocols Handbooks,
https://doi.org/10.1007/978-1-0716-5348-7_17,

2 Aim

To evaluate the cytotoxic and morphological effects of doxorubicin on 2D monolayer and 3D spheroid cultures of MDA-MB-231 cells using MTT assay, spheroid size analysis, and histological staining.

3 Materials

- MDA-MB-231 cells (ATCC HTB-26).
- Dulbecco's modified Eagle's medium (DMEM).
- Fetal bovine serum (FBS).
- Penicillin–streptomycin (1%).
- Agarose (1.5%).
- Phenol red-free DMEM.
- 96-well flat-bottom and U-bottom plates (TPP).
- Doxorubicin (Sigma).
- MTT reagent (Sigma).
- Dimethyl sulfoxide (DMSO).
- Paraformaldehyde (4%).
- Phosphate-buffered saline (PBS).
- Leica microscope and LEICA D-LUX 3 camera.
- ImageJ software.
- Microplate reader (Cytation 3, BioTek).
- GraphPad Prism 8.3.0.
- Tissue processing cassettes and sponges.
- Hematoxylin and eosin staining kit.

4 Detailed Procedures [2, 3] (Fig. 1)

4.1 Cell Culture of MDA-MB-231 Cells

1. Thaw the MDA-MB-231 (ATCC HTB-26) cells rapidly in a 37°C water bath.
2. Transfer the contents to a 15 mL conical tube containing 9 mL of pre-warmed complete DMEM medium (DMEM + 10% FBS + 1% penicillin/streptomycin).
3. Centrifuge at 200 × *g* for 5 min to remove DMSO.
4. Discard the supernatant and resuspend the pellet in 10 mL of fresh complete DMEM.

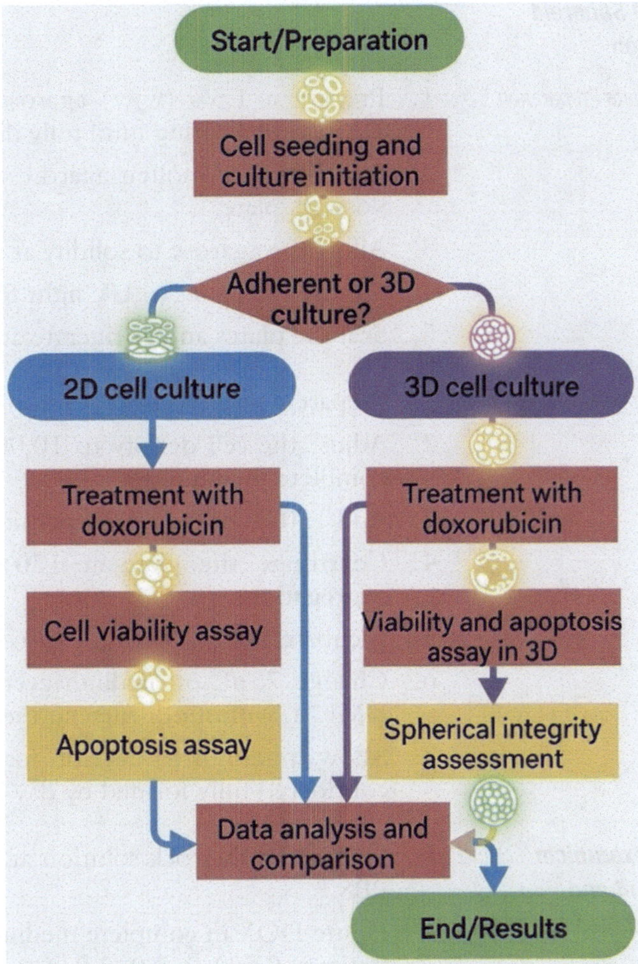

Fig. 1 Overall flowchart for the evaluation of doxorubicin efficacy on 2D and 3D cultures of triple-negative breast cancer cells (MDA-MB-231)

5. Seed the cells into a T-25 flask and incubate at 37°C in a humidified incubator with 5% CO_2.
6. Subculture the cells upon reaching 70%–80% confluency using standard trypsinization protocol (0.25% trypsin–EDTA).

4.2 2D Monolayer Culture

1. Harvest MDA-MB-231 cells using trypsinization and count using a hemocytometer or automated cell counter.
2. Prepare a cell suspension at 1000 cells per 100 μL in complete DMEM.
3. Plate 100 μL (1000 cells) into each well of a flat-bottom 96-well tissue culture plate (TC Plate 96 Well Standard d.F).
4. Incubate the plate at 37°C, 5% CO_2 for 24 h to allow cell adherence before drug treatment.

4.3 3D Spheroid Formation

4.3.1 Plate Preparation

1. Prepare a 1.5% (w/v) agarose solution in phenol red-free DMEM by heating until fully dissolved.
2. Add 50 μL of molten agarose into each well of a U-bottom 96-well plate.
3. Allow the agarose to solidify at room temperature (~30 min).
4. Expose the plates to UV light for 60 min for sterilization.
5. Seal the plates and refrigerate at 4°C for 24 h before use.

4.3.2 Spheroid Seeding

1. Prepare a single-cell suspension of MDA-MB-231 cells.
2. Adjust the cell density to 10,000–15,000 cells per 150 μL of complete medium.
3. Add 150 μL of the cell suspension to each agarose-coated well.
4. Centrifuge the plate at 170 × *g* for 60 s to facilitate cell aggregation.
5. Incubate at 37°C with 5% CO_2 for 72 h.
6. Change 75 μL of medium every 3 days with fresh complete DMEM, without disturbing the spheroids.
7. Allow spheroids to develop for up to 13 days. Spheroids are considered fully formed by day 7.

4.4 Doxorubicin Treatment and Spheroid Size Analysis

1. Prepare DOX stock solution at 200 μg/mL in sterile water or PBS.
2. Dilute DOX in complete medium to desired working concentrations: 0.5, 1.0, 2.0, 3.0, 4.0, 5.0, and 10.0 μg/mL.
3. On day 7 of spheroid culture, gently remove 75 μL of medium from each well and add 75 μL of DOX solution to reach a final volume of 150 μL.
4. Incubate treated spheroids for 24 h and 48 h on an orbital shaker at 90 rpm.
5. After incubation, remove DOX-containing medium and replace it with fresh supplemented medium.
6. Capture images of spheroids using a Leica Wetzlar microscope equipped with a LEICA D-LUX 3 camera.
7. Measure the 2D area (μm^2) of spheroids using ImageJ software:
   - Open image in ImageJ.
   - Set scale using known scale bar.
   - Outline spheroid boundary using freehand or threshold tool.
   - Measure area using "Measure" (Analyze > Measure).

4.5 MTT Cell Viability Assay

4.5.1 Treatment and Dissociation (3D Spheroids)

1. Treat 3D spheroids on day 7 with 2, 3, and 4 μg/mL DOX for 24 h and 48 h as described above.
2. After incubation, collect three spheroids per treatment into 1.5 mL Eppendorf tubes.
3. Pipette up and down repeatedly to dissociate spheroids into single cells.
4. Centrifuge at 1300 rpm for 3 min.
5. Discard supernatant and resuspend in 200 μL phenol red-free DMEM.
6. Count viable cells and seed into flat-bottom 96-well plates.

4.5.2 Treatment (2D Monolayers)

1. After 24 h of initial seeding, treat monolayer cultures with 2, 3, and 4 μg/mL DOX for 24 h and 48 h.

4.5.3 MTT Assay

1. After treatment, discard the media and wash gently with PBS (optional).
2. Add 100 μL of MTT solution (0.5 mg/mL in DMEM) to each well.
3. Incubate at 37°C for 2 h, protected from light.
4. Remove MTT solution and add 100 μL DMSO to dissolve the formazan crystals.
5. Gently shake the plate for 5 min to ensure complete dissolution.
6. Measure absorbance at 570 nm using a microplate reader.
7. Calculate percentage viability relative to untreated control (set at 100%).

4.6 Immunohistochemical (H&E) Analysis of 3D Spheroids

1. Treat 3D spheroids with 4 μg/mL DOX for 24 h and 48 h.
2. Wash spheroids three times with 1× PBS to remove residual media.
3. Fix spheroids in 4% paraformaldehyde (PFA) for 30 min or overnight at room temperature.
4. Wash spheroids three times with PBS to remove fixative.
5. Transfer spheroids to tissue cassettes containing sponge pads on both sides.
6. Submerge cassettes in PFA and submit for paraffin embedding and sectioning.
7. Section spheroids at 4 μm thickness.
8. Stain sections with hematoxylin and eosin (H&E) following standard histology protocols.
9. Analyze morphology and tissue architecture under a light microscope.

4.7 Statistical Analysis

1. Compile absorbance and image data from replicate experiments.
2. Perform two-way ANOVA using GraphPad Prism 8.3.0 to compare treatments and time points.
3. Use Dunnett's multiple comparisons test to determine statistical significance against control.
4. Present results as mean ± standard deviation (SD).
5. Consider $p < 0.05$ as statistically significant.

References

1. Huang Z, Yu P, Tang J (2020) Characterization of triple-negative breast cancer MDA-MB-231 cell spheroid model. Onco Targets Ther 13:5395–5405
2. Januškevičienė I, Petrikaitė V (2024) Exploring doxorubicin transport in 2D and 3D models of MDA-MB-231 sublines: impact of hypoxia and cellular heterogeneity on doxorubicin accumulation in cells. Am J Cancer Res 14(7):3584
3. Muguruma M, Teraoka S, Miyahara K, Ueda A, Asaoka M, Okazaki M et al (2020) Differences in drug sensitivity between two-dimensional and three-dimensional culture systems in triple-negative breast cancer cell lines. Biochem Biophys Res Commun 533(3):268–274

Check for updates

Chapter 18

Generation and Analysis of SK-MEL-28 Melanoma Spheroids for 3D Co-Culture and Drug Testing Models

Abstract

This protocol describes a methodology for generating SK-MEL-28 melanoma spheroids using agarose micromolds (MicroTissues® 3D Petri Dish®) and establishing 3D co-culture models with human umbilical vein endothelial cells (HUVECs) on bacterial nanocellulose (BNC) and BNC-collagen scaffolds. Spheroids are formed by seeding 1×10^6 cells into 81-well micromolds, allowing aggregation for 3 h and maturation for 48–72 h with daily medium changes. Harvested spheroids are characterized by MTS viability assay and live/dead staining (calcein AM/ethidium homodimer-1) with confocal microscopy. Co-cultures are established by sequential seeding of HUVECs followed by SK-MEL-28 spheroids onto BNC-COL scaffolds and maintained for up to 7 days. The models are validated for drug testing by exposing 2D monolayers, 3D spheroids, and co-cultures to doxorubicin (25–100 μM) for 24 h, with cytotoxicity assessed via MTS assay at 490 nm. Fixation with 4% paraformaldehyde and staining with phalloidin (Alexa Fluor 546) and DAPI enables visualization of the actin cytoskeleton and nuclei by confocal microscopy.

Keywords Melanoma spheroids, HUVEC, Co-culture, Bacterial nanocellulose, Doxorubicin, Drug testing

1 Introduction

Three-dimensional (3D) spheroid models provide a more physiologically relevant environment for studying cancer cell behavior, drug response, and cell–cell interactions compared to traditional two-dimensional (2D) monolayers. This protocol details the methods for generating and characterizing SK-MEL-28melanoma spheroids, their subsequent culture on bacterial nanocellulose (BNC)-based scaffolds, and their use in establishing co-culture models with human umbilical vein endothelial cells(HUVECs) [1]. These 3D models are ultimately applied to assess the cytotoxic effects of chemotherapeutic agents such as doxorubicin.

Karuppusamy Arunachalam et al., *Advanced Protocols in Cancer Research*, Springer Protocols Handbooks,
https://doi.org/10.1007/978-1-0716-5348-7_18,

2 Aim

To establish a standardized *in vitro* 3D model using SK-MEL-28 melanoma spheroids co-cultured with HUVECs on BNC scaffolds for the purpose of mimicking tumor microenvironmental interactions and evaluating drug efficacy in a more representative context.

3 Materials

- **Cell Lines:** SK-MEL-28 (human melanoma), HUVEC (human umbilical vein endothelial cells).
- **Culture Media:** DMEM (for SK-MEL-28), RPMI-1640 (for HUVEC), both supplemented with 10% fetal bovine serum (FBS), 1% penicillin/streptomycin, and sodium bicarbonate.
- **Reagents:** Trypsin, phosphate-buffered saline (PBS), paraformaldehyde (4%), agarose, sodium chloride (NaCl), MTS reagent, calcein AM, ethidium homodimer-1, DAPI, phalloidin (Alexa Fluor 546 conjugate), and doxorubicin (DOX).
- **Supplies and Equipment:** MicroTissues® 3D Petri Dish® micromolds, tissue culture plates (12-well, 24-well, 96-well), Neubauer chamber, centrifuge, CO_2 incubator (37°C, 5% v), autoclave, microwave, laminar flow hood, inverted light microscope, confocalmicroscope, spectrophotometer (for 490 nm absorbance).
- **Scaffolds:** Bacterial nanocellulose (BNC) and BNC-collagen (BNC-COL) membranes.

4 Working Procedure [2]

4.1 Cell Culture Maintenance

4.1.1 Culturing SK-MEL-28 Cells

1. Culture SK-MEL-28 cells (passages 3-23) in T–75 flasks with DMEM supplemented with:
   - 10% (v/v) fetal bovine serum (FBS).
   - 3.7 g/L sodium bicarbonate.
   - 1% (v/v) penicillin/streptomycin.
2. Maintain cells in a humidified incubator at 37°C with 5% CO_2.
3. Subculture upon reaching 70%–80% confluence.

1. Aspirate medium.
2. Wash monolayer with 5 mL PBS.
3. Add 1 mL of 0.25% trypsin–EDTA and incubate at 37°C for 3–5 min.
4. Neutralize with 5 mL complete DMEM.
5. Centrifuge at 300 × *g* for 5 min. Resuspend pellet in fresh medium for counting or seeding.

4.1.2 Culturing HUVECs

1. Culture HUVECs (passages 57–77) in T-75 flasks with RPMI-1640 supplemented with:
   - 10% (v/v) FBS.
   - 1.5 g/L sodium bicarbonate.
   - 1% (v/v) penicillin/streptomycin.
2. Maintain cells under the same conditions as above (37°C, 5% CO_2).
3. Subculture using the same trypsinization protocol as described in 4.1.1.

4.2 Production of SK-MEL-28 Spheroids [3]

4.2.1 Preparation of Agarose Micromolds

1. Wash MicroTissues® 3D Petri Dish® micromolds with ultrapure water.
2. Autoclave for 20 min at 120°C, 1 atm. Dry in an oven at 60°C.
3. Prepare 0.9% NaCl saline: Dissolve 0.9 g NaCl in 100 mL distilled water.
4. Prepare 2% Agarose Solution: Dissolve 2 g UltraPure™ Agarose in 100 mL of the 0.9% NaCl saline. Heat in a microwave in 10-s intervals until completely dissolved and clear.
5. Place a sterile micromold into one well of a 12-well plate.
6. Pipette 600 μL of the molten agarose solution into the mold. Let it solidify for 10 min at room temperature.
7. Using sterile forceps, carefully lift the agarose mold out and place it into a new well.
8. Pipette 700 μL of molten agarose around the base of the mold to secure it. Let solidify.
9. Sterilize the assembled mold under UV light in the laminar flow hood for 30 min.

10. Equilibrate the mold by adding 1.5 mL of complete DMEM and incubating (37°C, 5% CO_2) for ≥15 min. Aspirate medium and repeat equilibration once.

4.2.2 Seeding Cells into Molds

1. Trypsinize a confluent flask of SK-MEL-28 cells as described in 4.1.1.
2. Count cells using a Neubauer chamber.
3. For one 81-well micromold, centrifuge 1×10^6 cells. Aspirate supernatant.
4. Resuspend the cell pellet in 120 μL of complete DMEM.
5. Carefully pipette the 120 μL cell suspension evenly over the surface of the equilibrated agarose mold.
6. Incubate the plate (37°C, 5% CO_2) for 3 h to allow cell aggregation at the bottom of each microwell.
7. After 3 h, gently add 1 mL of complete DMEM to the well surrounding the mold.
8. Continue incubation. Change the medium every 24 h. Spheroids are typically mature and ready for use after 48–72 h.

4.2.3 Harvesting Spheroids

1. Using a P1000 pipette, gently wash spheroids out of the micromold with a jet of 1× PBS.
2. Collect the PBS containing spheroids in a 1.5 mL microcentrifuge tube.
3. Let spheroids settle by gravity or brief, low-speed centrifugation ($50 \times g$ for 1 min).
4. Carefully aspirate the PBS, leaving the spheroid pellet intact.

4.3 Spheroid Characterization Assays [4]

4.3.1 MTS Viability Assay

1. Transfer three spheroids per well into a 96-well plate.
2. Add 100 μL of complete DMEM to each well.
3. Add 20 μL of MTS reagent to each well. Mix gently by swirling the plate.
4. Incubate for 2 h (37°C, 5% CO_2).
5. Pipette to mix, then transfer 100 μL from each well to a fresh 96-well plate.
6. Measure the absorbance at 490 nm using a plate reader.

4.3.2 Live/Dead Staining (for Confocal Microscopy)

1. Harvest spheroids and place them in a microcentrifuge tube.
2. Prepare staining solution: Dilute 2 μL calcein AM (4 mM) and 4 μL ethidium homodimer-1 (2 mM) in 4 mL PBS (or as per manufacturer's instructions).
3. Remove PBS from spheroids and add 500 μL of the staining solution.
4. Incubate for 45 min at room temperature, protected from light.
5. Wash spheroids once with PBS.
6. Transfer to a glass-bottom dish for imaging. Image using a confocalmicroscope (Ex/Em: Calcein ~494/517 nm; EthD-1 ~528/617 nm).

4.4 Co-Culture on BNC/BNC-COL Scaffolds

4.4.1 Monoculture on Scaffolds

1. Cut BNC or BNC-COL membranes to fit a 24-well plate.
2. For HUVECs: Seed 100,000 cells in a small volume (e.g., 50 μ L) onto the top or bottom surface of the membrane placed in a well.
   - After 4 h, add 500 μL of complete RPMI.
3. For SK-MEL-28 Spheroids: Seed 50 spheroids in a small volume onto the membrane.
   - After 6 h, add 500 μL of complete DMEM.
4. Incubate cultures for 3 days (37°C, 5% CO_2), changing medium every 48 h.

4.4.2 Sequential Co-Culture Setup (for Invasion Assay)

1. Place a BNC-COL membrane in a 24-well plate (lower side facing up).
2. Seed HUVECs at 5.2×10^4 cells/cm^2 in a small volume of RPMI.
3. After 4 h, add 500 μL RPMI. Incubate for 24 h.
4. After 24 h, add SK-MEL-28 spheroids at a density of 28 spheroids/cm^2 in a small volume of DMEM.
5. After 6 h, replace medium with 500 μL of fresh complete DMEM.
6. Maintain co-culture for up to 7 days, changing medium every 48 h. Fix and analyze at desired time points (e.g., days 1, 3, 7).

4.5 Drug Treatment and Cytotoxicity Testing

4.5.1 Preparation of Doxorubicin (DOX) Solutions

1. Prepare a stock solution of DOX in DMSO or water as per manufacturer's instructions.
2. Dilute stock in the appropriate complete medium (DMEM for spheroids, DMEM for co-culture) to create working concentrations of 25, 50, and 100 μM.

4.5.2 Treatment of 2D SK-MEL-28 Monolayers

1. Seed 10,000 SK-MEL-28 cells/well in a 96-well plate. Incubate for 24 h.
2. Aspirate medium. Add 100 μL of DOX working solutions (25, 50, 100 μM) to respective wells. Include a negative control (medium only).
3. Incubate for 24 h (37°C, 5% CO_2).
4. Perform MTS assay as described in 4.3.1.

4.5.3 Treatment of 3D Spheroids

1. Harvest 48-h spheroids.
2. Distribute nine spheroids/well in a 96-well plate (low-attachment plate is ideal).
3. Add 100 μL of DOX working solutions (25, 50, 100 μM) to respective wells. Include a negative control.
4. Incubate for 24 h.
5. Perform MTS assay.

4.5.4 Treatment of 3D Co-Culture Model [5]

1. Establish the 7-day HUVEC-SK-MEL-28 spheroid co-culture on BNC-COL as described in 4.1.2.
2. On day 7, aspirate the old medium.
3. Add 500 μL of DOX working solutions (25, 50, 100 μM in DMEM) to the respective wells. Include a negative control.
4. Incubate for 24 h.
5. To assess viability, transfer the entire membrane with co-culture to a new well, add 120 μL of fresh DMEM + 20 μL MTS reagent directly onto the membrane, and incubate for 2 h.
6. Transfer 100 μL of the reacted medium to a 96-well plate and read absorbance at 490 nm.

4.6 Fixation and Staining for Microscopy

4.6.1 Fixation

- For Spheroids/HUVECs on Scaffolds: Aspirate medium, wash with PBS. Add 4% paraformaldehyde (PFA).
  - Fix spheroids for 12 h at 4°C.
  - Fix HUVEC monolayers for 30 min at room temperature.
- Wash fixed samples three times for 5 min with PBS.

4.6.2 Actin/Nuclei Staining (for Confocal)

1. Permeabilize samples with 0.1% Triton X-100 in PBS for 10 min.
2. Wash 2× with PBS.
3. Incubate with phalloidin (e.g., Alexa Fluor 546, 1:200 dilution) in PBS for 45–60 min, protected from light.
4. Wash 3× with PBS.
5. Incubate with DAPI (1 μg/mL) for 10 min.
6. Wash 3× with PBS.
7. Mount on slides or image directly in plates using a confocalmicroscope.

References

1. Friedrich J, Seidel C, Ebner R, Kunz-Schughart LA (2009) Spheroid-based drug screen: considerations and practical approach. Nat Protoc 4(3):309–324. https://doi.org/10.1038/nprot.2008.226
2. Meierjohann S (2021) What's new in melanoma? - the use of 3D models to understand immunotherapy-resistance. Pigment Cell Melanoma Res 34(2):236–247. https://doi.org/10.1111/pcmr.12941
3. Vantangoli MM, Madnick SJ, Huse SM, Weston P, Boekelheide K (2016) MCF-7 human breast cancer cells form differentiated microtissues in scaffold-free hydrogels. PLoS One 11(7):e0159446. https://doi.org/10.1371/journal.pone.0159446
4. Kenny HA, Lal-Nag M, White EA, Shen M, Chiang CY, Mitra AK et al (2015) Quantitative high throughput screening using a primary human three-dimensional organotypic culture predicts in vivo efficacy. Nat Commun 6:6220. https://doi.org/10.1038/ncomms7220
5. Smalley KS, Haass NK, Brafford PA, Lioni M, Flaherty KT, Herlyn M (2006) Multiple signaling pathways must be targeted to overcome drug resistance in cell lines derived from melanoma metastases. Mol Cancer Ther 5(5):1136–1144. https://doi.org/10.1158/1535-7163.MCT-06-0084

Chapter 19

In Vitro Development and Evaluation of Reconstructed Human Skin Models Using HaCat, MRC5, and CAL27 Cell Lines

Abstract

This protocol describes the generation and comprehensive characterization of three-dimensional reconstructed human skin models using HaCat keratinocytes, MRC5 fibroblasts, and CAL27 squamous carcinoma cells. Three distinct models are established: normal HaCat-Skin (keratinocytes on fibroblast-populated collagen dermis), tumorigenic CCE-Skin (co-seeded CAL27 and HaCat cells), and in situ carcinoma CCEinsitu-Skin (CAL27 spheroids transferred onto HaCat-Skin). Spheroids are generated via agarose-coated 96-well plates (500–3000 cells/well, 10 days) or micromold arrays ($50–100 \times 10^4$ cells, 7 days) and characterized for growth kinetics, viability (Alamar Blue), and necrotic centers (acridine orange/ethidium bromide staining). Skin models are evaluated by histology (hematoxylin and eosin staining), MTT viability assay following compound exposure, in vitro caffeine permeation by HPLC, and matrix metalloproteinase activity via polyacrylamide gel and in situ gelatin zymography. Statistical analysis is performed using GraphPad Prism with significance at $p < 0.05$.

Keywords Reconstructed skin, HaCat, CAL27, Spheroids, Zymography

1 Introduction

Three-dimensional (3D) in vitro reconstructed human skin models serve as advanced systems for dermatological and oncology research. These models mimic the architecture and physiology of normal and diseased human skin and are useful for evaluating drug cytotoxicity, skin permeability, and tumor progression [1]. In this protocol, HaCat keratinocytes, MRC5 fibroblasts, and CAL27 squamous carcinoma cells are employed to create normal (HaCat-Skin), tumorigenic (CCE-Skin), and in situ carcinoma (CCEinsitu-Skin) skin models [2]. Comprehensive evaluation of these models includes histology, cell viability, permeation assays, spheroid analysis, and matrix metalloproteinase activity.

Karuppusamy Arunachalam et al., *Advanced Protocols in Cancer Research*, Springer Protocols Handbooks, https://doi.org/10.1007/978-1-0716-5348-7_19,

2 Aim

- To establish and characterize HaCat-Skin, CCE-Skin, and CCEinsitu-Skin models.
- To generate tumor spheroids and assess their growth and viability.
- To evaluate skin model permeability and cytotoxic response to drugs.
- To examine tissue morphology and MMP activity through zymography.

3 Materials

3.1 Cell Lines

- HaCat (keratinocyte).
- MRC5 (fibroblast).
- CAL27 (squamous cell carcinoma).

3.2 Culture Media and Supplements

- Dulbecco's modified Eagle medium (DMEM).
- HAM-F12 Nutrient Mixture.
- Fetal bovine serum (FBS).
- Penicillin–streptomycin (100 U/mL and 100 μg/mL).
- Cholera toxin (1 μM).
- Insulin (5 μg/mL).
- Apo-transferrin (5 μg/mL).
- Hydrocortisone-21 (0.1 μg/mL).
- Epidermal growth factor (EGF) (2 μg/mL).
- Transforming growth factor-α (TGF-α) (100 ng/mL).

3.3 Reagents

- Type I Collagen (Gibco).
- PBS, MTT, isopropanol, and Alamar Blue.
- Ethidium bromide, acridine orange, and DQ-gelatin.
- Caffeine, cisplatin, and 22-β-hydroxytingenone.

3.4 Equipment

- CO_2 incubator.
- Inverted microscope (Zeiss Axio Vert.A1).
- ELISA plate reader (DTX 800).
- HPLC with XTerra MSC18 column.

- Microplate reader (fluorescence detection).
- Paraffin embedding station and microtome.
- Fluorescence microscope with FITC filter.
- Software: ImageJ, AxioVision, NIS-Elements.

4 Detailed Procedures [3–7]

4.1 Cell Culture

1. Thaw frozen vials of HaCat, MRC5, and CAL27 cells in a 37°C water bath.
2. Transfer contents to 15 mL tubes containing 10 mL pre-warmed DMEM with 10% FBS and 1% Pen/Strep.
3. Centrifuge at 1200 rpm for 5 min. Discard supernatant.
4. Resuspend cells in fresh complete medium and transfer to a T-75 flask.
5. Incubate at 37°C with 5% CO_2 and change medium every 2–3 days.
6. Subculture cells upon reaching 80%–90% confluence using 0.05% trypsin–EDTA.

4.2 Preparation of Reconstructed Human Skin Models

4.2.1 Dermis Formation

1. On ice, prepare dermal mix per insert: 700 μL of 3 mg/mL collagen I, 50 μL FBS, 108 μL 10× reconstitution buffer (0.05 M NaOH, 2.2% $NaHCO_3$, 200 mM HEPES), and 108 μL HAM-F12.
2. Add 2.5×10^4 MRC5 cells and gently mix.
3. Immediately pipette 800 μL into 12-mm Transwell inserts.
4. Incubate at 37°C for 30 min to allow collagen polymerization.
5. Rinse with PBS to stabilize pH.

4.2.2 Epidermis Formation

1. Seed 5×10^4 HaCat cells atop each dermal layer.
2. For CCE-Skin, co-seed 1.5×10^4 CAL27 cells.
3. Submerge in complete medium for 24 h to promote adhesion.
4. Remove apical medium to expose tissues to air–liquid interface.
5. Maintain for 10 days at 37°C, 5% CO_2, changing basolateral medium every 2 days.

4.3 Tumor Spheroid Generation

4.3.1 96-Well Plate Method

1. Add 50 μL of 1.5% sterile agarose to each well and allow to solidify.
2. Seed CAL27 cells at 500, 1000, 1500, 2000, or 3000 cells/well in 200 μL DMEM.
3. Incubate for 10 days at 37°C, 5% CO_2.
4. Replace 100 μL medium every 3–4 days.

4.3.2 Micromold Method

1. Pipette 500 μL of 2% autoclaved agarose into 9 × 9 micromold arrays.
2. Allow gel to polymerize for 6–8 min.
3. Transfer molds to 24-well plates and equilibrate with 1 mL DMEM.
4. Seed 50×10^4 or 100×10^4 CAL27 cells in 150 μL over molds.
5. Incubate at 37°C, 5% CO_2 for up to 7 days.

4.4 Spheroid Analysis

1. Capture spheroid images on days 1, 2, 6, and 10 (96-well) or days 1, 3, and 7 (micromolds).
2. Use calibrated AxioVision software to determine spheroid area and mean diameter.

4.5 Spheroid Growth Kinetics

1. Measure diameters on day 1 and the final day.
2. Calculate growth percentage:

$$\begin{aligned}&\%\ \text{Diameter increase}\\&\quad= [(\text{Final} - \text{Initial diameter}) \times 100]/\text{Initial diameter}\end{aligned}$$

4.6 Cell Viability in Spheroids (Alamar Blue Assay)

1. Prepare 60 μM Alamar Blue solution in DMEM.
2. Add 150 μL to each well containing spheroids.
3. Incubate for 2 h at 37°C.
4. Measure fluorescence: Ex 465 nm, Em 540 nm.

4.7 Necrotic Center Staining

1. Wash spheroids with PBS.
2. Stain with 5 μg/mL acridine orange/ethidium bromide for 10 min.
3. Wash with PBS and image under fluorescence microscopy (4×).

4.8 Generation of CCEinsitu-Skin Model

1. Follow HaCat-Skin protocol.
2. After 24 h of HaCat adhesion, transfer CAL27 spheroids (three to five per insert) onto tissue surface.
3. Incubate 10 more days at air–liquid interface.
4. Fix tissues in 10% formalin, embed in paraffin, and section for histological analysis.

4.9 In Vitro Skin Permeation Test

1. Prepare 0.1% caffeine stock in sterile PBS and store at 4°C.
2. Apply 50 μL of 500 μg/mL caffeine on tissue surface (22.32 μg/cm^2).
3. Maintain diffusion chamber at 32 ± 1°C.
4. Collect 1 mL receptor fluid at 0, 15, 30, 45, 60, 120, 180, and 240 min.
5. Analyze caffeine by HPLC:
   - Column: XTerra MSC18, 50 × 2.1 mm, 5 μm.
   - Mobile phase: 10 mM phosphate buffer (pH 3.5)/acetonitrile.
   - Flow: 0.6 mL/min; gradient: 5%–95% MeCN (0–5 min).
   - Inject 10 μL/sample.
6. Calculate permeation rate and % dose:
   - % Dose = (Sample peak area/Std. peak area) × 100.
   - Permeation rate (μg/cm^2/h) = Total μg/1.12 cm^2/4 h.

4.10 Cell Viability Assay (MTT)

1. Expose skin models to 10 μL of test compounds for 15 min.
2. Wash with PBS and incubate for 42 h.
3. Add 300 μL MTT (1 mg/mL) to each tissue insert.
4. Incubate 3 h, remove excess MTT, and wash with PBS.
5. Extract formazan with 2 mL isopropanol (2 h).
6. Transfer 200 μL of solution to 96-well plate and measure absorbance at 570 nm.

4.11 Morphological Analysis of Tissues

1. Fix tissues in 10% formalin overnight.
2. Dehydrate, embed in paraffin, and section at 3.5 μm.
3. Stain with hematoxylin and eosin.
4. Capture images using Nikon Eclipse and analyze with NIS-Elements.

4.12 Polyacrylamide Gel Zymography

1. Measure protein in supernatants using the Bradford assay.
2. Load 30 μg protein per lane on 10% SDS-PAGE + gelatin.
3. Run: 70 V for 30 min, then 120 V for 90 min.

4. Wash gel in 2.5% Triton X-100 (2×, 30 min).
5. Incubate overnight at 37°C in buffer (0.05 M Tris-HCl, pH 8, 5 mM $CaCl_2$, 5 μM $ZnCl_2$).
6. Stain with 0.5% Coomassie Brilliant Blue; destain until bands appear.
7. Quantify gelatinolytic bands with ImageJ.

4.13 In Situ Zymography

1. Dissolve 1 mg DQ-gelatin in 1 mL PBS.
2. Apply 80 μL to each tissue.
3. Incubate 2 h in a humidified chamber.
4. Visualize with FITC filter (Ex 460–500 nm; Em 512–542 nm).

4.14 Statistical Analysis

1. Perform analysis using GraphPad Prism 6.
2. Use Student's *t*-test, one-way, or two-way ANOVA as appropriate.
3. $p < 0.05$ is considered significant.

References

1. OECD (2015) Test No. 439: in vitro skin irritation: reconstructed human epidermis test method. OECD guidelines for the testing of chemicals, section 4. OECD Publishing, Paris, https://doi.org/10.1787/9789264242845-en
2. OECD (2004) Test No. 428: skin absorption: in vitro method. OECD guidelines for the testing of chemicals, section 4. OECD Publishing, Paris, https://doi.org/10.1787/9789264071087-en
3. Brohem CA, da Silva Cardeal LB, Tiago M, Soengas MS, de Moraes Barros SB, Maria-Engler SS (2011) Artificial skin in perspective: concepts and applications. Pigment Cell Melanoma Res 24(1):35–50. https://doi.org/10.1111/j.1755-148X.2010.00786.x
4. Friedrich J, Seidel C, Ebner R, Kunz-Schughart LA (2009) Spheroid-based drug screen: considerations and practical approach. Nat Protoc 4(3):309–324. https://doi.org/10.1038/nprot.2008.226
5. Ivanov D, Shuleva M, Pashov A, Heiner T (2014) A two-step acute toxicity study for the prioritization of antitumor drugs in the Ehrlich ascites carcinoma model. Toxicol Rep 1:1024–1032. https://doi.org/10.1016/j.toxrep.2014.10.009
6. Aranha MP, dos Santos RS, Muthu MS, Hwang J-H (2021) Evaluation of in vitro and in vivo antitumor activity of plant-derived essential oils in Ehrlich ascites carcinoma model. Biomed Pharmacother 138:111523. https://doi.org/10.1016/j.biopha.2021.111523
7. Vandooren J, Geurts N, Martens E, Van den Steen PE, Opdenakker G (2013) Zymography methods for visualizing hydrolytic enzymes. Nat Methods 10(3):211–220. https://doi.org/10.1038/nmeth.2371

Check for updates

Chapter 20

Multi-Elemental Analysis Using X-Ray Microfluorescence in 3D Cultures of Human Neuroblastoma Cells

Abstract

This protocol describes the generation and multi-elemental analysis of three-dimensional (3D) neuroblastoma spheroids using SH-SY5Y and SK-N-BE(2) cell lines combined with X-ray microfluorescence (MicroXRF) spectroscopy for spatially resolved elemental mapping and quantification. Spheroids are formed via the agarose-coated U-bottom 96-well plate method (1% agarose, 50 μL/well) with seeding densities of 1250 cells/well for SH-SY5Y (6-day culture) and 750 cells/well for SK-N-BE(2) (5-day culture), maintained at 37°C, 5% CO_2 with medium replacement on day 3. Following culture, spheroids are washed with PBS, fixed in 4% paraformaldehyde (20 min, 4°C), rinsed with Milli-Q water, and air-dried on 4 μm Ultralene® film for analysis. Elemental analysis is performed using a Bruker M4 Tornado MicroXRF spectrometer with a rhodium anode X-ray tube (30 W, 50 kV, 600 μA) and polycapillary focusing optics. Elemental mapping employs a 100 μm aluminum filter, 15 μm step size, and 300 ms/pixel dwell time. Point quantification for light elements (P, S, K, Ca) uses a 12.5 μm Al filter (40 kV, 600 μA, 100 s), and for heavy elements (Fe, Cu, Zn) a 630 μm Al filter (40 kV, 600 μA, 250 s). Spectral deconvolution and quantification are performed using PyMCA software with an ICRU-44 soft tissue matrix model. System validation utilizes NIST-traceable multi-element standards (10 μg/g) dried on Ultralene® film with an accuracy acceptance within ±15%.

Keywords Neuroblastoma, 3D spheroids, X-ray microfluorescence, Elemental mapping, Trace elements

1 Introduction

Three-dimensional (3D) cell cultures have emerged as advanced in vitro models that better mimic the in vivo tumor microenvironment compared to traditional two-dimensional (2D) monolayer cultures. Among these, multicellular spheroids are particularly effective in recapitulating the structural and functional features of solid tumors, including gradients of oxygen, nutrients, and cellular proliferation. Neuroblastoma, a pediatric extracranial solid tumor derived from neural crest cells, presents significant clinical challenges, especially in its high-risk forms. Cell lines such as SH-SY5Y and SK-N-BE(2) are commonly employed as in vitro models for neuroblastoma due to their distinct morphological and biochemical characteristics [1]. Multi-elemental analysis in 3D tumor spheroids can offer valuable

Karuppusamy Arunachalam et al., *Advanced Protocols in Cancer Research*, Springer Protocols Handbooks,
https://doi.org/10.1007/978-1-0716-5348-7_20,

insights into trace elemental composition, cellular metabolism, and drug interactions. X-ray microfluorescence (MicroXRF) spectroscopy is a powerful non-destructive technique capable of spatially resolved elemental mapping and quantification. This study describes the detailed methodology for the formation of SH-SY5Y and SK-N-BE(2) neuroblastoma cell spheroids and their elemental profiling using a Bruker M4 Tornado MicroXRF system [2].

2 Aim

To establish and characterize 3D spheroid cultures of human neuroblastoma cell lines (SH-SY5Y and SK-N-BE(2)) and to perform multi-elemental spatial analysis using X-ray microfluorescence (MicroXRF) to identify and quantify trace elements relevant to tumor biology and cellular homeostasis.

3 Materials

3.1 Cell Culture and Spheroid Formation

- SH-SY5Y cell line (ATCC CRL-2266).
- SK-N-BE(2) cell line (ATCC HTB-11).
- Dulbecco's modified Eagle medium (DMEM, Sigma-Aldrich).
- Fetal bovine serum (FBS, Gibco or equivalent).
- Penicillin–streptomycin (100 U/mL and 100 μg/mL).
- 96-well U-bottom plates (non-adherent or coated with 1% agarose).
- 1% Agarose solution (for coating wells).
- Phosphate-buffered saline (PBS, pH 7.4).
- Paraformaldehyde (PFA) 4%.
- Milli-Q water.
- Ultralene® film (4 μm thickness).
- Incubator (37°C, 5% CO_2).
- Confocal microscope (e.g., Olympus IX71S8F-3).

3.2 X-Ray Microfluorescence Analysis

- Bruker M4 Tornado MicroXRF spectrometer.
- Rhodium (Rh) anode X-ray tube (30 W, 50 kV, 600 μA).
- Polycapillary focusing optics.
- Silicon drift detector (SDD, 30 mm^2).
- Aluminum filters (12.5, 100, 630 μm).
- Titanium and copper filter combinations.

- Sample holders with triaxial geometry.
- ESPRIT software (Bruker).
- PyMCA software (ESRF, version 3.9.4).

3.3 Reference Standard for Validation

- NIST-certified multi-element solution.
- Milli-Q water for dilution.

4 Methods

4.1 Cell Culture and Three-Dimensional Spheroid Formation [1]

4.1.1 Cell Lines and Authentication

- **SH-SY5Y(ATCC® CRL-226™):** Human neuroblastoma cell line derived from a metastatic bone tumor (SK-N-SH subclone). Use cells between passages 15 and 25.
- **SK-N-BE(2)(ATCC® HTB-1™):** Human neuroblastoma cell line derived from a bone marrow metastasis post-therapy. Use cells between passages 10 and 20.
- **Quality Control:** Perform regular mycoplasma testing (e.g., monthly via PCR). Authenticate cell lines annually using short tandem repeat (STR) profiling.

4.1.2 Two-Dimensional Monolayer Culture (Pre-Spheroid Expansion)

- **Culture Medium:** High-glucose Dulbecco's modified Eagle medium (DMEM, e.g., Sigma-Aldrich D6429) supplemented with 10% (v/v) heat-inactivated fetal bovine serum (FBS) and 1% (v/v) penicillin–streptomycin (optional, but recommended for maintenance).
- **Culture Conditions:** Maintain cells in a humidified incubator at 37°C with 5% CO_2.
- **Subculturing:** Passage cells at ~80%–90% confluence using 0.25% trypsin–EDTA. Neutralize trypsin with complete medium, centrifuge (300 × *g*, 5 min), resuspend, and seed at an appropriate density (e.g., 1:5 to 1:10 split ratio). Renew culture medium every 48 h.

4.1.3 Three-Dimensional Spheroid Formation via Hanging Drop or Agarose-Coated Plates [2]

- **Method Selection:** For consistent, single-spheroid-per-well formation, the agarose-coated plate method is specified.
- **Preparation of Agarose-Coated Plates:**

1. Prepare a 1% (w/v) agarose solution in sterile, serum-free DMEM or PBS.
2. Microwave to dissolve completely and allow to cool to ~50–60°C (touchable but warm).
3. Pipette 50 µL of the agarose solution into each well of a sterile, U-bottom 96-well plate.
4. Swirl gently to coat the bottom and lower walls. Allow to solidify at room temperature under a laminar flow hood for 30–60 min.
5. *Optional:* Before use, pre-wet wells with 100 µL of culture medium for 1 h to prevent initial osmotic shock, then aspirate (Fig. 1).

- **Cell Seeding for Spheroids:**
  1. Harvest monolayer cells as described in Sect. 4.1.2. Obtain a viable single-cell suspension by gentle pipetting and passing through a 40 µm cell strainer if needed.
  2. Count cells using a hemocytometer or automated counter.
  3. Prepare cell suspensions in complete DMEM at the following densities:
     - **SH-SY5Y:** 25,000 cells/mL → 50 µL/well containing 1250 cells (Note: Original protocol states 5000/200 µL; this adjustment standardizes volume. Confirm optimal density for final 300–600 µm spheroid).
     - **SK-N-BE(2):** 15,000 cells/mL → 50 µL/well containing 750 cells (Original: 3000/200 µL).
  4. Carefully pipette 50 µL of the cell suspension into the center of each agarose-coated well.
  5. Gently add an additional 150 µL of complete medium to the side of the well, bringing the total volume to 200 µL, without disturbing the cell droplet.

- **Spheroid Incubation:**
  1. Carefully transfer the plate to the incubator (37°C, 5% CO_2). Avoid shaking or vibration.
  2. Incubate for:
     - **SH-SY5Y:** 6 days.
     - **SK-N-BE(2):** 5 days.
  3. Monitor spheroid formation daily using an inverted microscope. A single, compact spheroid should form in the center of each well within 24–48 h.

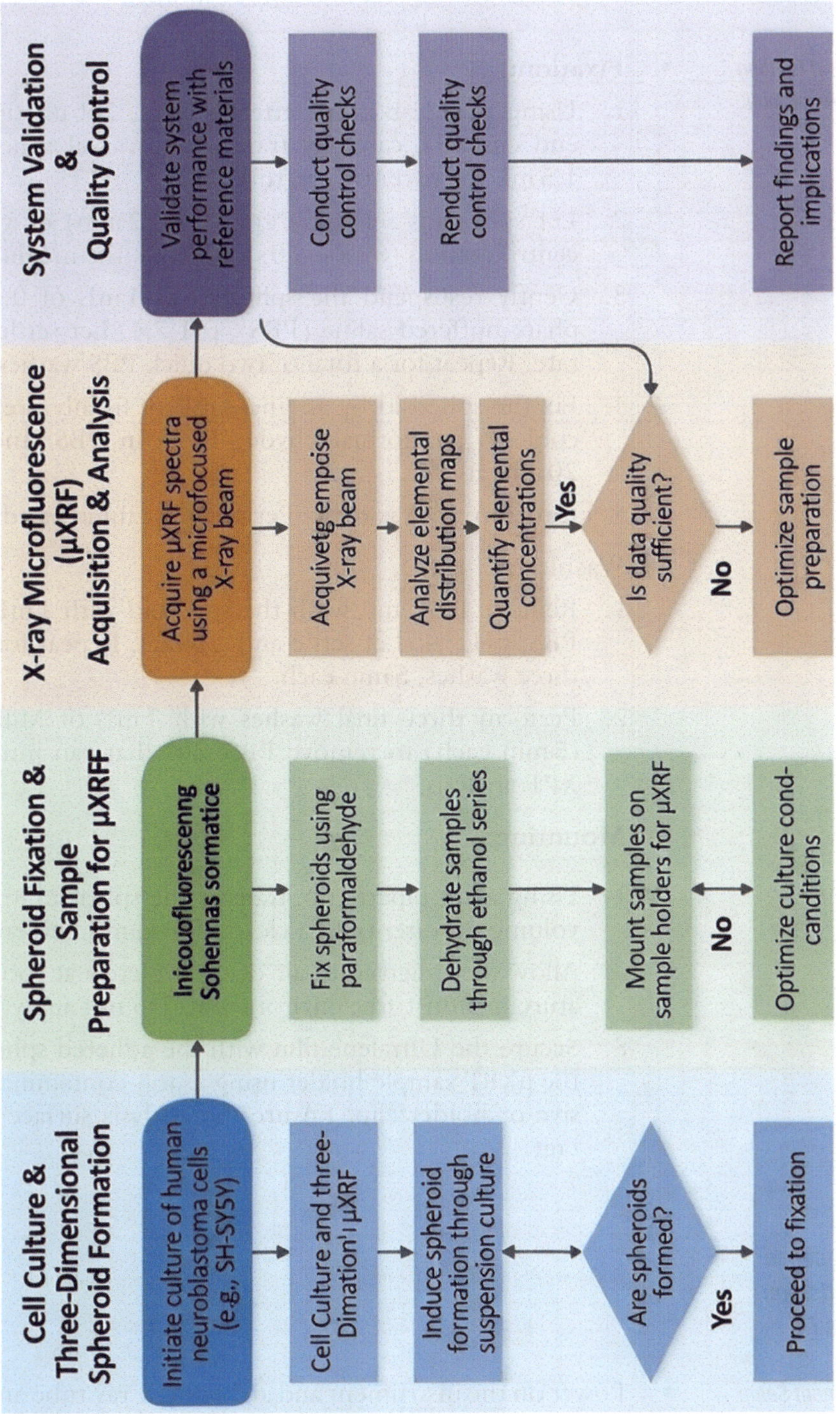

Fig. 1 The flowchart represents the sequential logic, critical parameters, and quality controls

4. On day 3, carefully aspirate 100 µL of medium from the side of the well and replace with 100 µL of fresh, pre-warmed complete medium to nourish the spheroid.

4.1.4 Spheroid Fixation and Sample Preparation for µXRF [3]

- **Fixation:**
  1. Using a wide-bore pipette tip (e.g., 200 µL tip with the end cut off), carefully transfer individual spheroids to a 1.5 mL microcentrifuge tube.
  2. Let spheroids settle by gravity (1–2 min) or very gentle centrifugation (50 × *g*, 30 s). Aspirate the medium.
  3. Gently resuspend the spheroid in 1 mL of 0.1 M phosphate-buffered saline (PBS), pH 7.4. Let settle and aspirate. Repeat for a total of two quick PBS washes.
  4. Fix the spheroid by adding 1 mL of freshly prepared, ice-cold 4% paraformaldehyde (PFA) in PBS. Incubate for 20 min at 4°C.
  5. **Caution**: PFA is toxic. Perform in a fume hood.
- **Washing:**
  1. Remove PFA and wash the spheroid with 1 mL of 0.1 M PBS, pH 7.4. Let settle and aspirate. Repeat for a total of three washes, 5 min each.
  2. Perform three final washes with 1 mL of Milli-Q water (5 min each) to remove PBS salts that can interfere with XRF analysis.
- **Mounting:**
  1. Using a cut pipette tip, transfer the spheroid in a minimal volume of water onto a clean, dry 4 µm Ultralene® film.
  2. Allow the spheroid to air-dry completely at room temperature in a dust-free environment. Do not apply heat.
  3. Secure the Ultralene film with the adhered spheroid onto the µXRF sample holder using a non-contaminating adhesive or holder clip. Ensure the analysis surface is flat and taut.

4.2 X-Ray Microfluorescence (µXRF) Acquisition and Analysis [4]

4.2.1 Instrument Setup (Bruker M4 Tornado)

- Power on the instrument and allow the X-ray tube and detector to stabilize (minimum 30 min).
- Load the mounted sample onto the motorized stage.

- In the ESPRIT software, define the sample holder and set the working distance according to the instrument manual.
- Select the silicon drift detector (SDD).
- Set the X-ray source with the rhodium (Rh) anode to a maximum power of 30 W.

4.2.2 Preliminary Imaging and Region of Interest (ROI) Selection

1. Using the optical camera in the software, navigate to locate the dried spheroid on the Ultralene film.
2. Perform a quick, low-resolution/low-time scout scan (e.g., 50 ms/pixel, 50 μm step size) in air (no filter) to visualize the spheroid's elemental distribution (primarily P, S, K) and confirm its integrity. This helps define the exact ROI for detailed mapping.

4.2.3 Elemental Mapping of the Entire Spheroid

- **Objective:** Obtain quantitative distribution maps of key elements (P, S, K, Ca, Fe, Cu, Zn).
- **Acquisition Parameters:**
  - **X-Ray Conditions:** 50 kV, 600 μA (30 W), "White Beam" (no monochromator).
  - **Primary Filter:** 100 μm aluminum to attenuate low-energy Rh L-lines and improve signal-to-background for mid-Z elements.
  - **Beam Spot Size:** ~25 μm (defined by polycapillary optics).
  - **Scan Geometry:** Raster scan with a step size of 15 μm (oversampling relative to beam size for smooth maps).
  - **Dwell Time:** 300 ms/pixel (Note: Original 1300 ms is very high; 300–500 ms is often sufficient and reduces total scan time drastically. Adjust based on signal).
  - **Atmosphere:** Measurement in vacuum (if available) to enhance sensitivity for light elements (P, S, K). If not, use helium flush.
- **Procedure:**
  1. In ESPRIT, draw a rectangular ROI encompassing the entire spheroid based on the scout scan.
  2. Input the above parameters and start the mapping run. The software will automatically control the stage and acquisition.
  3. Save the spectral data cube (.bcf or .h5 format).

4.2.4 Point Analysis for Quantification and Detection Limit Determination [5]

- **Objective:** Acquire high-count spectra at specific points (center, periphery) for accurate quantification and to determine method detection limits (MDLs).
- Acquisition Parameters (Two-Step per Point):
  - **For Light Elements (P, S, K, Ca):**

    Filter: 12.5 μm Al.

    Voltage/Current: 40 kV, 600 μA.

    Live Time: 100 s.

    Atmosphere: Vacuum or He.
  - **For Heavy Elements (Fe, Cu, Zn):**

    Filter: 630 μm Al (strong attenuation of Rh lines to reduce background and pile-up).

    Voltage/Current: 40 kV, 600 μA.

    Live Time: 250 s.

    Atmosphere: Air is acceptable.
- **Procedure:**
  1. Using the optical image or elemental map, select 10–20 representative points across different spheroids (e.g., 5 points in the spheroid core, 5 in the rim, 5 on the Ultralene background).
  2. Move the stage to the first point. Acquire the "light element" spectrum with the 12.5 μm Al filter settings.
  3. Without moving the stage, switch to the 630 μm Al filter and acquire the "heavy element" spectrum.
  4. Repeat for all points. The software will co-add or store spectra separately.

4.2.5 Data Processing and Quantitative Analysis

1. **Spectral Import:** Export sum spectra from maps and point analyses, or import the raw data cube into quantitative software such as PyMCA (v6.0 or higher) as mentioned in Notes 1,2 and 3.
2. **Spectral Deconvolution:** Fit the spectra using a fundamental parameters (FP) approach in PyMCA. The model includes:
   - The Rh tube spectrum (bremsstrahlung and lines).
   - Filter transmission profiles.
   - Detector efficiency and response function.
   - Matrix absorption effects.
3. **Quantification:**
   - Use the ICRU-44 soft tissue model as the default matrix composition (density ~1.06 g/cm^3, composition: H 10.2%, C 25.6%, N 2.4%, O 60.2%, Na 0.1%, other 1.5%).

- The FP software iteratively calculates element concentrations (typically in μg/g or ppm) that best fit the measured spectrum.
- Generate quantitative elemental maps from the raster scan data cube.

4. **Background Subtraction and ROI Analysis:** For point analyses, subtract the average background signal from the Ultralene film. For maps, define spatial ROIs (e.g., core vs. shell) to extract average concentrations for each region.

4.3 System Validation and Quality Control [6]

4.3.1 Preparation of Calibration/Validation Standard (Fig. 1)

1. Obtain a NIST-traceable multi-element standard solution (e.g., Inorganic Ventures IV-28 or equivalent containing Ag, Al, B, Ba, Bi, Ca, Cd, Co, Cr, Cu, Fe, Ga, In, K, Li, Mg, Mn, Na, Ni, Pb, Sr, Tl, Zn).
2. Prepare a 10 μg/g (ppm) working solution by diluting the stock in Milli-Q water.
3. Pipette 5–10 μL of this solution onto a clean Ultralene film and allow to dry completely, forming a thin, homogeneous residue spot.

4.3.2 Validation Measurement

1. Analyze the dried standard spot using the identical parameters established for the spheroid point analysis (Sect. 4.2.4): two acquisitions per point (light/heavy filters) at 40 kV.
2. Perform the measurement on at least five different spots on the standard residue.
3. Process the spectra using the same FP quantification method and tissue model as for the samples.

4.3.3 Validation Criteria

- **Accuracy**: For elements present in the standard (e.g., Ca, K, Fe, Cu, Zn), the quantified value should be within ±15% of the known concentration (10 μg/g), accounting for the thin film morphology.
- **Detection Limit (MDL)**: Calculate for each element as three times the standard deviation of the background (from multiple measurements on a blank Ultralene film) divided by the sensitivity (counts per second per μg/g). The MDL should be below the expected physiological concentrations.
- **System Stability**: The measured net counts for a Rh Compton or Rayleigh scatter peak from a constant reference (e.g., a pure PET sample) should vary by <5% over a weekly period.

4.3.4 Documentation

Maintain a log for each analysis session recording: Instrument conditions, operator, sample IDs, acquisition parameters, standard validation results, and any deviations from the protocol.

5 Notes

1. Ensure uniform spheroid size before μXRF analysis to minimize matrix effects.
2. Drying on ultralene film is critical for minimizing background noise.
3. PyMCA software is recommended for peak deconvolution and background subtraction.

References

1. Biedler JL, Roffler-Tarlov S, Schachner M, Freedman LS (1978) Multiple neurotransmitter synthesis by human neuroblastoma cell lines and clones. Cancer Res 38(11 Pt 1):3751–3757
2. Pampaloni F, Reynaud EG, Stelzer EHK (2007) The third dimension bridges the gap between cell culture and live tissue. Nat Rev Mol Cell Biol 8(10):839–845
3. Sole VA, Papillon E, Cotte M, Walter P, Susini J (2007) A multiplatform code for the analysis of energy-dispersive X-ray fluorescence spectra. Spectrochim Acta B 62(1):63–68
4. ICRU Report 44 (1989) Tissue substitutes in radiation dosimetry and measurement. International Commission on Radiation Units and Measurements, Bethesda, MD
5. Becker JS (2007) Inorganic mass spectrometry: principles and applications. Wiley
6. Vekemans B, Janssens K, Vincze L, Adams F, Van Espen P (1994) Analysis of X-ray spectra by iterative least squares (AXIL): new developments. X-Ray Spectrom 23(6):278–285

Chapter 21

Integrated Computational and Cellular Analysis of Triterpenoid Compounds: Target Prediction, Pharmacokinetic Profiling, and Antimelanoma Activity in 2D and 3D Models

Abstract

This protocol describes an integrated computational and experimental pipeline for evaluating the antimelanoma activity of triterpenoid compounds, combining in silico target prediction and pharmacokinetic profiling with comprehensive biological validation in two-dimensional (2D) and three-dimensional (3D) culture models. The computational workflow begins with target prediction using SwissTargetPrediction and ADMET profiling via SwissADME, admetSAR, and pKCSM servers based on compound SMILES notation. Molecular docking against predicted targets (e.g., AKR1B1, AKR1B10) is performed using AutoDock Vina or DockThor following protein preparation (PDB2PQR-PropKa) and ligand energy minimization. Biological validation employs Alamar Blue viability assays (excitation 530–560 nm/emission 590 nm) in human melanoma cell lines (SKMEL-19, SKMEL-28, SKMEL-103) and non-cancerous MRC5 fibroblasts to determine IC_{50} values and selectivity. Three-dimensional spheroids are generated using 2.0% agarose micromolds (MicroTissues® 3D Petri Dish®) with seeding densities of $50–150 \times 10^4$ cells per chip, cultured for 3–5 days with medium changes every 2–3 days. Metabolic disruption is assessed through glucose uptake measurement (enzymatic-colorimetric assay, 450 nm), intracellular and released lactate dehydrogenase (LDH) activity (kinetic absorbance at 340 nm), and ATP level quantification (luciferase-based luminescence). Cell death in spheroids is visualized by acridine orange/ethidium bromide (AO/EB) staining (10 μg/mL) with fluorescence microscopy. Statistical analysis is performed using GraphPad Prism with Student's t-test or ANOVA ($p < 0.05$ significance). This integrated approach bridges computational hypothesis generation with experimental validation in physiologically relevant 3D tumor models.

Keywords Triterpenoid, Molecular docking, ADMET, Melanoma spheroids, Metabolic disruption

1 Introduction

The discovery of novel anticancer agents requires a multi-faceted approach that integrates computational predictions with robust biological validation. Triterpenoid compound, a natural compound, shows promise, but its mechanism of action and pharmacokinetic profile are not fully characterized. This protocol outlines a pipeline beginning with in silico prediction of molecular targets (e.g., aldose reductase isoforms AKR1B1/1B10) and key Absorption, Distribution, Metabolism, Excretion, and Toxicity (ADMET) parameters

Karuppusamy Arunachalam et al., *Advanced Protocols in Cancer Research*, Springer Protocols Handbooks,
https://doi.org/10.1007/978-1-0716-5348-7_21,

using established databases and servers [1]. These computational insights are then experimentally tested through a series of cellular assays. The biological evaluation is conducted in both traditional 2D monolayers and more physiologically relevant 3D spheroid models of melanoma, focusing on viability, metabolic disruption (glucose uptake, lactate dehydrogenase activity, ATP levels), and induction of cell death. This integrated methodology efficiently bridges computational hypothesis generation with experimental confirmation in cancer models [2].

2 Aim

To employ a combined in silico and in vitro strategy to: (1) predict the biological targets, molecular interactions, and drug-like properties of triterpenoid compounds; (2) evaluate its cytotoxic, metabolic, and antiproliferative effects on human melanomacell lines in two-dimensional (2D) and three-dimensional (3D) spheroid cultures; and (3) assess its potential selectivity by comparing activity against non-cancerous human fibroblast (MRC5) cells.

3 Materials and Methods

3.1 In Silico Prediction and Molecular Docking

1. **Predictionof Biological Targets and ADMET Parameters**
   - **Software and Servers:**SwissTargetPrediction, SwissADME, admetSAR, pKCSM, Pred-hERG, Pred-Skin.
   - **Input:** The SMILES (Simplified Molecular Input Line Entry System) notation of triterpenoid compound, generated using chemical drawing software (e.g., MarvinSketch).
   - **Procedure:** The SMILES string is submitted to the listed web servers to predict:
     - **Targets:** Potential protein targets ranked by probability.
     - **Pharmacokinetics:** Key parameters including Lipinski's Rule of Five (molecular weight, logP, H-bond donors/acceptors), gastrointestinal absorption, blood–brain barrier penetration, and cytochrome P450 interactions.
     - **Toxicity:** Ames mutagenicity, hepatotoxicity, hERG channel inhibition, and skin sensitization potential. Results are often expressed as "+" (risk detected) or "−" (no risk detected).
2. **Protein and Ligand Preparation**
   - **Data Source:** The RCSB Protein Data Bank (PDB) is used to download high-resolution (<2.0Å) 3D structures

of target proteins (e.g., AKR1B1 PDB: 5OU0, AKR1B10 PDB: 1ZUA).

- **Protein Preparation (Using PyMol and PDB2PQR Server):**
  1. Remove non-essential molecules (crystallographic water, original ligands).
  2. Add hydrogen atoms and assign protonation states at physiological pH (7.4) using the PDB2PQR-PropKa server.
- **Ligand Preparation:** The 3D structure of triterpenoid compound is energy-minimized using molecular mechanics force fields (e.g., MMFF94 in ChemBioDraw or Avogadro).

3. **Molecular Docking Simulation**

   - **Software:** AutoDock Vina or the DockThor server.
   - **Method:** Perform docking using a "flexible ligand, rigid receptor" approach.
   - **Grid Definition:** Define a search box (grid) centered on the protein's active site with dimensions sufficient to allow ligand binding (e.g., 20 × 20 × 20 Å). Spacing is typically 1.0 Å.
   - **Output Analysis:** Docking poses are ranked by binding affinity (kcal/mol). The best poses are analyzed in Discovery Studio Visualizer or PyMol to identify key interactions (hydrogen bonds, hydrophobic contacts).

3.2 In Vitro Cellular Assays

- **Cell Lines:** Human melanoma (SKMEL-19, SKMEL-28, SKMEL-103) and non-cancerous human lung fibroblast (MRC5).
- **Culture Conditions:** Maintain in DMEM + 10% FBS at 37°C, 5% CO_2.
- **Compound:** Test compound, Rotenone (positive control for metabolic inhibition).

3.2.1 Cell Viability Assay (Alamar Blue) [1–5]

- **Day 1:** Seed cells in a 96-well plate (0.5×10^4 cells/well in 100 μL medium). Incubate for 24 h for adhesion.
- **Day 2:** Prepare serial dilutions of 22-HTG (e.g., 46–0.71 μM) in medium. Aspirate old medium from wells and add 100 μL of compound solutions. Include untreated control and vehicle control wells. Incubate for 24, 48, or 72 h.
- **Endpoint:** Add 10 μL of 0.02% Alamar Blue solution directly to each well. Incubate for 2–4 h at 37°C.

- **Measurement:** Read fluorescence (excitation: 530–560 nm, emission: 590 nm). Calculate cell viability as a percentage of the untreated control. Determine the half-maximal inhibitory concentration (IC_{50}) using non-linear regression in GraphPad Prism.

3.2.2 Generation of 3D Melanoma Spheroids

- **Agarose Chip Fabrication:**
  1. Prepare a 2.0% (w/v) agarose solution in PBS and autoclave.
  2. While liquid, pipette 550 μL into a polydimethylsiloxane (PDMS) micromold (e.g., MicroTissues® 3D Petri Dish®).
  3. Let it gelify at room temperature, then gently separate the solid agarose chip from the mold.
  4. Place the chip into a well of a 12- or 24-well plate and store in sterile PBS at 37°C until use.
- **Spheroid Formation:**
  1. Trypsinize, count, and resuspend monolayer cells.
  2. Remove PBS from the plate well containing the agarose chip.
  3. Seed a calculated cell number (e.g., 50×10^4 to 150×10^4 cells) in a minimal volume (190 μL) directly onto the chip surface.
  4. Allow cells to settle into the microwells by gravity for 30 min.
  5. Carefully add 500 μL of fresh culture medium around (not directly on top of) the chip. Change medium every 2–3 days. Spheroids typically form within 3–5 days.

3.2.3 Metabolic and Functional Assays (Can Be Performed in 2D or 3D Cultures) [2–8]

- **Glucose Uptake Measurement:**
  1. Treat cells/spheroids with triterpenoid compound (e.g., at IC_{50}) for 24 h in medium with a known glucose concentration.
  2. Collect conditioned medium and centrifuge to remove debris.
  3. Measure glucose concentration in the supernatant using a commercial enzymatic-colorimetric assay kit (e.g., Labtest® Glucose Liquiform). Follow kit instructions (typically incubating sample with reagent and reading absorbance at 450 nm).

4. Calculate glucose consumption by comparing to the glucose level in fresh, unused medium.

- **Lactate Dehydrogenase (LDH) Activity Assay (Cellular Releaseor Intracellular):**
  1. **For released LDH (cytotoxicity):** Collect conditioned medium after treatment. Follow kit instructions to mix with LDH reaction mixture. Monitor the increase in absorbance at 340 nm over time.
  2. **For intracellular LDH (metabolic activity):** Lyse cells with 0.1%–1.0% Triton X-100 for 30–45 min at 37°C. Centrifuge and use the supernatant for the same enzymatic assay.
- **ATP Level Quantification:**
  1. After treatment, lyse cells with an ATP-compatible lysis buffer.
  2. Use a luciferase-based ATP assay kit. Mix cell lysate with luciferin/luciferase reagent.
  3. Measure luminescence immediately. Prepare an ATP standard curve to convert luminescence readings to ATP concentration (nM or μM), normalized to total protein or cell number.
- **Cell Death Staining (AO/EB) for Spheroids:**
  1. After treating spheroids, carefully recover them (e.g., by inverting and centrifuging the agarose chip).
  2. Resuspend spheroids in PBS containing acridine orange (AO, 10 μg/mL) and ethidium bromide (EB, 10 μg/mL). Incubate for 20–30 min at 37°C.
  3. Wash with PBS, place in a well of a black-walled plate, and image using a fluorescence microscope. Viable cells stain green (AO), early apoptotic cells show condensed green chromatin, and late apoptotic/necrotic cells stain orange/red (EB).

3.2.4 Statistical Analysis [9]

- Perform all experiments in at least triplicate and repeat three times independently.
- Express data as mean ± standard deviation (SD).
- Use GraphPad Prism for analysis. For comparisons between two groups, use an unpaired Student's *t*-test. For multiple comparisons (e.g., different doses, time points), use one-way or two-way ANOVA followed by an appropriate post-hoc test (e.g., Tukey's, Bonferroni).
- A p-value <0.05 is considered statistically significant.

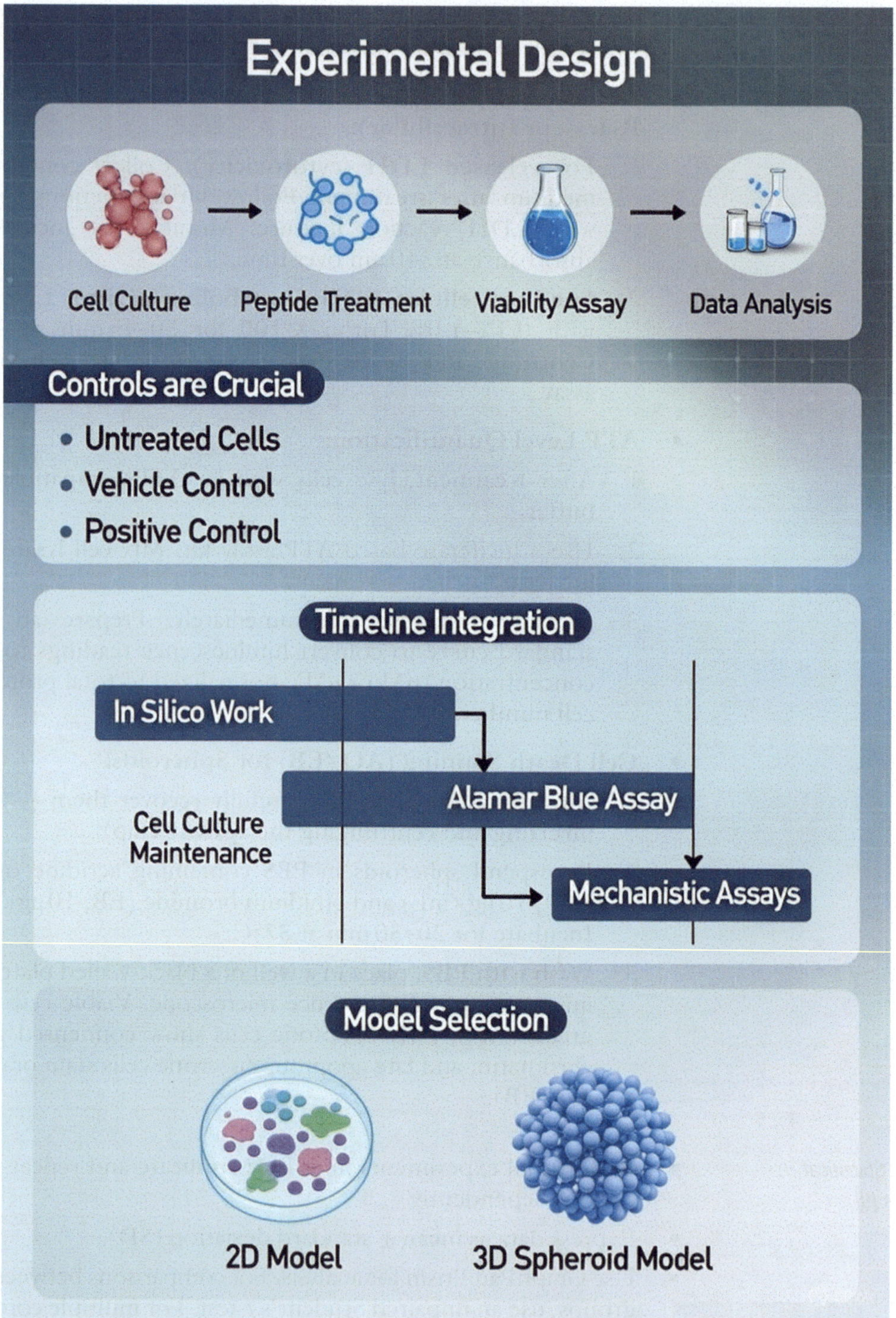

Fig. 1 Schematic representation of experimental design

4 Key Points for Experimental Design (Fig. 1)

1. Controls are Crucial: Always include untreated cells (negative control), vehicle-only treated cells (e.g., DMSO at the highest concentration used), and relevant positive controls (e.g., Rotenone for metabolic assays, a known chemotherapeutic for viability).
2. Timeline Integration: The in silico work (Part I) can proceed in parallel with initial cell culture maintenance. The cellular IC_{50} determined in the Alamar Blue assay (Step A) informs the concentrations used for the detailed mechanistic assays (Steps B–D).
3. Model Selection: Use both 2D (for high-throughput screening) and 3D spheroid models (for assessing compound penetration and activity in a more tissue-like environment) to obtain comprehensive data.

References

1. Gfeller D, Michielin O, Zoete V (2014) Shaping the interaction landscape of bioactive molecules. Bioinformatics 30(17):i615–i621. https://doi.org/10.1093/bioinformatics/btu469
2. Daina A, Michielin O, Zoete V (2017) SwissADME: a free web tool to evaluate pharmacokinetics, drug-likeness and medicinal chemistry friendliness of small molecules. Sci Rep 7:42717. https://doi.org/10.1038/srep42717
3. Yang H, Lou C, Sun L, Li J, Cai Y, Wang Z, Li W, Liu G, Tang Y (2019) admetSAR 2.0: web-service for prediction and optimization of chemical ADMET properties. Bioinformatics 35(6):1067–1069. https://doi.org/10.1093/bioinformatics/bty707
4. Trott O, Olson AJ (2010) AutoDock Vina: improving the speed and accuracy of docking with a new scoring function, efficient optimization, and multithreading. JComput Chem 31(2):455–461. https://doi.org/10.1002/jcc.21334
5. Berman HM, Westbrook J, Feng Z, Gilliland G, Bhat TN, Weissig H, Shindyalov IN, Bourne PE (2000) The protein data bank. Nucleic Acids Res 28(1):235–242. https://doi.org/10.1093/nar/28.1.235
6. Jurrus E, Engel D, Star K, Monson K, Brandi J, Felberg LE, Brookes DH, Wilson L, Chen J, Liles K, Chun M, Li P, Gohara DW, Dolinsky T, Konecny R, Koes DR, Nielsen JE, Head-Gordon T, Geng W et al (2018) Improvements to the APBS biomolecular solvation software suite. Protein Sci 27(1):112–128. https://doi.org/10.1002/pro.3280
7. Durand-Herrera D, Moreno-Jiménez I, Duarte S, Hernández-Cruz E, Castro-Muñozledo F, Kuri-Harcuch W (2018) In vitro three-dimensional (3D) skin models for wound healing and cancer studies. J Vis Exp 135:e57619. https://doi.org/10.3791/57619
8. Ahmed SA, Gogal RM Jr, Walsh JE (1994) A new rapid and simple non-radioactive assay to monitor and determine the proliferation of lymphocytes: an alternative to [3H] thymidine incorporation assay. J Immunol Methods 170(2):211–224. https://doi.org/10.1016/0022-1759(94)90396-4
9. Motulsky HJ (2018) Intuitive. Biostatistics: a nonmathematical guide to statistical thinking, 4th edn. Oxford University Press

Part IV

Evaluation of Specific Compounds and Natural Products

Chapter 22

In Vitro Evaluation of Biflorin's Antitumor Activity

Abstract

This protocol describes a comprehensive in vitro evaluation of biflorin, a naturally derived naphthoquinone, for its antitumor activity against cancer cell lines (ACP02, AGP01, PG100) and normal fibroblasts (MRC-5). Cytotoxicity is assessed via Alamar Blue assay (excitation 465 nm/emission 540 nm) over 24–72 h to determine IC_{50} values, complemented by trypan blue exclusion for viability quantification. Long-term proliferative effects are evaluated through clonogenic assays (7–10 days, crystal violet staining) with calculation of plating efficiency and survival fraction. Morphological changes (nuclear condensation, fragmentation, vacuolization) are examined by panoptic staining following cytocentrifugation. Cell migration is assessed via wound healing (scratch) assay with wound closure quantified at 24 and 48 h using ImageJ. Differentiation potential is measured by nitro blue tetrazolium (NBT) reduction assay (37°C, 1 h) with safranin counterstaining. Molecular cytogenetic analysis employs fluorescence in situ hybridization (FISH) using Poseidon® MYC probe and StarFISH® pantelomeric probe following hypotonic KCl treatment (0.075 M, 20 min, 37°C) and methanol:acetic acid (3:1) fixation. MYC amplification (red foci) and telomere length (fluorescence intensity) are quantified in ≥ 200 nuclei using fluorescence microscopy and TFL-TELO software. Statistical analysis uses one-way/two-way ANOVA with appropriate post-tests ($p < 0.05$ significance). This integrated approach enables a comprehensive assessment of biflorin's antitumor mechanisms from cytotoxicity through molecular cytogenetic alterations.

Keywords Biflorin, Naphthoquinone, Cytotoxicity, FISH, Telomere

1 Introduction

Biflorin is a naturally derived naphthoquinone with reported anticancer properties. This protocol outlines a comprehensive in vitro assessment of biflorin's effects on cancer cell lines, focusing on cytotoxicity, viability, proliferation, morphology, migration, differentiation, and MYC gene and telomere alterations [1].

2 Aim

To evaluate the biological effects of biflorin on cancer cell lines using cytotoxicity, clonogenic, migration, differentiation, and FISH assays.

Karuppusamy Arunachalam et al., *Advanced Protocols in Cancer Research*, Springer Protocols Handbooks,
https://doi.org/10.1007/978-1-0716-5348-7_22,

3 Materials and Reagents

3.1 Cell Lines

- ACP02, AGP01, PG100 (cancer cell lines).
- MRC-5 (normal fibroblast cell line).

3.2 Reagents

- RPMI-1640 medium (with 5.6% $NaHCO_3$, 25 mM HEPES).
- Fetal bovine serum (FBS), 10%–20%.
- Streptomycin (0.005 mg/L), Penicillin (0.001 U/L).
- Trypsin-EDTA, PBS.
- Biflorin (prepared in DMSO).
- Doxorubicin (positive control).
- TPA (positive control for differentiation).
- Alamar Blue reagent (0.02%).
- Trypan Blue dye.
- Crystal violet, Methanol.
- Nitro blue tetrazolium (NBT).
- Safranin, DAPI/Antifade.
- FISH Probes: Poseidon® (MYC), StarFISH® (Telomeres).
- Cytoclear Procell®.

3.3 Equipment

- CO_2 incubator (37°C, 5% CO_2).
- Microplate reader (Ex: 465 nm, Em: 540 nm).
- Fluorescence and inverted microscopes.
- Cytocentrifuge.
- Neubauer counting chamber.
- Image analysis software: TFL-TELO and Applied Spectral Imaging.

3.4 Procedure [1]

1. Thaw cryopreserved cells rapidly in a 37°C water bath (1–2 min).
2. Transfer the thawed suspension into a 15 mL tube with 10 mL pre-warmed RPMI-1640 medium.
3. Centrifuge at 1500 rpm for 5 min at room temperature.
4. Discard the supernatant and resuspend the pellet in 5 mL fresh complete medium (RPMI + 10%–20% FBS + antibiotics).

5. Transfer cells to a culture flask and incubate at 37°C with 5% CO_2.
6. Observe cell morphology and confluence daily using an inverted microscope.
7. Replace media every 48–72 h.
8. When cells reach 70%–80% confluence, aspirate the medium and wash once with PBS.
9. Add 1–2 mL trypsin-EDTA, incubate at 37°C for 2–3 min.
10. Once cells detach, neutralize with complete medium, and transfer to a 15 mL tube.
11. Centrifuge at 1500 rpm for 5 min, resuspend and re-seed at $0.5–1.0 \times 10^6$ cells/mL.

4 Alamar Blue Cytotoxicity Assay [2]

Objective

To determine the IC_{50} of biflorin by assessing mitochondrial activity as a marker of cell viability.

Materials

- 96-well flat-bottom plates (sterile).
- Alamar Blue reagent (0.02%).
- Biflorin (dissolved in DMSO).
- Doxorubicin (positive control).
- RPMI medium (complete).
- Microplate reader (465 nm excitation, 540 nm emission).

Procedure

1. Harvest exponentially growing cells and count using a hemocytometer or automated counter.
2. Adjust the cell density to 5×10^3 cells per 100 µL medium.
3. Dispense 100 µL of cell suspension into each well of a 96-well plate.
4. Incubate the plate for 24 h at 37°C in a 5% CO_2 incubator to allow cell attachment.
5. Prepare serial dilutions of biflorin (25, 12.5, 6.25, 3.125, 1.56, 0.78, 0.39 µg/mL) in RPMI.
6. Remove the culture medium from wells and add 100 µL of each biflorin concentration in triplicate.
7. Include DMSO-only wells as negative controls and doxorubicin (5 µg/mL) as a positive control.

8. Incubate for 24 or 72 h, depending on the experimental endpoint.
9. Add 10 μL of 0.02% Alamar Blue solution to each well.
10. Incubate for 2 h at 37°C, protected from light.
11. Read fluorescence at 465 nm excitation and 540 nm emission.
12. Calculate IC_{50} using non-linear regression in GraphPad Prism 5.

5 Trypan Blue Exclusion Assay [3]

Objective

To measure the percentage of viable cells after biflorin treatment.

Materials

- 12-well culture plates.
- Trypan Blue (0.4%).
- Biflorin solutions (1.0, 2.5, 5.0 μg/mL).
- DMSO (vehicle control).
- Neubauer counting chamber.

Procedure

1. Seed 1×10^5 cells per well in 12-well plates in 1 mL complete medium.
2. Incubate for 24 h at 37°C.
3. Treat cells with biflorin at three concentrations (1.0, 2.5, 5.0 μg/mL) in triplicate.
4. Include a DMSO-treated group (final concentration 0.1%).
5. After 24, 48, and 72 h, collect both floating and adherent cells by trypsinization.
6. Pool the contents into 1.5 mL tubes and centrifuge at 1500 rpm for 5 min.
7. Resuspend the pellet in 200 μL of PBS.
8. Mix 90 μL of cell suspension with 10 μL of Trypan Blue dye.
9. Incubate for 2 min at room temperature.
10. Load 10 μL onto a Neubauer chamber and count cells in four corners.
11. Calculation of Cell Viability

The percentage of viable cells was calculated using the following formula:

$$\text{Viability}(\%) = \frac{N_{\text{live}}}{N_{\text{live}} + N_{\text{dead}}} \times 100$$

Where:

- N_{live} = Number of live (unstained) cells.
- N_{dead} = Number of dead (stained) cells.
- $N_{\text{live}} + N_{\text{dead}}$ = Total cells counted.

For assays based on fluorescence (e.g., using calcein-AM/ethidium homodimer or acridine orange/propidium iodide), the equivalent formula is:

$$\text{Viability}(\%) = \frac{\text{Mean Fluorescence Intensity}(\text{MFI})_{\text{sample}}}{\text{MFI}_{\text{untreated control}}} \times 100$$

12. Analyze statistical differences using one-way ANOVA with Tukey's post-test.

6 Morphological Analysis [4]

Objective

To observe cellular morphological changes induced by biflorin treatment.

Materials

- 12-well plates.
- Trypsin-EDTA.
- PBS.
- Cytocentrifuge.
- Panoptic staining kit (Laborclin®).
- Microscope with 40× and 100× objectives.

Procedure

1. Seed 5×10^4 ACP02 cells per well in 12-well plates.
2. Treat cells with biflorin (1.0, 2.5, 5.0 μM), DMSO, or TPA (0.16 μM).

3. After 72 h, collect supernatant and trypsinized cells in 1.5 mL tubes.
4. Centrifuge at 3000 rpm for 5 min.
5. Resuspend pellet in 200 μL PBS and cytospin 100 μL at 1000 rpm for 5 min.
6. Fix and stain slides using the panoptic kit.
7. Examine slides under an optical microscope.
8. Capture images and document nuclear condensation, fragmentation, vacuolization, and cell shrinkage.

7 Clonogenic Assay [5]

Objective
To assess the long-term proliferative capacity of single cells after biflorin treatment.

Materials

- 6-well culture plates.
- Biflorin (1.0, 2.5, 5.0 μM).
- DMSO (0.1%).
- Methanol (100%).
- Crystal violet solution (0.5% w/v in 25% methanol).
- PBS.
- Microscope.
- ImageJ (or manual counter).

Procedure

1. Harvest and count cells during the logarithmic growth phase.
2. Plate 400 viable cells per well in 2 mL of complete RPMI medium in a 6-well plate.
3. Incubate for 24 h to allow cell attachment.
4. Treat wells in triplicate with biflorin at 1.0, 2.5, and 5.0 μM. Include DMSO (0.1%) as the negative control.
5. Incubate for 7–10 days under standard conditions, replacing the medium every 3 days without disturbing colonies.
6. Observe under the microscope. When colonies reach >50 cells:
    - Gently aspirate medium.
    - Rinse wells once with PBS.
    - Fix cells by adding 1 mL of ice-cold methanol per well for 15 min at room temperature.
    - Discard methanol and allow to air-dry.

- Stain with 1 mL of 0.5% crystal violet for 20 min.
- Rinse thoroughly with tap water until background clears and air-idry.

7. Count visible colonies manually or using ImageJ.
8. Perform one-way ANOVA with Dunnett's post-test for statistical comparison.

8 Data Expression

8.1 Plating Efficiency (PE)

The Plating Efficiency for a given condition (control or treated) was calculated as follows:

$$PE(\%) = \frac{\text{Number of Colonies Counted}}{\text{Number of Cells Seeded}} \times 100$$

8.2 Survival Fraction (SF)

The Surviving Fraction for each treatment group was then calculated relative to the control group's plating efficiency:

$$SF = \frac{PE_{treated}}{PE_{control}}$$

Where:

- $PE_{control}$ is the plating efficiency of the untreated control group.
- $PE_{treated}$ is the plating efficiency of the group treated with the test agent.

9 Wound Healing (Scratch) Assay [5]

Objective

To evaluate the migratorycapacity of adherent cells following biflorin treatment.

Materials

- 12-well plates.
- Sterile 200 μL pipette tips.
- Biflorin (1.0, 2.5, 5.0 μM).
- DMSO.
- Inverted microscope with imaging system.
- ImageJ or equivalent analysis software

Procedure

1. Seed 1×10^5 cells per well in 12-well plates. Allow cells to grow until ~90% confluent.
2. Treat cells with biflorin (1.0–5.0 µM) or DMSO in serum-free medium for 24 h.
3. After treatment, create a straight scratch across each well using a sterile pipette tip.
4. Gently wash each well twice with PBS to remove detached cells.
5. Replace medium with biflorin-containing or control medium.
6. Immediately capture phase-contrast images at 0 h.
7. Return plates to the incubator and acquire images at 24 and 48 h from the same position.
8. Measure the wound area at each time point using ImageJ.
9. Calculation of Wound Closure.
   The percentage of wound closure at time point t was calculated relative to the initial wound area ($t = 0$) using the following formula:

$$\text{Wound Closure}(\%) = \frac{A_0 - A_t}{A_0} \times 100$$

   Where:

10. A_0 = Wound area at time zero (0 h).
11. A_t = Wound area at the measured time point t (e.g., 12, 24, 48 h).
12. Analyze migration rates using one-way ANOVA with Dunnett's post-test.

10 NBT (Nitro Blue Tetrazolium) Differentiation Assay

Objective

To evaluate biflorin-induced cell differentiation via NBT reduction.

Materials

- NBT (2 mg/mL in PBS).
- TPA (2 µg/mL).
- 12-well plates.
- Biflorin (1.0, 2.5, 5.0 µM).
- Safranin (0.5%).
- Methanol (PA grade).

- PBS.
- Microscope.
- Cytocentrifuge and slides.

Procedure

1. Seed 2.5×10^4 cells/well in 12-well plates.
2. After 24 h, treat cells with biflorin (1.0–5.0 μM), TPA (0.16 μ M, positive control), and DMSO.
3. At 24 h and 72 h post-treatment, collect supernatant and trypsinized cells into 15 mL tubes.
4. Centrifuge at 1500 rpm for 5 min.
5. Resuspend the pellet in 100 μL PBS and add 100 μL of NBT + TPA solution.
6. Incubate at 37°C in a water bath for 1 h, protected from light.
7. Stop the reaction by adding 3 mL of cold PBS and centrifuge again.
8. Discard supernatant, resuspend the pellet in 200 μL PBS.
9. Cytospin 50 μL onto slides at 1000 rpm for 5 min.
10. Fix cells with methanol for 1 min, rinse in tap water.
11. Counterstain with 0.5% safranin for 1 min, rinse, air-dry, and mount in xylene.
12. Under the microscope, count 200 cells per sample.
    - Blue/purple cells = differentiated.
    - Pink cells = undifferentiated.
13. Calculate % differentiation and compare using two-way ANOVA with Bonferroni post-test.

11 Fluorescence In Situ Hybridization (FISH): MYC and Telomere Analysis

Objective

To assess MYC gene amplification and telomere length changes after biflorin treatment.

Materials

- Biflorin (1.0, 2.5, 5.0 μM).
- KCl (0.075 M, hypotonic solution).
- Fixative (methanol:acetic acid 3:1 with Cytoclear®).
- Poseidon® MYC probe (directly labeled).
- StarFISH® pantelomeric probe.
- DAPI/Antifade mounting medium.
- Pre-cleaned microscope slides.

- Fluorescence microscope.
- Hybridization chamber.
- Water bath (37°C, 75°C).
- TFL-TELO analysis software.

Procedure

1. Treat ACP02 cells (5 × 104 cells/mL) with biflorin or DMSO for 24 and 72 h in 12-well plates.
2. Collect and centrifuge cells at 1500 rpm for 5 min.
3. Resuspend the pellet in 5 mL of 0.075 M KCl and incubate at 37°C for 20 min.
4. Centrifuge and resuspend cells in 5 mL cold fixative (3:1 methanol:acetic acid + 5 μL/mL Cytoclear®).
5. Repeat wash and fixation steps 3× until pellet is clean.
6. Drop 20 μL of cell suspension onto slides and allow to air-dry.
7. Examine slides under phase contrast to confirm nuclear quality.
8. Apply 10–20 μL of probe (MYC or telomeric), cover with 22 × 22 mm coverslip, and seal with parafilm.
9. Denature DNA and probe at 75°C for 10 min.
10. Incubate slides overnight at 37°C in a humidified dark chamber.
11. Carefully remove coverslip and apply DAPI/Antifade. Add a clean coverslip.
12. Store slides at −20°C for at least 20 min before imaging.
13. Analyze at least 200 nuclei per treatment using a fluorescence microscope.
14. Quantify MYC amplification (red foci) and telomere intensity (blue).
15. Use TFL-TELO software for telomere length quantification.
16. Report average signal intensity and number of foci per nucleus.

References

1. Pinto AV, de Castro SL, Pinto MCFR (1997) The cytotoxicity of 1,4-naphthoquinones against Trypanosoma cruzi and mammalian cells. Mem. Inst. Oswaldo Cruz 92(Suppl. II):273–277. https://doi.org/10.1590/S0074-02761997000800039
2. Lemos AB, de Oliveira TB, de Sá JC, dos Santos MH, de Paula SO (2019) Biflorin induces apoptosis and cell cycle arrest in human leukemia cells via p53-mediated signaling. Chem-Biol Interact 308:332–339. https://doi.org/10.1016/j.cbi.2019.05.049
3. Riss TL, Moravec RA, Niles AL, Duellman S, Benink HA, Worzella TJ, Minor L (2013) Cell viability assays. in assay guidance manual [Internet]. Eli Lilly & Company and the National Center for Advancing Translational

Sciences. https://www.ncbi.nlm.nih.gov/books/NBK144065/
4. Franken NA, Rodermond HM, Stap J, Haveman J, van Bree C (2006) Clonogenic assay of cells in vitro. Nat Protoc 1(5):2315–2319. https://doi.org/10.1038/nprot.2006.339
5. Canela A, Vera E, Klatt P, Blasco MA (2007) High-throughput telomere length quantification by FISH and its application to human population studies. Proc Natl Acad Sci U S A 104(13):5300–5305. https://doi.org/10.1073/pnas.0609367104

Chapter 23

In Vitro Evaluation of Cytotoxic Activity and Mechanisms of Action of Compounds in Human Cancer Cell Lines

Abstract

This protocol describes a comprehensive methodology for evaluating the cytotoxic activity and underlying mechanisms of action of metal-based compounds, including copper(II) and platinum(II) complexes, against a panel of human cancer cell lines representing solid tumors (H460, A549, MDA-MB-231, PC3) and hematologic malignancies (U937, MOLT-4, THP-1). Initial cytotoxicity screening is performed using the MTT colorimetric assay following 48-h compound exposure across concentration gradients (H31: 0–20 μmol/L; H39: 0–200 μmol/L; H36 ligand: 0–2 μmol/L) to determine half-maximal inhibitory concentrations (IC_{50}) via non-linear regression in GraphPad Prism. Mechanistic investigations employ flow cytometry-based assays: cell cycle analysis with propidium iodide (PI) staining (50 μg/mL) to quantify Sub-G_1 apoptotic populations following 70% ethanol fixation and RNase A treatment (100 μg/mL); mitochondrial membrane potential (ΔΨm) assessment using JC-1 dye (25 μg/mL, 15 min incubation) with FL1 (monomers) and FL2 (aggregates) channel detection; and reactive oxygen species (ROS) measurement via DCFH-DA fluorescence (2.5 μmol/L, 30 min incubation, FL1 channel). All flow cytometry acquisitions are performed on a BD FACSCalibur™ instrument with 10,000 events per sample and analyzed using WinMDI software. Statistical significance is determined by one-way ANOVA with Tukey's post-hoc test ($p < 0.05$). This integrated workflow enables comprehensive characterization of compound-induced cytotoxicity from initial potency determination through detailed mechanistic investigation of apoptosis, mitochondrial dysfunction, and oxidative stress.

Keywords Metal-based compounds, Cytotoxicity, Apoptosis, Mitochondrial membrane potential

1 Introduction

Metal-based compounds, particularly synthetic complexes, have emerged as promising chemotherapeutic agents due to their ability to interfere with cellular redox balance and DNA integrity [1]. While cisplatin remains a cornerstone in cancer treatment, novel complexes with improved selectivity and reduced toxicity are being investigated. This study focuses on the cytotoxic effects and underlying mechanisms of action—including apoptosis induction, cell cycle

Karuppusamy Arunachalam et al., *Advanced Protocols in Cancer Research*, Springer Protocols Handbooks,
https://doi.org/10.1007/978-1-0716-5348-7_23,

arrest, mitochondrial dysfunction, and reactive oxygen species (ROS) production—of synthetic complexes against a panel of human cancer cell lines representing solid and hematologic tumors.

2 Aim

To analyze the cytotoxic activity and elucidate the mechanism of action of copper(II) (H31), platinum(II) (H39), and ligand (H36) compounds in various human neoplastic cell lines using viability, apoptosis, cell cycle, mitochondrial membrane potential, and ROS assays.

3 Objectives

1. To evaluate the cytotoxic activity of copper(II) and platinum(II) compounds in various human cancer cell lines using the MTT assay.
2. To investigate mechanisms of cell death induced by the compounds through cell cycle arrest, Mitochondrial membrane potential disruption, and reactive oxygen species (ROS) generation using flow cytometry.

4 Materials and Reagents

4.1 Cell Lines

- H460 (non-small cell lung carcinoma).
- A549 (lung adenocarcinoma).
- MDA-MB-231 (breast adenocarcinoma).
- PC3 (prostate carcinoma).
- U937 (histiocytic lymphoma).
- MOLT-4 (acute lymphoblastic leukemia).
- THP-1 (acute monocytic leukemia).

4.2 Culture Media and Supplements

- D-MEM/F12 (Gibco or equivalent).
- Fetal Bovine Serum (FBS), heat-inactivated (10%).
- Gentamicin (20 μg/mL).
- Trypsin-EDTA (0.25%).
- PBS (1×), sterile.

4.3 Compounds and Reagents

- Ligand (H36).
- Cisplatin (standard drug).

- MTT (5 mg/mL, Sigma-Aldrich).
- Isopropanol with 0.04% HCl.
- RNase A (100 μg/mL).
- Propidium iodide (PI, 50 μg/mL).
- JC-1 dye (25 μg/mL, Sigma).
- DCFH-DA (2.5 μmol/L).
- NAC (5 mmol/L, N-acetyl cysteine).

4.4 Equipment

- Cell culture incubator (37°C, 5% CO_2).
- 96-well, 6-well, and 12-well tissue culture plates.
- Hemocytometer or automated cell counter.
- Spectrophotometer (570 nm).
- Flow cytometer (BD FACSCalibur™).
- Centrifuge.
- Vortex mixer.
- Micropipettes and tips.
- Sterile conical tubes and microtubes.

5 Experimental Procedures [2–4]

5.1 Cell Culture and Maintenance

1. Thaw and culture cell lines under sterile conditions in D-MEM/F12 supplemented with 10% FBS and 20 μg/mL gentamicin.
2. Incubate cells in a humidified incubator at 37°C with 5% CO_2.
3. Change medium every 48 h.
4. Subculture when cells reach ~80% confluency using trypsin-EDTA for adherent lines and centrifugation for suspension lines.

5.2 MTT Cytotoxicity Assay

Objective: Determine IC_{50} of compounds in H460 cells.

1. Seed H460 cells in a 96-well plate at 2×10^5 cells/mL (100 μL/well).
2. Incubate overnight to allow cell attachment.
3. Treat cells with varying concentrations:
   - H31: 0–20 μmol/L.
   - H39: 0–200 μmol/L.
   - H36 (ligand): 0–2 μmol/L.
   - Include untreated control (media only) and cisplatin-treated positive control.

4. Incubate for 48 h at 37°C, 5% CO_2.
5. Add 20 µL of MTT (5 mg/mL) per well and incubate for 4 h.
6. Remove 170 µL supernatant and add 120 µL isopropanol with 0.04% HCl to solubilize formazan crystals.
7. Centrifuge at 300 × *g* for 5 min; transfer 100 µL of supernatant to new plate.
8. Read absorbance at 570 nm.
9. Calculate % viability:

$$\text{Viability} = (\text{Abscontrol}/\text{Abstreated}) \times 100$$

10. Determine IC_{50} using GraphPad Prism.

5.3 Cell Cycle Analysis (Sub-G1 Population)

Objective: Evaluate apoptotic cell death via Sub-G1 peak

1. Seed H460 cells at 3×10^5 cells/mL in 12-well plates (500 µL/well).
2. Treat with 2× IC_{50} concentrations of H31 and cisplatin.
3. Incubate for 48 h.
4. Harvest cells, centrifuge (200 × *g*, 5 min), and wash twice with PBS.
5. Fix cells with 1 mL cold 70% ethanol at 4°C for 30 min.
6. Wash twice with phosphate-citrate buffer (0.2 M, pH 7.8).
7. Resuspend pellet in 50 µL RNase A (100 µg/mL), incubate 15 min.
8. Add 400 µL of PI (50 µg/mL).
9. Analyze DNA content in a flow cytometer (FACSCalibur™, FL2 channel).
10. Acquire 10,000 events/sample; analyze Sub-G1population with WinMDI software.

5.4 JC-1 Mitochondrial Membrane Potential Assay [5]

Objective: Evaluate $\Delta\Psi m$ loss as an apoptosis indicator.

1. Treat H460 cells in 12-well plates with 2× IC_{50} of H31 and cisplatin for 48 h.
2. Centrifuge and wash twice with warm D-MEM F12.
3. Resuspend in 500 µL JC-1 solution (25 µg/mL in D-MEM F12).
4. Incubate 15 min at 37°C.
5. Wash twice and resuspend in 500 µL of unsupplemented medium.

6. Analyze in a flow cytometer using FL1 (green, monomer) and FL2 (red, aggregate).
7. Quantify % of cells with depolarized mitochondria using WinMDI.

5.5 ROS Detection by DCFH-DA Fluorescence

Objective: Detect oxidative stress induced by H31.

1. Seed H460 cells in 6-well plates at 3×10^5 cells/mL (500 μL/well).
2. Group treatments:
   - H31 ($2\times IC_{50} = 1.8\,\mu M$).
   - H31 + NAC (5 mM).
   - Cisplatin ($2\times IC_{50} = 50\,\mu M$).
   - Untreated control.
3. Incubate for 48 h.
4. Add DCFH-DA (final 2.5 μmol/L), incubate 30 min at 37°C.
5. Wash and resuspend in PBS.
6. Acquire fluorescence in the FL1 channel of the flow cytometer (10,000 events/sample).
7. Express results as fold increase over control fluorescence.

6 Data Analysis

- IC_{50} values calculated by non-linear regression.
- GraphPad Prism 5.1 was used for statistical analysis.
- One-way ANOVA followed by Tukey's test was used to determine significance.
- Significance is defined as:
  - $*P < 0.05$
  - $**P < 0.01$
  - $***P < 0.001$

7 Safety and Waste Disposal

- Handle all chemicals, especially PI, JC-1, and metal compounds, in a fume hood.
- Wear a lab coat, gloves, and safety goggles.
- Dispose of all biohazardous and chemical waste in accordance with institutional biosafety protocols [5].

References

1. Wang D, Lippard SJ (2005) Cellular processing of platinum anticancer drugs. Nat Rev Drug Discov 4(4):307–320. https://doi.org/10.1038/nrd1691
2. Riss TL, Moravec RA, Niles AL, Duellman S, Benink HA, Worzella TJ, Minor L (2013) Cell viability assays. In assay guidance manual [Internet]. Eli Lilly & Company and the National Center for Advancing Translational Sciences. https://www.ncbi.nlm.nih.gov/books/NBK144065/
3. Wlodkowic D, Skommer J, Darzynkiewicz Z (2009) Flow cytometry-based apoptosis detection. Methods Mol Biol 559:19–32. https://doi.org/10.1007/978-1-60327-017-5_2
4. Kalyanaraman B, Darley-Usmar V, Davies KJ, Dennery PA, Forman HJ, Grisham MB et al (2012) Measuring reactive oxygen and nitrogen species with fluorescent probes: challenges and limitations. Free Radic Biol Med 52(1):1–6. https://doi.org/10.1016/j.freeradbiomed.2011.09.030
5. Santini C, Pellei M, Gandin V, Porchia M, Tisato F, Marzano C (2014) Advances in copper complexes as anticancer agents. Chem Rev 114(1):815–862. https://doi.org/10.1021/cr400135x

Chapter 24

Evaluation of Antitumor Potential of Phytocompound Fractions

Abstract

This protocol describes a comprehensive experimental approach for evaluating the antitumor potential of phytocompound fractions from *plant species*, integrating in vitro cytotoxicity profiling, mechanistic studies of anti-metastatic activity, and in vivo efficacy validation in a syngeneic 4T1 murine breast cancer model. Initial screening employs MTT, trypan blue, and neutral red viability assays across human (HeLa, MCF-7, MDA-MB-231, BT-20) and murine (4T1) cancer cell lines, with selectivity assessed against primary human PBMCs and murine splenocytes. Apoptosis induction is evaluated by acridine orange/propidium iodide (AO/PI) fluorescence microscopy. Anti-metastatic potential is assessed through wound healing (scratch) assays (0–48 h, ImageJ quantification), Boyden chamber migration, Matrigel invasion assays (18–48 h, crystal violet staining), and gelatin zymography for MMP-2/MMP-9 activity (10% SDS-PAGE with 1 mg/mL gelatin, Coomassie staining). For in vivo studies, female BALB/c mice (n = 8–10/group) are inoculated subcutaneously with 4T1 cells (5×10^4-1×10^5 cells), randomized upon tumor reach 50–100 mm^3 (Day 7–9), and treated daily for 14 days with test fractions, vehicle control, or positive control (e.g., 5-FU 25 mg/kg). Tumor volume is monitored by caliper measurement ($V = L \times W^2/2$) every 2–3 days. At study termination (Day 22), primary tumors, lungs, and livers are excised, weighed, and surface lung metastases quantified. Histopathological analysis of H&E-stained sections (5 μm) quantifies tumor necrosis, metastatic foci, and inflammatory infiltration using ImageJ. Statistical analysis employs one-way/two-way ANOVA with appropriate post-hoc tests ($p < 0.05$ significance) in GraphPad Prism 9.0.

Keywords Phytocompounds, Cytotoxicity, Metastasis, 4T1 model, MMP activity

1 Introduction

Breast cancer is a leading cause of cancer-related mortality worldwide, with metastatic disease representing the primary cause of death. Despite advances in therapy, drug resistance and toxicity remain significant challenges, underscoring the need for novel therapeutic agents. Plants of the genus *Ficus* have been used in traditional medicine and have demonstrated promising bioactive properties. This study aims to perform a comprehensive in vitro and in vivo

Karuppusamy Arunachalam et al., *Advanced Protocols in Cancer Research*, Springer Protocols Handbooks, https://doi.org/10.1007/978-1-0716-5348-7_24,

evaluation of cytotoxic fractions from *Ficus* sp., focusing on their mechanisms of action (including apoptosis induction, anti-migratory, and anti-invasive effects) and their efficacy in a murine model of metastatic breast cancer.

2 Aim

To characterize the anticancer potential of selected *Ficus* fractions through:

1. Assessment of cytotoxicity and selectivity in a panel of human and murine cancer cell lines versus normal immune cells.
2. Investigation of mechanisms, including apoptosis, inhibition of migration, invasion, adhesion, and modulation of key proteases.
3. Evaluation of in vivo antitumor and anti-metastatic efficacy in a syngeneic 4T1 murine breast cancer model.

3 Materials

3.1 Chemical Reagents & Kits

- Culture Media: DMEM, RPMI-1640 (Gibco®).
- Supplements: Fetal Bovine Serum (FBS, heat-inactivated), Penicillin-Streptomycin (10,000 U/mL), L-Glutamine.
- Cell Dissociation: Trypsin-EDTA (0.25%), Phosphate-Buffered Saline (PBS), pH 7.4.
- Viability & Staining: MTT (3-(4,5-dimethylthiazol-2-yl)-2,5-diphenyltetrazolium bromide), MTS reagent (Promega), Neutral Red dye, Trypan Blue (0.4%), Acridine Orange, Propidium Iodide, Toluidine Blue O, Coomassie Brilliant Blue R-250.
- Apoptosis & Protein Analysis: RIPA Lysis Buffer, Protease & Phosphatase Inhibitor Cocktail, Bradford Protein Assay Kit, SDS-PAGE reagents, Nitrocellulose/PVDF membranes, ECL Substrate. Primary antibodies: Cleaved PARP, Caspase-7, Caspase-8, β-Actin. HRP-conjugated secondary antibodies.
- Migration/Invasion: Matrigel® Basement Membrane Matrix (Corning), Transwell inserts (5.0 μm pore, polycarbonate).
- Adhesion: Purified proteins: Collagen Type I, Collagen Type IV, Fibronectin, Laminin. Bovine Serum Albumin (BSA).
- Nitric Oxide: Nitrate/Nitrite Colorimetric Assay Kit (Cayman Chemical) or equivalent.
- Tissue Processing: 10% Neutral Buffered Formalin, Ethanol series (70%, 95%, 100%), Xylene, Paraffin wax, Hematoxylin & Eosin (H&E) stain.

- Solvents & Others: Dimethyl Sulfoxide (DMSO, cell culture grade), Methanol, Acetic Acid, Glacial Acetic Acid, Sodium Dodecyl Sulfate (SDS), Triton X-100, Ficoll-Paque Plus.

3.2 Biological Materials

- **Cell Lines:**
  - Human: HeLa (cervical adenocarcinoma), MCF-7 (breast adenocarcinoma, ER+), MDA-MB-231 (breast adenocarcinoma, triple-negative), BT-20 (breast carcinoma).
  - Murine: 4T1 (mammary carcinoma, highly metastatic).
- **Primary Cells:** Human Peripheral Blood Mononuclear Cells (PBMCs) from healthy donors, Murine Splenocytes from BALB/c mice.
- **In Vivo Model:** Female BALB/c mice, 6–8 weeks old, ~20–25 g.

3.3 Equipment

- **Cell Culture:** Class II Biological Safety Cabinet, CO_2 Incubator (37°C, 5% CO_2, humidified), Inverted Phase-Contrast Microscope, Water Bath (37°C).
- **Centrifugation:** Benchtop Centrifuge with swing-bucket rotor for microplates and 15/50 mL tubes.
- **Spectroscopy:** Microplate Reader capable of absorbance measurements at 490 nm (MTS), 540 nm (Neutral Red), 570 nm (MTT), and 620 nm.
- **Imaging:** (with FITC/TRITC filters), Gel Documentation System, Chemiluminescence Imager (e.g., ImageQuant LAS 4000).
- **Electrophoresis:** Mini-PROTEAN Tetra Cell system (Bio-Rad) or equivalent for SDS-PAGE and Western Blot.
- **In Vivo:** Digital Caliper, Analytical Balance, Microtome, Tissue Embedding Station, Syringes (1 mL) with 27-30G needles.
- **Software:** GraphPad Prism 9.0, ImageJ/FIJI, Statistical analysis software.

4 Detailed Step-by-Step Experimental Protocol

4.1 In Vitro Cytotoxicity and Selectivity Profiling

4.1.1 Cell Culture Maintenance

1. **Thawing and Subculture:** Rapidly thaw cryovials. Dilute in complete medium (DMEM/RPMI-1640 + 10% FBS + 1% P/S), centrifuge (300 × *g*, 5 min), resuspend, and culture in T-25 flasks. Subculture at 80%–90% confluence using trypsin-EDTA.

2. **Primary Cell Isolation:**
   * **Human PBMCs:**) (ratio 2:1). Centrifuge at 400 × *g* for 30 min at room temperature (brake off). Harvest the PBMC ring, wash twice with PBS (250 × *g*, 10 min). Resuspend in complete RPMI-1640. For monocyte-derived macrophages, plate cells and allow adherence for 2 h before removing non-adherent cells (lymphocytes) [1].
   * **Murine Splenocytes:** Aseptically remove spleen from euthanized BALB/c mouse. Gently homogenize through a 70 μm cell strainer into cold PBS. Centrifuge (300 × *g*, 5 min). Lyse red blood cells using ACK lysis buffer (5 min on ice). Wash twice with PBS and resuspend in complete RPMI-1640 [2].

4.1.2 Cell Viability Assays (MTT/Trypan Blue/ Neutral Red)

1. **Seeding:** Seed cells in 96-well plates at optimal densities (e.g., 5×10^3 - 2×10^4 cells/well) in 100 μL complete medium. Incubate 24 h for adherence.
2. **Treatment:** Prepare serial dilutions of *Bauhinia* fractions (ID7, IA19, IID10) from DMSO stocks in serum-free or low-serum (0.5%-2% FBS) medium. Final DMSO ≤0.5%. Aspirate medium from wells and add 100 μL of treatment per well. Include controls: vehicle (0.5% DMSO), blank (medium only), and positive control (e.g., 10 μM cisplatin).
3. **Incubation:** Incubate for 24, 48, and 72 h.
4. **MTT Assay Endpoint:** Add 10 μL of MTT solution (5 mg/mL in PBS) per well. Incubate 3–4 h. Carefully aspirate medium, add 100 μL DMSO to dissolve formazan. Shake for 10 min. Read absorbance at 570 nm (ref. 630 nm) [3].
5. **Data Analysis:** Calculate % cell viability = [(At - Ab)/(Ac - Ab)] × 100. Determine IC_{50} values using non-linear regression (log(inhibitor) vs. normalized response).
6. **Selectivity Index (SI):** SI = IC_{50} (normal cell, e.g., PBMC)/IC_{50} (cancer cell, e.g., 4T1). SI >2 is typically considered selective.

4.1.3 Apoptosis Detection by Acridine Orange/Propidium Iodide (AO/PI) Staining

1. Treat cells (e.g., 4T1) with fractions at their IC_{50} in 6-well plates for 72 h.
2. Harvest cells (supernatant + trypsinized), wash with PBS.
3. Resuspend ~1×10^5 cells in 100 μL PBS. Add 1 μL each of AO (100 μg/mL) and PI (100 μg/mL).
4. Incubate in dark for 5–10 min. Place 10 μL on a slide, cover.
5. Immediately visualize under fluorescence microscope (FITC filter for AO/green, TRITC for PI/red).
6. Count >200 cells per sample and categorize: viable (green nucleus), early apoptotic (bright green nucleus with condensed chromatin), late apoptotic (orange/red nucleus with condensed chromatin), necrotic (uniformly red nucleus)

4.2 Anti-Metastatic Potential In Vitro

4.2.1 Wound Healing (Scratch) Assay

1. Seed 5×10^5 4T1 cells/well in a 24-well plate. Grow to 100% confluence.
2. Create a uniform "scratch" down the center of each well using a sterile 200 µL pipette tip.
3. Wash gently 3× with PBS to remove debris.
4. Add fresh medium containing fractions at IC_{50} or sub-IC_{50} (non-cytotoxic) concentrations.
5. Image the same wound locations at 0, 12, 24, and 48 h using an inverted microscope (40× objective).
6. Quantify wound area using ImageJ: % Wound Closure = [(Area_t=0 - Area_t=x)/Area_t=0] × 100.

4.2.2 Boyden Chamber Migration & Matrigel Invasion Assays

1. **Migration:** Pre-wet Transwell inserts (5 µm pores) with serum-free medium. Place in a 24-well plate.
2. **Invasion:** Coat inserts with 50–100 µL of diluted Matrigel (1:8 in cold serum-free medium). Incubate at 37°C for 4–6 h to gel.
3. **Cell Preparation:** Serum-starve cells (4×10^4 cells in 200 µL serum-free medium) with or without treatment (IC_{50}) for 30 min.
4. **Assay Setup:** Add cell suspension to the upper chamber. Add 500 µL of medium with 10% FBS (chemoattractant) to the lower chamber.
5. **Incubation:** Incubate for 18–24h (migration) or 24–48 h (invasion) at 37°C.
6. **Staining & Quantification:** Remove non-migrated/invaded cells from the upper side with a cotton swab. Fix cells on the lower membrane with 4% paraformaldehyde (10 min), stain with 0.1% Crystal Violet (20 min), wash. Air-dry, capture images (5 random fields/membrane at 100×). Count cells manually or extract dye with 10% acetic acid and read absorbance at 590 nm [4].

4.2.3 Gelatin Zymography for MMP-2/MMP-9 Activity

1. Collect conditioned serum-free media from treated 4T1 cells (24–48 h). Concentrate if necessary.
2. Prepare samples with non-reducing Laemmli buffer (no β -mercaptoethanol, no boiling).
3. Load equal protein amounts on a 10% SDS-PAGE gel co-polymerized with 1 mg/mL gelatin.
4. Run electrophoresis at 4°C.
5. **Gel Processing:** Wash gels 2× in 2.5% Triton X-100 (30 min each) to remove SDS, then incubate in zymography development buffer (50 mM Tris-HCl, pH 7.5, 5 mM $CaCl_2$, 0.02% NaN_3) at 37°C for 36–48 h.

6. Stain with 0.5% Coomassie Blue R-250 for 1 h, destain. Proteolytic activity appears as clear bands against a blue background.
7. Quantify band intensity using ImageJ. % Inhibition = 100 - [(Band Intensity_Treated / Band Intensity_Control) × 100].

4.3 In Vivo Antitumor Efficacy Study

4.3.1 4T1 Syngeneic Breast Cancer Model

1. **Ethics & Housing:** Obtain IACUC approval. House female BALB/c mice (n = 8–10/group) under SPF conditions (12 h light/dark, 22 ± 2°C) with free access to food/water.
2. **Tumor Inoculation:** Harvest log-phase 4T1 cells, resuspend in sterile PBS. Inject 5×10^4 - 1×10^5 cells (in 100 μL) subcutaneously into the 4th mammary fat pad or left flank of each mouse [5–7].
3. **Randomization & Treatment:** When tumors reach ~50–100 mm^3 (Day 7–9), randomize mice into groups: Vehicle (saline or 2% DMSO/saline), Positive Control (e.g., 5-FU, 25 mg/kg), and Treatment (ID7, e.g., 30 mg/kg). Administer i.p. daily for 14 days.
4. **Monitoring:** Measure body weight and tumor dimensions (Length (L) and Width (W)) with calipers every 2–3 days. Calculate tumor volume: $V = (L \times W^2)/2$.
5. **Termination & Sample Collection:** On Day 22, euthanize via CO_2 overdose/cervical dislocation. Excise primary tumors, lungs, and livers. Weigh organs. Count surface lung metastases under a dissecting microscope. Fix tissues in 10% formalin for 24 h, then transfer to 70% ethanol for histology.

4.3.2 Histopathological Analysis [8]

1. Process fixed tissues through an ethanol-xylene series, and embed in paraffin.
2. Section at 5 μm thickness using a microtome.
3. H&E Staining: Deparaffinize, rehydrate. Stain with Harris Hematoxylin (5 min), differentiate, blue. Counterstain with Eosin Y (2 min). Dehydrate, clear, mount.
4. Quantification: Capture 5–10 random, non-overlapping fields per tissue section (400× for tumors/lungs, 200× for liver). Analyze using ImageJ:
   * Tumor Necrosis: % Necrotic area per field.
   * Lung Metastasis: Number of metastatic foci per field or per whole lung section.
   * Liver Inflammation: Quantify infiltrating leukocyte clusters or areas of immune infiltration.

4.4 Statistical Analysis

1. Perform all experiments in triplicate (minimum) and repeat independently at least twice.
2. Express data as mean ± standard deviation (SD) or standard error of the mean (SEM).

3. For in vitro data (IC_{50}, % inhibition), use one-way ANOVA with Dunnett's post-hoc test for multiple comparisons vs. control.
4. For in vivo data (tumor volume, weight), analyze using two-way ANOVA for repeated measures (time × treatment) followed by Tukey's post-hoc test.
5. For single comparisons (e.g., final tumor weight, metastasis count), use unpaired Student's t-test.
6. Set statistical significance at $p<0.05$. Conduct analysis using GraphPad Prism 9.0 [8].

References

1. Cossarizza A et al (2017) Guidelines for the use of flow cytometry and cell sorting in immunological studies. Eur J Immunol 47(10):1584–1797
2. Justus CR, Leffler N, Ruiz-Echevarria M, Yang LV (2014) In vitro cell migration and invasion assays. J Vis Exp 88:51046
3. Mosmann T (1983) Rapid colorimetric assay for cellular growth and survival: application to proliferation and cytotoxicity assays. J Immunol Methods 65(1–2):55–63
4. Pulaski BA Ostrand-Rosenberg S (2001) Mouse 4T1 breast tumor model. Curr Protoc Immunol 39:20.2.1–20.2.16
5. Ribble D et al (2005) A simple technique for quantifying apoptosis in 96-well plates. BMC Biotechnol 5:12
6. Varghese E, Samuel SM, Sadiq Z et al (2016) Anti-cancer agents from natural products: a review. Curr Top Med Chem 16(22):2412–2427
7. Yong WK et al (2019) Mechanism of action of plant-derived natural compounds in cancer: a review. Int J Mol Sci 20(6):1451
8. Boyum A (1974) Isolation of mononuclear cells and granulocytes from human blood. Scand J Clin Lab Invest Suppl 21:77–89

Chapter 25

Comprehensive Protocol for Evaluating Antiproliferative and Pro-Apoptotic Effects of Novel Compounds

Abstract

This protocol provides a comprehensive and standardized workflow for evaluating the antiproliferative and pro-apoptotic effects of novel compounds, integrating cytotoxicity screening, mechanistic cell death studies, and biophysical interaction analyses. The methodology begins with cell culture maintenance of human tumor cell lines (A2780, HCT116, A549, MCF-7) and normal human dermal fibroblasts, followed by MTS metabolic viability assays (CellTiter 96® AQueous) to determine half-maximal inhibitory concentrations (IC_50) and calculate selectivity indices (SI = IC_50 fibroblasts/IC_50 tumor cells; SI >3 considered selective). Apoptosis is comprehensively assessed through three complementary approaches: (1) nuclear morphological analysis by Hoechst 33258/propidium iodide (PI) dual staining (5 µg/mL Hoechst + 25 µg/mL PI, fluorescence microscopy) to visualize chromatin condensation and fragmentation; (2) quantitative flow cytometry using Annexin V-FITC/PI staining (10,000 events/sample) to distinguish viable, early apoptotic, late apoptotic, and necrotic populations; and (3) mitochondrial membrane potential ($\Delta\Psi m$) evaluation using JC-1 dye (2–5 µM, 20–30 min incubation) with dual-wavelength fluorescence measurement (red aggregates: 560/595 nm; green monomers: 485/535 nm), where decreased red/green ratio indicates depolarization. For mechanistic insights into DNA targeting, UV-Vis absorption spectroscopy titrations are performed with calf thymus CT-DNA (ε_260 = 6600 $M^{-1}cm^{-1}$) to determine DNA-binding constants (Kb) via McGhee-von Hippel analysis, with hypochromism at the compound's λmax indicating intercalative binding. This integrated approach enables comprehensive characterization from initial potency through detailed mechanistic and biophysical investigations.

Keywords Cytotoxicity, Apoptosis, Mitochondrial membrane potential, DNA binding, Selectivity index

1 Introduction

This document provides detailed methodologies for the in vitro evaluation of novel compounds for potential anticancer activity. The protocol encompasses cell culture maintenance, cytotoxicity screening, mechanistic studies on apoptosis and autophagy, and biophysical interaction studies with biomolecules. The integrated approach allows for the determination of antiproliferative potency (IC_50), selectivity for tumor over non-tumor cells, and initial insights into the compound's mechanism of action, including induction of programmed cell death, oxidative stress, and DNA interaction [1, 2].

Karuppusamy Arunachalam et al., *Advanced Protocols in Cancer Research*, Springer Protocols Handbooks,
https://doi.org/10.1007/978-1-0716-5348-7_25,

2 Aim

To establish a standardized, reproducible workflow for:

1. Determining the half-maximal inhibitory concentration (IC_50) of compounds against a panel of human tumor cell lines and a non-tumor fibroblast line.
2. Calculating a Selectivity Index (SI) to identify compounds with preferential toxicity toward cancer cells.
3. Investigating the mechanistic pathways of cell death, including apoptosis (via morphology, phosphatidylserine externalization, and caspase activation), autophagy, and mitochondrial dysfunction.
4. Assessing the compound's ability to interact with key biological targets such as genomic DNA and serum transport proteins.

3 Detailed Experimental Procedures [3]

3.1 Cell Culture and Maintenance

- **Objective:** To propagate and maintain the human cell lines in optimal, consistent conditions for experimentation.
- **Materials:**
  - Cell lines: A2780, HCT116, A549, MCF-7, Human Dermal Fibroblasts.
  - Complete Growth Media:

    For HCT116, A549, MCF-7, Fibroblasts: DMEM + 10% (v/v) FBS + 1% (v/v) Penicillin-Streptomycin-Antimycotic + 1× MEM Non-Essential Amino Acids.

    For A2780: RPMI-1640 + 10% FBS + 1% Pen/Strep/Antimycotic + 1× MEM NEAA.
  - Reagents: Tryple™ Express, Dulbecco's Phosphate Buffered Saline (DPBS).
  - Consumables: T25 & T75 tissue culture flasks, 15 mL conical centrifuge tubes.
  - Equipment: CO_2 incubator (37°C, 5% CO_2, >95% humidity), biological safety cabinet, inverted microscope, centrifuge.
- Procedure:

1. **Thawing:** Rapidly thaw a cryovial in a 37°C water bath. Transfer contents to a 15 mL tube containing 9 mL of pre-warmed complete medium. Centrifuge at 200×*g*

for 5 min. Aspirate supernatant, resuspend pellet in 5 mL medium, and transfer to a T25 flask.

2. **Maintenance:** Incubate cultures, checking confluence daily. Refresh medium every 2–3 days.
3. **Subculturing (Passaging):**
   a. Aspirate medium from a ~80% confluent flask.
   b. Wash the cell monolayer gently with 3–5 mL of DPBS.
   c. Add pre-warmed Tryple™ Express (3 mL for T75, 2 mL for T25).
   d. Incubate at room temperature for ~5 min or until cells detach (monitor under microscope).
   e. Neutralize trypsin by adding an equal volume of complete medium.
   f. Transfer cell suspension to a 15 mL tube and centrifuge at 200 × *g* for 5 min.
   g. Aspirate supernatant, resuspend pellet in fresh complete medium.
   h. Perform a cell count using the Trypan Blue exclusion method (see 4.1.1).
   i. Seed new flasks at the appropriate seeding density (e.g., 1:3 to 1:10 split ratio).
4. **Cell Counting (Trypan BlueMethod):**
   a. Mix 10 μL of cell suspension with 10 μL of 0.4% Trypan Blue solution.
   b. Load 10 μL of the mixture into a hemocytometer.
   c. Count live (unstained) and dead (blue-stained) cells in the four corner quadrants.
   d. Calculate cell concentration: Cells/mL = (Total live cells counted/4) × Dilution Factor (2) × 104
   e. Viability (%) = (Total live cells/Total cells) × 100.

3.2 Metabolic Viability Assay (MTS - CellTiter 96® AQueous)

- **Objective:** To **determine** the concentration-dependent antiproliferative effect of compounds and calculate IC_50 values.
- **Materials:** CellTiter 96® AQueous One Solution Reagent (MTS), 96-well flat-bottom tissue culture plates, DMSO, and a microplate reader.
- **Procedure:**

1. **Cell Seeding:** Trypsinize, count, and dilute cells to 7.5 × 104 cells/mL in complete medium. Seed 100 μL/well (7500 cells/well) in a 96-well plate. Include medium-only wells as background control. Incubate for 24 h.

2. **Compound Treatment:**
   a. Prepare a serial dilution of the test compound in complete medium (e.g., 100 μM, 50 μM, 25 μM... 0.5 μM). Ensure final DMSO concentration is ≤0.1%.
   b. After 24 h, aspirate the old medium from the plate.
   c. Add 100 μL/well of the compound dilutions. Test each concentration in at least triplicate wells.
   d. Include controls: "Cell Control" wells (medium + 0.1% DMSO), "Background" wells (medium only).
3. **Incubation:** Incubate the plate for 48 h.
4. **MTS Assay Development:**
   a. Add 20 μL of MTS reagent directly to each well.
   b. Return plate to incubator for 45 min–4 h (until color develops).
5. **Absorbance Measurement:** Record absorbance at 490 nm using a microplate reader. Subtract the average absorbance of background wells from all readings.
6. **Data Analysis:**
   a. Calculate % Cell Viability for each well: Viability (%) = (Abs_sample - Abs_background)/(Abs_cell_control - Abs_background) × 100
   b. Plot % Viability vs. Log[Compound]. Fit a sigmoidal dose-response curve (variable slope) using GraphPad Prism.
   c. The IC_50 is the concentration at which viability is reduced to 50%.
7. **Selectivity Index (SI) Calculation:**

   SI = IC_50 (Non-tumor fibroblasts)/IC_50 (Tumor cell line)

   An SI >3 is typically considered indicative of selective toxicity toward the tumor cell line.

3.3 Apoptosis Analysis by Hoechst 33258/Propidium Iodide (PI) Staining [4, 5]

- **Objective:** To observe nuclear morphological changes characteristic of apoptosis (chromatin condensation, nuclear fragmentation) and distinguish early/late apoptotic and necrotic cells.
- **Materials:** Hoechst 33258 stock (1 mg/mL in H_2O), 4% Paraformaldehyde (PFA), sterile glass coverslips, 24-well plate, fluorescence microscope with DAPI and TRITC filters.
- **Procedure:**

1. Place sterile coverslips in a 24-well plate. Sterilize with 70% ethanol and wash with PBS.

2. Seed cells on coverslips at 7.5×104 cells/mL (500 μL/well). Incubate 24 h.
3. Treat cells with $IC_5$0 concentration of compound or 0.1% DMSO control for 48 h.
4. **Fixation & Staining:**
   a. Aspirate medium. Wash cells gently with 1× PBS.
   b. Fix cells with 4% PFA (500 μL/well) for 20 min at RT, in the dark.
   c. Wash 3× with PBS.
   d. Prepare staining solution: 5 μg/mL Hoechst 33258 + 25 μg/mL PI in PBS.
   e. Add 200 μL of staining solution to each well. Incubate for 15 min at RT, in the dark.
   f. Wash 3× with PBS.
5. **Mounting & Imaging:**
   a. Place a drop of mounting medium (e.g., glycerol) on a microscope slide.
   b. Using forceps, place the coverslip (cell-side down) onto the mounting medium.
   c. Seal edges with clear nail polish.
   d. Visualize immediately under a fluorescence microscope:

      Hoechst (Blue/UV filter): All nuclei stain blue. Apoptotic nuclei show bright, condensed, or fragmented chromatin.

      PI (Red/TRITC filter): Only cells with compromised membranes (late apoptotic/necrotic) stain red.
6. **Interpretation:** Viable cells = normal blue nuclei. Early apoptotic = condensed bright blue nuclei (PI−). Late apoptotic = condensed/fragmented red nuclei (PI+). Necrotic = normal shaped red nuclei (PI+).

3.4 Apoptosis Analysis by Annexin V-FITC/PI Staining (Flow Cytometry)

- **Objective:** To quantitatively assess the percentage of cells in early apoptosis, late apoptosis, and necrosis.
- **Materials:** Annexin V-FITC Apoptosis Detection Kit, flow cytometer with 488 nm laser, FITC (530/30 nm) and PI (> 670 nm) detectors, 35 mm dishes or 6-well plates.
- **Procedure:**

1. Seed HCT116 cells in 35 mm dishes at 1×10⁵ cells/mL (2 mL/dish). Incubate 24 h.
2. Treat with $IC_5$0 of compound or control for 48 h.

3. Cell Harvest & Staining (Perform steps on ice or at 4°C where possible):
   a. Collect both floating and adherent cells (by trypsinization). Pool in a 15 mL tube.
   b. Centrifuge at 300 × *g* for 5 min. Wash pellet with 1 mL of cold 1× PBS. Centrifuge again.
   c. Resuspend pellet in 100 μL of 1× Annexin Binding Buffer.
   d. Add 5 μL of FITC-conjugated Annexin V and 2 μL of PI (100 μg/mL) working solution.
   e. Incubate for 15 min at RT in the dark.
   f. Add 400 μL of 1× Annexin Binding Buffer to each tube.
4. **Flow Cytometry Analysis:**
   a. Analyze samples within 1 h. Acquire at least 10,000 events per sample.
   b. Use unstained and single-stained controls to set up compensation and quadrants.
5. **Gating Strategy (Dot Plot: FITC vs. PI):**
   - Lower Left (FITC−/PI−): Viable cells.
   - Lower Right (FITC+/PI−): Early apoptotic cells (Annexin V+, membrane intact).
   - Upper Right (FITC+/PI+): Late apoptotic/necrotic cells (Annexin V+, membrane compromised).
   - Upper Left (FITC−/PI+): Necrotic cells or debris.

3.5 Assessment of Mitochondrial Membrane Potential (ΔΨm) using JC-1

- **Objective:** To detect early apoptosis via the loss of mitochondrial membrane potential, a hallmark event.
- **Materials:** JC-1 dye, black-walled, clear-bottom 96-well plates or 8-well chamber slides, fluorescence plate reader or microscope.
- **Procedure:**

1. Seed A2780 cells at 7.5 × 104 cells/mL and incubate 24 h.
2. Treat with IC_50 of compound for 48 h. Include a positive control (e.g., 50 μM Carbonyl cyanide m-chlorophenyl hydrazone (CCCP) for 20 min) to induce depolarization.
3. **JC-1 Staining:**
   a. Prepare JC-1 working solution (2–5 μM) in serum-free medium or assay buffer.
   b. Aspirate treatment medium and wash cells with PBS.

   c. Add JC-1 working solution. Incubate for 20–30 min at 37°C, 5% CO_2.
   d. Wash cells gently with JC-1 assay buffer or warm PBS.
4. **Measurement & Analysis:**
   a. For microplate reader: Read fluorescence intensity with dual wavelengths:
      – Red (Aggregates): Ex/Em = 560/595 nm.
      – Green (Monomers): Ex/Em = 485/535 nm.
   b. For microscopy: Image using TRITC (red aggregates) and FITC (green monomers) filters.
5. **Data Interpretation:** A decrease in the Red/Green fluorescence ratio indicates mitochondrial depolarization (loss of $\Delta\Psi m$). Calculate ratio for each treatment relative to the control.

3.6 DNA Interaction Studies via UV-Vis Absorption Spectroscopy

- **Objective:** To determine the binding affinity (Kb) of the compound for calf thymus DNA (CT-DNA) and infer the binding mode (intercalation, groove binding).
- **Materials:** Calf Thymus DNA (CT-DNA), Tris-HCl buffer (5 mM Tris, 50 mM NaCl, pH 7.0), UV-transparent cuvettes (e.g., quartz), UV-Vis spectrophotometer.
- **Procedure:**

1. **DNA Preparation:** Dissolve CT-DNA in buffer and determine its concentration using ε_{260} = 6600 $M^{-1}cm^{-1}$ (per nucleotide phosphate). Ensure A_{260}/A_{280} ratio is ~1.8–1.9 for protein-free DNA.
2. **Compound Solution:** Prepare a stock solution of the test complex in DMSO. Dilute in buffer to a working concentration (e.g., 25 μM). Keep final DMSO constant (<1%).
3. **Titration Experiment:**
   a. Place 2 mL of the compound solution in both the sample and reference cuvettes. Record baseline spectrum (250–800 nm).
   b. To the sample cuvette, add increasing aliquots (2–10 μL) of the concentrated CT-DNA stock solution. Mix gently.
   c. To the reference cuvette, add equal aliquots of buffer to compensate for volume and dilution effects.
   d. After each addition, allow 3–5 min for equilibration, then record the spectrum.

4. **Data Analysis (for Intercalative Binding):**
   a. Monitor the change in absorbance (hypochromism) at the compound's λ_max.
   b. Process data using the McGhee-von Hippel equation or a double reciprocal plot: $[DNA]/(\varepsilon\_a - \varepsilon\_f) = [DNA]/(\varepsilon\_b - \varepsilon\_f) + 1/[K\_b (\varepsilon\_b - \varepsilon\_f)]$ where: $[DNA]$ = DNA concentration, $\varepsilon\_a = A\_obs/[Compound]$, ε_f = molar absorptivity of free compound, ε_b = molar absorptivity of bound compound.
   c. Plot $[DNA]/(\varepsilon\_a - \varepsilon\_f)$ vs. $[DNA]$. The slope = $1/(\varepsilon\_b - \varepsilon\_f)$ and Y-intercept = $1/[K\_b(\varepsilon\_b - \varepsilon\_f)]$.
   d. Calculate the DNA-binding constant, K_b, from: K_b = Slope/Intercept.

References

1. Gloeckner H, Jonuleit T, Lemke HD (2001) Monitoring of cell viability and cell growth in a hollow-fiber bioreactor by use of the dye Alamar Blue™. J Immunol Methods 252(1-2):131–138
2. Elmore S (2007) Apoptosis: a review of programmed cell death. Toxicol Pathol 35(4):495–516
3. Sirajuddin M, Ali S, Badshah A (2013) Drug–DNA interactions and their study by UV–Visible, fluorescence spectroscopies and cyclic voltametry. J Photochem Photobiol B 124:1–9
4. Novak MS, Büchel GE, Keppler BK, Jakupec MA (2016) Biological properties of novel ruthenium-and osmium-nitrosyl complexes with azole heterocycles. J Biol Inorg Chem 21(3):347–356
5. Brumatti G, Ma C, Lalaoui N, Nguyen NY, Navarro M, Tanzer MC et al (2016) The caspase-8 inhibitor emricasan combines with the SMAC mimetic birinapant to induce necroptosis and treat acute myeloid leukemia. Sci Transl Med 8(339):339ra69

Part V

In Vivo Efficacy and Pharmacological Evaluation

Check for updates

Chapter 26

In Vivo Biological Assays

Abstract

This protocol describes a comprehensive in vivo experimental approach for evaluating the antitumor efficacy and mechanistic effects of phytocompounds, alone and in combination with sodium ascorbate, using the Ehrlich Ascites Tumor (EAT) model in male Balb/C mice (20 ± 2 g, n = 108 total, 12 per group). Following intraperitoneal inoculation of 5×10^6 viable EAT cells (Day 0), treatments are administered intraperitoneally daily for 9 consecutive days (Days 1–9) at 1 mg/kg for phytocompounds and 100 mg/kg for ascorbate, with doxorubicin (1.2 mg/kg) as a positive control. Tumor progression is monitored by body weight and abdominal circumference measurements on Days 1 and 10, with tumor growth inhibition (% ICT) calculated. Survival analysis employs the Kaplan-Meier method with daily monitoring. Mechanistic studies on Day 9 include: (1) DNA fragmentation assessment via alkaline comet assay (ethidium bromide staining, 100 nuclei/sample, damage index 0–400); (2) cell cycle analysis by flow cytometry (PI/RNase staining, BD FACSCanto II); (3) glucose uptake measurement using [^{14}C]-2-deoxy-D-glucose (0.1 μCi/mL, 1 h incubation, liquid scintillation counting); (4) cell death classification by acridine orange/ethidium bromide (AO/EB) fluorescence microscopy (300 cells/sample); and (5) Western blot analysis of protein expression (RIPA lysis, SDS-PAGE, chemiluminescent detection). Statistical analysis uses one-way ANOVA with Bonferroni or Tukey-Kramer post-hoc tests ($p < 0.05$ significance).

Keywords Ehrlich ascites tumor, In vivo, Comet assay, Cell cycle, Glucose uptake

1 Introduction

In vivo studies are essential for validating the antitumor efficacy and systemic toxicity of novel therapeutic candidates identified in vitro. This study utilized the Ehrlich Ascites Tumor (EAT) model in Balb/C mice to investigate the antineoplastic effects of phytocompounds, individually and in combination with sodium ascorbate [1]. This model was chosen due to its reproducibility and ability to mimic the aggressive proliferative behavior of solid tumors in vivo. The assay monitored parameters such as tumor volume, survival rate, DNA fragmentation, and protein expression to assess therapeutic outcomes [2].

Karuppusamy Arunachalam et al., *Advanced Protocols in Cancer Research*, Springer Protocols Handbooks, https://doi.org/10.1007/978-1-0716-5348-7_26,

2 Aim

To evaluate the in vivo antitumor activity of phytocompounds, alone and in combination with sodium ascorbate, using the Ehrlich ascites tum or model in Balb/C mice through assessment of tumor growth inhibition and animal survival.

3 Methods

3.1 Animal Preparation

3.1.1 Materials

- Male Balb/C mice (20 ± 2 g, ~60 days old).
- Polycarbonate cages with filter tops.
- Commercial rodent diet and water (ad libitum).
- Controlled room conditions: 12 h light/dark cycle, 25 ± 2°C, 60% humidity.
- Institutional animal ethics approval.

3.1.2 Procedure

1. A total of 108 Balb/C mice were housed in groups of 12 per treatment group.
2. Mice were acclimatized for at least 1 week before experimentation.
3. Ethical approval for animal use was obtained from the Institutional Ethics Committee, in compliance with national guidelines for the care and use of laboratory animals.

3.2 Ehrlich Ascites Tumor (EAT) Model and Experimental Protocol

3.2.1 Materials

- Ehrlich carcinoma cells were maintained via serial transplantation in mice.
- Phytocompounds.
- Sodium ascorbate.
- Doxorubicin (positive control, 1.2 mg/kg).
- Sterile saline solution (0.9%).
- Intraperitoneal (i.p.) injection equipment (syringes, needles).
- Electronic scale and measuring tape.

- Laminar flow hood for aseptic handling.
- Centrifuge, PBS, and sample collection tools.

3.2.2 Procedure

1. **Cell Preparation**:
   - Collect Ehrlich ascites tumor cells from donor mice.
   - Resuspend in sterile saline to achieve a concentration of 5×10^6 viable cells/0.2 mL.
   - Assess viability via trypan blue exclusion (>95% required).
2. **Tumor Induction:**
   - Inject each experimental mouse intraperitoneally with 0.2 mL of the prepared EAT cell suspension.
   - Designate the day of injection as Day 0.
3. **Group Allocation (n = 12 per group):**
   - **Group a:** Negative control (saline only).
   - **Group b:** Positive control (doxorubicin, 1.2 mg/kg).
   - **Group c:** Ascorbate alone (100 mg/kg).
   - **Group d:** Phytocompound 1 (1 mg/kg).
   - **Group e:** Phytocompound 2 (1 mg/kg).
   - **Group f:** Phytocompound 3 (1 mg/kg).
   - **Group g:** Juglone + Ascorbate (1 mg/kg + 100 mg/kg).
   - **Group h:** Phytocompound 2 + Ascorbate (1 mg/kg + 100 mg/kg).
   - **Group i:** Phytocompound 3 + Ascorbate (1 mg/kg + 100 mg/kg).
4. **Treatment Regimen:**
   - Treatments began 24 h post-inoculation (Day 1).
   - All compounds were administered intraperitoneally (i.p.) once daily for 9 consecutive days (Days 1–9).
   - Naphthoquinone/ascorbate combinations were freshly prepared immediately prior to each administration.
5. **Sample Collection:**
   - On Day 9, 2 h after the last treatment:
     - Six mice per group were euthanized under anesthesia.
     - Samples were collected for DNA fragmentation, cell cycle analysis, and protein expression via immunodetection.
   - The remaining six mice in each group were maintained for tumor progression and survival analysis.

3.3 Tumor Growth Inhibition and Animal Survival

3.3.1 Materials

Digital scale.

- Flexible measuring tape.
- Data sheets or software for Kaplan–Meier survival analysis.

3.3.2 Procedure

1. **Tumor Growth Evaluation**:
   - Measure body weight (g) and abdominal circumference (cm) on:
     - **Day 1** (pre-treatment baseline).
     - **Day 10** (post-treatment).
   - Calculate change (Δ) for each parameter:
     - ΔWeight = Final weight – Initial weight
     - ΔCircumference = Final circumference – Initial circumference
2. **Tumor Growth Inhibition (% ICT)**:
   - Use the following formula (Kviecinski et al., 2011): ICT(%) = (Mean ΔCircumference of Test Group × 100 / Mean ΔCircumference of Control Group) – 100
3. **Survival Analysis:**
   - The survival time of remaining mice was monitored daily until death.
   - Results were expressed as mean survival time (days) using the Kaplan–Meier method [3].

3.4 DNA Fragmentation Index—Comet Assay

To evaluate the genotoxic effects of treatments on DNA in Ehrlich ascites tumor (EAT) cells, the alkaline comet assay was performed following the method of Lala et al. [4], with slight modifications to optimize for murine ascites cells.

Procedure:

1. Collect 500 μL of ascitic fluid (TAE) from each animal and centrifuge at 1000 × *g* for 10 min at 4 °C.
2. Discard the supernatant and resuspend the cell pellet in 1000 μL of ice-cold PBS.
3. Mix 5 μL of the resuspended cells with 95 μL of 0.5% low-melting-point agarose (at 37 °C).
4. Immediately pipette this mixture onto microscope slides pre-coated with 1% normal melting agarose and spread evenly.

5. Place the slides on a chilled flat surface or at 4°C for 5 min to solidify the agarose.
6. Immerse the slides in pre-chilled lysis buffer (2.5 M NaCl, 100 mM EDTA, 10 mM Tris-HCl, 1% Triton X-100, 10% DMSO; pH 10) and incubate at 4°C for 2 h in the dark.
7. Transfer slides to an electrophoresis chamber and incubate in alkaline buffer (300 mM NaOH, 1 mM EDTA; pH 13) for 20 min at 4°C to allow DNA unwinding.
8. Perform electrophoresis for 20 min at 25 V and 300 mA in the same buffer.
9. Neutralize the slides in 0.4 M Tris-HCl (pH 7.5) for 5 min and rinse with distilled water.
10. Stain each slide with 50 μL of ethidium bromide (0.25 mg/mL).
11. Visualize comets under a fluorescence microscope (Olympus Bx41) and analyze 100 randomly selected nuclei per slide.
12. Classify DNA damage into five classes (0–4), with 0 representing no damage and 4 indicating maximal fragmentation.
13. Calculate a DNA damage index (0–400) using the sum of cells multiplied by their respective damage class (Fig. 1).

3.5 Cell Cycle Analysis

To evaluate alterations in the cell cycle distribution of EAT cells after treatment, the PI/RNase staining method (Immunostep Kit) was used according to the manufacturer's protocol.

Procedure:

1. Harvest 5×10^5 EAT cells and centrifuge at $1000 \times g$ for 10 min.
2. Resuspend the pellet in 250 μL PBS; separate 200 μL into a new tube.
3. Centrifuge again at $1000 \times g$ for 10 min and discard the supernatant.
4. Add 200 μL of ice-cold 70% ethanol dropwise while vortexing to fix the cells.
5. Store fixed cells at −20°C for 24 h.
6. Wash cells by centrifugation (1000 × g for 10 min), resuspend in 1 mL PBS, and centrifuge again.
7. Remove PBS and stain the cells with 200 μL of PI/RNase solution.
8. Analyze cell cycle distribution using a BD FACSCanto II flow cytometer and process data with Flowing Software 2.5.

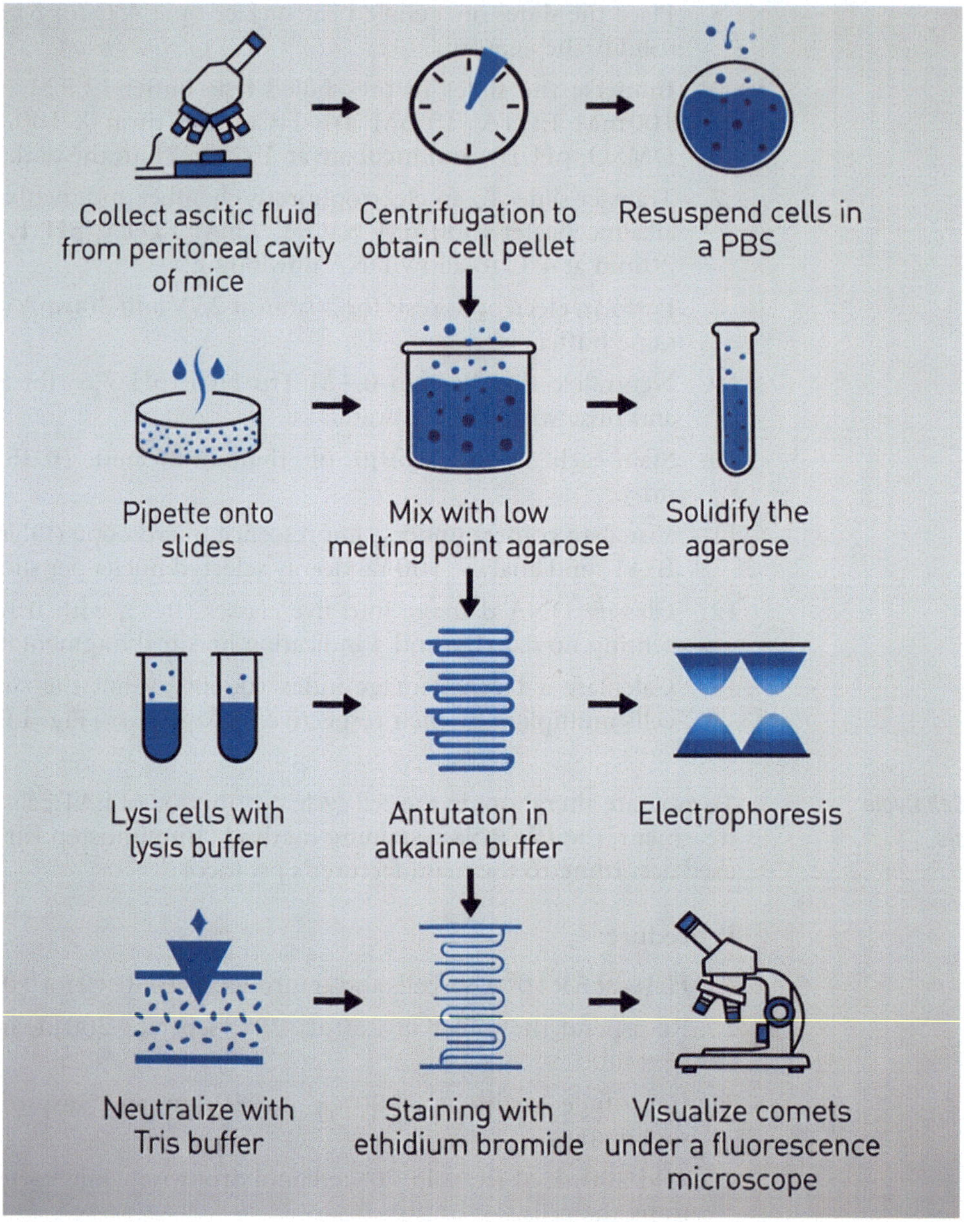

Fig. 1 Schematic representation of DNA Fragmentation Index—Comet Assay

3.6 Glucose Uptake Assay

The glucose uptake by EAT cells was evaluated using radiolabeled deoxyglucose ([14C]-2-deoxy-D-glucose, 14C-DG), following the protocol by Yamamoto et al. [5].

Procedure:

1. Collect 8×10^5 EAT cells and centrifuge at $1000 \times g$ for 8 min to remove ascitic fluid.

2. Resuspend cells in 200 μL of DMEM medium supplemented with 10% FBS, 100 U/mL penicillin, and 100 μg/mL streptomycin.
3. Pre-incubate cells for 2 h at 37 °C in a 5% CO2 incubator.
4. Discard supernatant and add 200 μL of medium containing the test compounds (juglone, Q7, or Q9 at 10 μM) with or without 1 mM ascorbate.
5. Add 14C-DG (0.1 μCi/mL) to each sample and incubate for 1 h.
6. Centrifuge at 1000 × *g* for 8 min, discard the supernatant, and wash cells twice with medium.
7. Add 200 μL of 0.5 M NaOH and measure radioactivity using a liquid scintillation spectrometer.
8. Normalize glucose uptake to total protein content (Lowry method) and express as nmol glucose/mg protein.

3.7 Cell Death Analysis (AO/EB Staining)

Cell viability and type of death (apoptosis/necrosis) were assessed by fluorescent staining with acridine orange(AO) and ethidium bromide (EB), following McGahon et al. [6].

Procedure:

1. Collect 125 μL of TAE and centrifuge at 1000 × *g* for 10 min.
2. Resuspend the cell pellet in 500 μL PBS.
3. Mix 25 μL of the cell suspension with 10 μL of AO/EB dye solution (1:1 mixture of 100 μg/mL each).
4. Place 10 μL of the stained sample on a microscope slide and observe under a fluorescence microscope (Olympus Bx41).
5. Count 300 cells per sample and classify as viable, apoptotic, or necrotic.
6. Perform three independent experiments in triplicate.

3.8 Immuno-electrophoresis (Western Blot) Assay

This assay was performed to detect specific protein expression in EAT cells after treatment.

Procedure:

1. Centrifuge 250 μL of TAE at 5000 × *g* for 5 min and discard the supernatant.
2. Wash cells with PBS three times.
3. Lyse cells using RIPA buffer (25 mM Tris-Cl, 150 mM NaCl, 1% NP40, 0.25% sodium deoxycholate, 1 mM PMSF, pH 7.4) supplemented with protease and phosphatase inhibitors.
4. Quantify protein using the Bradford assay (BioRad).

5. Mix protein samples (25 μg) with Laemmli buffer and denature.
6. Separate proteins by SDS-PAGE and transfer to nitrocellulose membranes.
7. Block membranes with skimmed milk, wash, and incubate overnight with primary antibodies.
8. Incubate with HRP-conjugated secondary antibodies.
9. Detect protein bands using ChemiDoc MP imaging system (Bio-Rad).

3.9 Statistical Analysis

All quantitative data are expressed as mean ± standard deviation (SD). In vitro and biochemical assays were performed in triplicate and repeated independently three times. Densitometric analysis of Western blot bands was performed using ImageJ software. Statistical significance was determined using one-way ANOVAStatistical , followed by Bonferroni or Tukey-Kramer post hoc tests as appropriate. A *p*-value <0.05 was considered statistically significant.

References

1. Samudrala PK, Augustine BB, Kasala ER, Bodduluru LN, Barua C, Lahkar M (2015) Evaluation of antitumor activity and antioxidant status of Alternanthera brasiliana against Ehrlich ascites carcinoma in Swiss albino mice. Pharmacognosy Res 7(1):66
2. Hossain MA, Hossain MT, Hossain MR, Ahmed T (2025) Assessment of the anticancer activity of Aegle marmelos leaf extracts against Ehrlich's Ascites Carcinoma (EAC) cell line in Swiss albino mice. J Phytochem Insights 2(01):1–10
3. Stalpers LJ, Kaplan EL (2018) Edward L. Kaplan and the Kaplan-Meier survival curve. BSHM Bull: J Br Soc Hist Math 33(2):109–135
4. Lala PK, Parhar RS, Singh P, Lala PK (1990) Cure of murine Ehrlich ascites tumors with chronic oral indomethacin therapy combined with intraperitoneal administration of LAK cells and IL-2. Cancer Lett 51(1):27–35
5. Yamamoto N, Ueda-Wakagi M, Sato T, Kawasaki K, Sawada K, Kawabata K, Ashida H (2015) Measurement of glucose uptake in cultured cells. Curr Protoc Pharmacol 71(1):12–14
6. McGahon AJ, Martin SJ, Bissonnette RP, Mahboubi A et al (1995) The end of the (cell) line: methods for the study of apoptosis in vitro. Methods Cell Biol 46:153–185

Chapter 27

Evaluation of Antitumor Action in Sarcoma 180 Solid Tumor Model (In Vivo)

Abstract

This protocol describes a comprehensive preclinical evaluation of the antitumor activity of three natural compounds—OEST (oxygenated sesquiterpene), α-pinene, and 3-carene—using both in vitro cytotoxicity assays against human cancer cell lines and in vivo efficacy studies in a Sarcoma 180 solid tumor model. Initial in vitro screening employs the MTT colorimetric assay (570 nm, 630 nm reference) following 72-h exposure of SNB-19 (glioblastoma), HCT-116 (colon carcinoma), and PC-3 (prostate carcinoma) cells to compound concentrations (0.5% DMSO vehicle control) to determine half-maximal inhibitory concentrations (IC_{50}) via non-linear regression in GraphPad Prism. For in vivo studies, male Swiss mice (n = 5–6/group) are inoculated subcutaneously with 2×10^6 Sarcoma 180 cells in the left groin (Day 0). Treatments are administered intraperitoneally daily for 7 consecutive days (Days 1–7) at selected doses, with 5-fluorouracil (5-FU, 25 mg/kg/day) as positive control and 2% DMSO/saline as vehicle control. On Day 8, animals are euthanized following blood collection via retro-orbital puncture; tumors, spleen, liver, kidneys, and heart are excised and weighed. Tumor inhibition rate (TIR%) is calculated as: [(Mean Tumor Weight_control - Mean Tumor Weight_treated) / Mean Tumor Weight_control] × 100. Relative organ weights are expressed as (organ weight/final body weight) × 100. Statistical analysis employs one-way ANOVA with Dunnett's post-hoc test ($p < 0.05$ significance). This integrated approach enables comprehensive assessment from in vitro potency through in vivo efficacy and preliminary toxicity evaluation.

Keywords Sarcoma 180, In vivo antitumor activity, MTT assay, Tumor inhibition rate, Swiss mice

1 Introduction

Natural product-derived compounds represent a significant source of novel anticancer agents. This study investigates the in vitro cytotoxicity and in vivo antitumor efficacy of three compounds, OEST (oxygenated sesquiterpene), α-pinene, and 3-carene, against human cancer cell lines and in a murine solid tumor model. The dual approach provides a comprehensive preclinical evaluation of their therapeutic potential.

Karuppusamy Arunachalam et al., *Advanced Protocols in Cancer Research*, Springer Protocols Handbooks,
https://doi.org/10.1007/978-1-0716-5348-7_27,

2 Aim

1. To evaluate the in vitro cytotoxic activity of OEST, α-pinene, and 3-carene against SNB-19 (glioblastoma), HCT-116 (colon carcinoma), and PC-3 (prostate carcinoma) cell lines using the MTT assay.
2. To assess the in vivo antitumor efficacy and systemic toxicity of these compounds against Sarcoma 180-induced solid tumors in Swiss mice.

3 Materials

3.1 For In Vitro Cytotoxicity Assay

- **Cell Lines:** SNB-19 (human glioblastoma), HCT-116 (human colon carcinoma), PC-3 (human prostate carcinoma).
- **Culture Reagents:** RPMI-1640 medium, Fetal Bovine Serum (FBS, heat-inactivated), Penicillin-Streptomycin solution (10,000 U/mL), 0.25% Trypsin-EDTA, Phosphate Buffered Saline (PBS), pH 7.4.
- **Test Compounds:** OEST, α-pinene, 3-carene. Prepare 10 mg/mL stock solutions in DMSO. Store at −20°C. Final working concentrations should not exceed 0.5% DMSO in culture media.
- **MTT Assay Reagents:** MTT powder (3-(4,5-dimethylthiazol-2-yl)-2,5-diphenyltetrazolium bromide), Dimethyl sulfoxide (DMSO, sterile filtered).
- **Equipment & Consumables:** Class II biological safety cabinet, CO_2 incubator (37°C, 5% CO_2, humidified), inverted phase-contrast microscope, water bath (37°C), centrifuge, 96-well flat-bottom tissue culture plates, multichannel pipettes, microplate reader capable of measuring absorbance at 570 nm with a reference filter of 630 nm.

3.2 For In Vivo Antitumor Assay

- **Animals:** Male Swiss albino mice (*Mus musculus*), 6–8 weeks old, weighing 25–35 g. House under standard conditions (12 h light/dark cycle, 22 ± 2°C, 50%–60% humidity) with *ad libitum* access to food and water. Acclimatize for 1 week prior to experimentation.
- **Tumor Model:** Sarcoma 180 (S180) ascitic cells, maintained by serial intraperitoneal passage in Swiss mice.
- **Test and Control Substances:**
  - **Test Compounds:** OEST, α-pinene, 3-carene. Prepare fresh daily in 2% DMSO + 0.9% saline (vehicle).
  - **Positive Control:** 5-Fluorouracil (5-FU, 25 mg/kg/day in saline).
  - **Vehicle Control:** 2% DMSO in 0.9% saline.
  - **Negative Control:** 0.9% saline.

- **Anesthesia & Euthanasia:** Isoflurane (3%–4% for induction, 1.5%–2% for maintenance), calibrated vaporizer, induction chamber.
- **Surgical & Analytical Tools:** Sterile surgical instruments (scissors, forceps), 1 mL syringes, 26-27G needles, microcapillary tubes for blood collection, precision analytical balance (0.1 mg), cryogenic vials.
- **Reagents:** Lactated Ringer's solution, Gentamicin sulfate (40 mg/mL), 10% neutral buffered formalin.
- **Approval:** Institutional Animal Ethics Committee approval.

4 Detailed Step-by-Step Protocol [1–5]

4.1 In Vitro Cytotoxicity Assay (MTT Protocol)

4.1.1 Cell Culture Maintenance

1. Rapidly thaw frozen cell vials in a 37°C water bath.
2. Transfer cells to a 15 mL tube containing 9 mL of pre-warmed complete medium (RPMI-1640 + 10% FBS + 1% Penicillin-Streptomycin).
3. Centrifuge at 300 × *g* for 5 min. Aspirate supernatant.
4. Resuspend the cell pellet in 5 mL of complete medium and transfer to a T-25 flask.
5. Incubate at 37°C in a 5% CO_2 humidified incubator.
6. Subculture cells at 80%–90% confluence using trypsin-EDTA.

4.1.2 Cell Seeding for Assay

1. Harvest exponentially growing cells and prepare a single-cell suspension.
2. Count cells using a hemocytometer or automated counter. Adjust cell density with complete medium to:
   - HCT-116: 0.7×10^5 cells/mL.
   - SNB-19 & PC-3: 1.0×10^5 cells/mL.
3. Seed 100 µL of cell suspension per well into a 96-well plate (resulting in 7000 HCT-116 or 10,000 SNB-19/PC-3 cells per well).
4. Incubate plates for 24 h to allow cell adhesion.

4.1.3 Compound Treatment

1. After 24 h, prepare serial dilutions of OEST, α-pinene, and 3-carene from stock solutions in complete medium. Ensure final DMSO concentration is ≤0.5%.

2. Aspirate the medium from the seeded plates.
3. Add 100 µL of fresh medium containing the desired final concentrations of compounds to respective wells. Include triplicate wells for each concentration.
4. Set up control wells: Cell control (medium with 0.5% DMSO), Blank control (medium only, no cells).
5. Return plates to the incubator for 72 h.

4.1.4 MTT Assay Execution

1. After 72 h, add 10 µL of MTT solution (5 mg/mL in PBS) directly to each well.
2. Incubate for 3–4 h at 37°C.
3. Carefully aspirate the medium without disturbing the purple formazan crystals.
4. Add 100 µL of DMSO to each well to dissolve the crystals.
5. Place the plate on an orbital shaker for 10 min in the dark to ensure complete dissolution.
6. Measure the absorbance at 570 nm, using 630 nm as a reference wavelength, on a microplate reader.

4.1.5 Data Analysis

1. Calculate the mean absorbance for each test group and the controls.
2. Determine cell viability: % Viability = [(At - Ab) / (Ac - Ab)] × 100, where At = Absorbance of test, Ac = Absorbance of cell control, Ab = Absorbance of blank.
3. Calculate % Growth Inhibition: 100 - % Viability.
4. Generate dose-response curves using non-linear regression (log(inhibitor) vs. normalized response) in GraphPad Prism 8.0.1 to determine the half-maximal inhibitory concentration (IC_{50}) for each compound/cell line.
5. Present data as Mean ± Standard Deviation (SD) from three independent experiments.

4.2 In Vivo Antitumor Assay (Sarcoma 180 Solid Tumor)

4.2.1 Preparation of Tumor Cell Inoculum (Fig. 1)

1. Euthanize a donor mouse bearing 7–10 days old S180 ascites under deep isoflurane anesthesia, followed by cervical dislocation.
2. Aseptically withdraw ascitic fluid using an 18G needle and transfer to a sterile tube containing ice-cold Lactated Ringer's solution with 1% gentamicin.
3. Centrifuge at 300 × *g* for 10 min at 4°C. Wash the cell pellet twice with Ringer's solution.
4. Resuspend the final pellet and count viable cells using Trypan Blue exclusion.

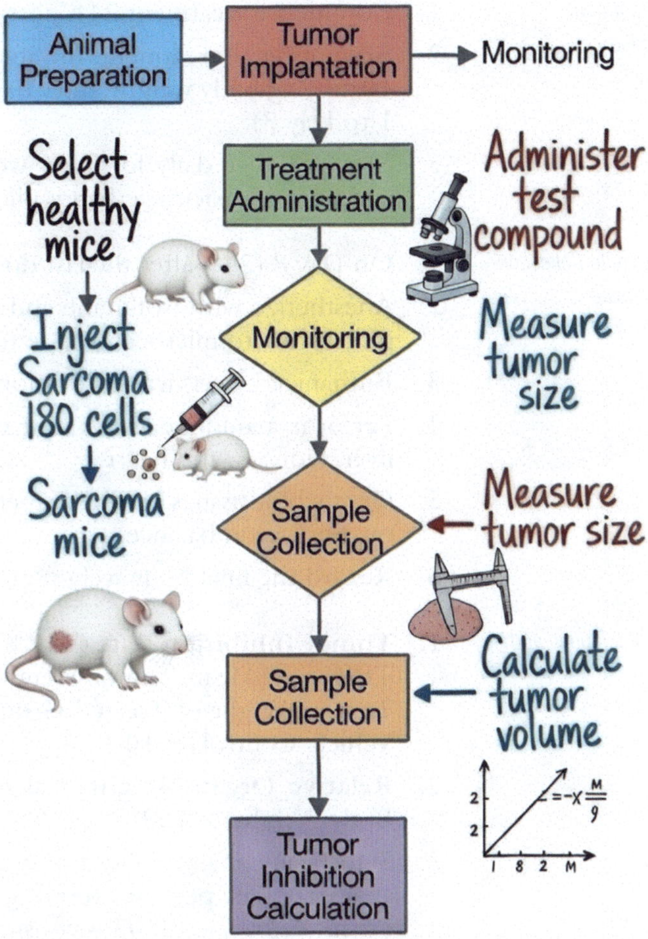

Fig. 1 Experimental representation of in vivo antitumor activity assay using the sarcoma 180 Model

5. Adjust cell concentration to 4×10^6 cells/mL in Ringer's solution. Keep on ice and use within 2 h.

4.2.2 Animal Grouping and Tumor Implantation

1. Randomly divide 30–35 Swiss mice into six groups (n = 5–6/group):
   - Group I: Normal Saline (Negative Control).
   - Group II: Vehicle Control (2% DMSO in Saline).
   - Group III: Positive Control (5-FU, 25 mg/kg/day, i.p.).
   - Groups IV–VI: Test Compounds (OEST, α-pinene, 3-carene at selected doses, i.p.).
2. On Day 0, restrain a mouse and disinfect the left groin area with 70% ethanol.
3. Subcutaneously inject 0.5 mL of the S180 cell suspension (containing 2×10^6 cells) into the left groin using a 27G needle.

4.2.3 Treatment Administration

1. Commence treatment 24 h post-implantation (Day 1).
2. Administer all treatments intraperitoneally (i.p.) in a volume of 10 mL/kg body weight, once daily for 7 consecutive days (Day 1 to Day 7).
3. Monitor mice daily for body weight changes, tumor growth, and signs of toxicity (lethargy, piloerection, abnormal behavior).

4.2.4 Sample Collection and Euthanasia

1. On Day 8 (24 h after the last dose), weigh each animal.
2. Anesthetize with isoflurane and collect blood via retro-orbital puncture into microcentrifuge tubes.
3. Euthanize by cervical dislocation while under deep anesthesia.
4. Perform a midline incision. Excise the solid tumor, spleen, liver, kidneys, and heart.
5. Gently blot tissues on filter paper and weigh them immediately on a precision balance.
6. Record the final body weight and organ weights.

4.2.5 Calculations and Analysis

1. **Tumor Inhibition Rate (TIR%):** Calculate using the formula: TIR% = [(Mean Tumor Weight of Vehicle Control - Mean Tumor Weight of Treated Group) / Mean Tumor Weight of Vehicle Control] × 100
2. **Relative Organ Weight:** Calculate as (Organ Weight/Final Body Weight) × 100.
3. Statistically analyze data using one-way ANOVA followed by an appropriate post-hoc test (e.g., Dunnett's test) in GraphPad Prism. A *p*-value <0.05 is considered significant.

4.2.6 Biosafety and Waste Disposal

1. All animal carcasses, tissues, and contaminated materials are to be treated as biohazardous waste.
2. Place waste in autoclave bags, sterilize by autoclaving, and then dispose of according to institutional biosafety protocols.

References

1. Mosmann T (1983) Rapid colorimetric assay for cellular growth and survival: application to proliferation and cytotoxicity assays. J Immunol Methods 65(1-2):55–63
2. Geran RI, Greenberg NH, MacDonald MM, Schumacher AM, Abbott BJ (1972) Protocols for screening chemical agents and natural products against animal tumors and other biological systems. Cancer Chemother Rep 3(2):1–103
3. Ozaslan M, Karagoz ID, Kilic IH, Guldur ME (2011) Ehrlich ascites carcinoma. Afr J Biotechnol 10(13):2375–2378
4. National Research Council (US) (2011). Guide for the care and use of laboratory animals, 8th edn. National Academies Press
5. Strese S, Fryknäs M, Larsson R, Gullbo J (2013) Effects of the sesquiterpene lactone on cancer cells and its potential use in combination therapy. Invest New Drugs 31(2):425–437.

Chapter 28

Evaluation of the Antitumor Activity in HL-60 Cells and TRAMP Mouse Model

Abstract

This protocol describes a comprehensive evaluation of the antitumor effects of phytocompounds using both in vitro assays in HL-60 and PC-3 cells and in vivo studies in TRAMP (transgenic adenocarcinoma of the mouse prostate) mice. In vitro, cytotoxicity and proliferation are assessed by alamarBlue® assay (12.5–100 μg/mL, 24–48 h, Ex/Em 570/585 nm), cell death quantified by Sytox® Green staining in RFP+ PC-3 cells, and apoptosis evaluated by annexin-V/7-AAD flow cytometry and cell cycle analysis (propidium iodide staining). Mechanistic studies include pre-treatment with apoptosis/necroptosis inhibitors (Z-VAD-FMK 25 μM, GSK'872 2 μM). In vivo, TRAMP mice are treated orally with EERP (50 mg/kg in PBS/1% Tween 80) from 8 to 12 weeks of age, with control groups euthanized at 8 weeks (T8) and 12 weeks (TC12). Ventral prostate tissues are analyzed by: (1) histopathology (H&E staining, classification into NT, LGPIN, HGPIN, adenocarcinoma); (2) immunohistochemistry for COX-2 (1:50) and PCNA (1:250) with DAB development; (3) TUNEL assay for apoptosis detection (DAPI counterstain, 10 fields/animal); and (4) Western blotting for COX-2 expression (RIPA lysis, SDS-PAGE, chemiluminescence, beta-actin normalization). Statistical analysis employs one-way/two-way ANOVA with Tukey/Bonferroni post-tests ($p < 0.05$ significance) in GraphPad Prism 5.0.

Keywords TRAMP mice, HL-60 cells, Apoptosis, Immunohistochemistry, COX-2

1 Introduction

Cancer remains a leading cause of morbidity and mortality worldwide. Despite the success of current chemotherapeutic agents, challenges such as adverse side effects and drug resistance limit their effectiveness. Phytocompounds, due to their structural diversity and multi-targeted mechanisms, have emerged as promising candidates in cancer therapy [1]. This study evaluates the antitumor effects of selected phytocompounds using both in vitro assays in HL-60 cells and in vivo models involving TRAMP (transgenic adenocarcinoma of the mouse prostate) animals.

Karuppusamy Arunachalam et al., *Advanced Protocols in Cancer Research*, Springer Protocols Handbooks,
https://doi.org/10.1007/978-1-0716-5348-7_28,

2 Aim

To assess the antitumor efficacy of phytocompounds in vitro using HL-60 cells and in vivo using TRAMP mice through cytotoxicity, morphological, genotoxic, immunohistochemical, apoptotic, and protein expression analyses.

3 Materials

- HL-60 and PC-3 cell lines.
- TRAMP mice (C57BL/6-Tg (TRAMP)8247Ng/JX FVB/Unib F1/J).
- RPMI-1640 medium, FBS, Penicillin-Streptomycin.
- DMSO, Tween 80, PBS (pH 7.0).
- MTT reagent, alamarBlue®, Trypan blue.
- AO/EB staining solutions, BrDU labeling kit.
- Hematoxylin, Eosin, May-Grünwald-Giemsa solutions.
- TUNEL assay kit (Dead-End™ Fluorometric TUNEL System).
- Primary and secondary antibodies (anti-COX-2, anti-PCNA, anti-beta-actin).
- DAB chromogen, DAPI, Rhodamine 123, Propidium Iodide, 7-AAD, Annexin V.
- Flow cytometer, fluorescence microscope, and microplate reader.
- Bouin's fixative, paraformaldehyde, paraffin (Paraplast), and microtome.
- RIPA buffer, protease inhibitor cocktail, SDS-PAGE, and Western blotting supplies.
- ImageJ, GraphPad Prism 5.0.

4 Experimental Procedures [2]

4.1 In Vivo Assays (Fig. 1)

4.1.1 Animal Treatments

Obtain TRAMP mice from CEMIB-UNICAMP and randomly divide them into three groups: T8 (euthanized at 8 weeks), TC12 (control, euthanized at 12 weeks), and TP12 (EERP-treated, euthanized at 12 weeks). Administer EERP orally at 50 mg/kg (dissolved in PBS with 1% Tween 80) from 8 to 12 weeks of age. Treat control animals

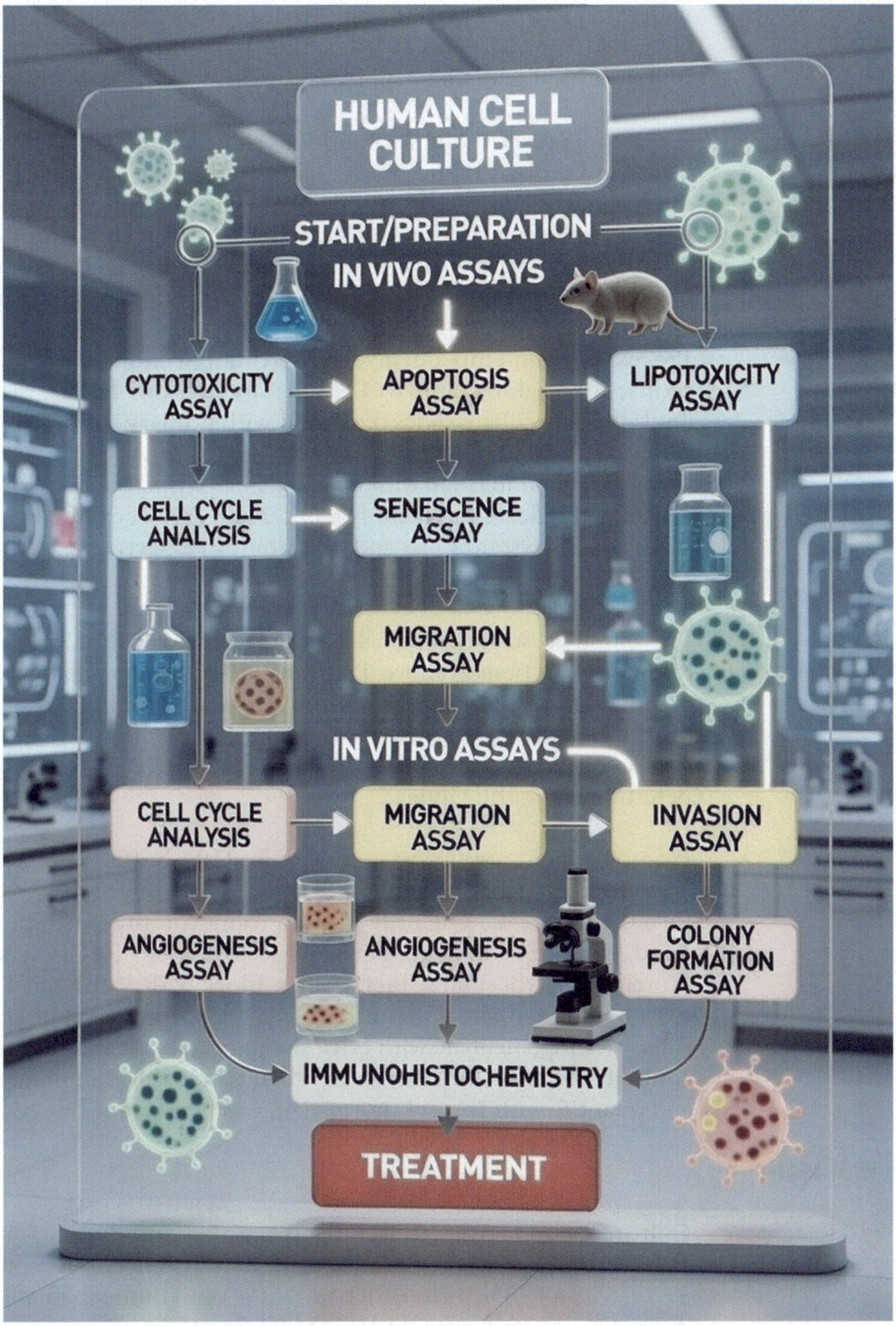

Fig. 1 Flowchart of the experimental design

with PBS (10 mL/kg). Perform euthanasia using 2% xylazine hydrochloride (5 mg/kg) and 10% ketamine hydrochloride (60 mg/kg). Follow ethical guidelines approved by the institutional committee.

4.1.2 Morphological Analysis

Fix ventral prostate samples in Bouin's solution for 24 h. Dehydrate, clear, and embed tissues in Paraplast. Cut 5 µm sections using a microtome. Stain sections with hematoxylin and eosin. Capture ten random fields per slide at 40× magnification using a Nikon Eclipse E-400 microscope. Classify quadrants according to Roy-Burman et al. (2004) into NT, LGPIN, HGPIN, and adenocarcinoma.

4.1.3 Immunohistochemistry

Process paraffin-embedded ventral prostate sections as above. Use mouse monoclonal anti-COX-2 (1:50) and anti-PCNA (1:250) antibodies. Incubate slides overnight with primary antibody. Apply HRP-conjugated goat anti-rabbit secondary antibody and develop with DAB. Counterstain with Harris' hematoxylin. Capture ten fields at 40× magnification. Quantify COX-2 and PCNA expression using a multipoint system (710 and 850 points, respectively). Calculate the relative frequency of positive cells.

4.1.4 Apoptosis Detection (TUNEL Assay)

Fix ventral prostate tissues in 4% paraformaldehyde for 12 h. Prepare histological sections as above. Perform TUNEL staining following the manufacturer's instructions. Counterstain with DAPI (0.5 µg/mL, 15 min). Capture 10 fields per animal using Olympus IX71-II fluorescence microscope. Analyze images using an 850-point grid to determine apoptotic index.

4.1.5 Western Blotting

Homogenize ventral prostate tissues in RIPA buffer with protease inhibitors using a Polytron homogenizer. Centrifuge at 14,000 rpm for 20 min at 4°C. Quantify protein using the Bradford method. Load 40 µg of protein per lane and perform SDS-PAGE. Transfer proteins to nitrocellulose membranes. Block with 3% BSA in TBS-T for 1 h and incubate with anti-COX-2 (1:350) overnight at 4°C. After washing, incubate with HRP-conjugated anti-rabbit secondary antibody (1:6000) for 2 h. Visualize bands using chemiluminescence and quantify with ImageJ, normalizing to beta-actin.

4.2 In Vitro Assays

4.2.1 Cell Culture and Treatment

Culture PC-3 cells in RPMI-1640 supplemented with 5% FBS, 100 U/mL penicillin, and 100 µg/mL streptomycin. Maintain at 37°C, 5% CO_2. Dissolve EERP in DMSO and dilute in medium to desired concentrations (≤0.1% DMSO final).

4.2.2 Proliferation Assay (alamarBlue®)

Seed PC-3 cells at 4.5×10^4 cells/mL in 96-well plates and incubate for 24 h. Treat with 12.5–100 µg/mL EERP or vehicle for 24 and 48 h. Add 20 µL alamarBlue® reagent and incubate for 4 h. Measure fluorescence at 570 nm excitation/585 nm emission. For apoptosis/necroptosis inhibition, pre-treat cells overnight with 25 μM Z-VAD-FMK or 2 μM GSK'872 before EERP exposure.

4.2.3 Cell Death Assay

Seed RFP+ PC-3 cells in 24-well plates and incubate for 24 h. Treat with EERP (12.5–50 μg/mL) for 24 h. Add 1 μM Sytox® Green for 20 min. Capture ten images/well using Nikon Eclipse 2000-U microscope. Quantify dead cells using ImageJ. Normalize death rates to vehicle control.

4.2.4 Cell Cycle and Phosphatidylserine (PS) Externalization

For cell cycle: Synchronize PC-3 cells via serum deprivation for 24 h. Treat with EERP (10, 25 μM) or colchicine (1 nM) for 24 h. Stain with PI and analyze DNA content by flow cytometry.

For PS exposure: Treat cells with EERP (25, 50 μM) for 24 h. Stain with annexin-V and 7-AAD. Analyze using flow cytometry to determine early apoptosis.

5 Data Analysis

Express results as mean ± SEM. Analyze data using one-way or two-way ANOVAtwo-way ANOVA followed by Tukey or Bonferroni post hoc tests. Consider $p < 0.05$ statistically significant. Perform statistical analysis using GraphPad Prism version 5.0.

References

1. Wang R, Li Y, Hu H, Persoons L, Daelemans D, De Jonghe S, Dehaen W (2021) Antibacterial and antitumoral properties of 1, 2, 3-triazolo fused triterpenes and their mechanism of inhibiting the proliferation of HL-60 cells. Eur J Med Chem 224:113727
2. Hseu YC, Lee CC, Chen YC, Kumar KS, Chen CS, Huang YC, Yang HL (2014) The anti-tumor activity of Antrodia salmonea in human promyelocytic leukemia (HL-60) cells is mediated via the induction of G1 cell-cycle arrest and apoptosis in vitro or in vivo. J Ethnopharmacol 153(2):499–510

Chapter 29

In Vivo Evaluation of Antitumor and Antimetastatic Activity Using Syngeneic and Xenograft B16F10 Melanoma Models

Abstract

This protocol describes a comprehensive in vivo evaluation of the antitumor and antimetastatic activity of peptide-based therapeutics (INKKI, Scramble, Mastoparan) using syngeneic (C57BL/6) and xenograft (NSG) B16F10 melanoma models. For primary tumor studies, C57BL/6 mice are inoculated subcutaneously with 1×105 B16F10 cells (right flank). When tumors reach ~100 mm^3 (Day 10–12), treatments are administered intraperitoneally (INKKI/Scramble 2.5 mg/kg, 5 consecutive days) or peritumorally (Mastoparan 5 mg/kg). Tumor growth is monitored by caliper measurement every other day using the volume formula $V = (L \times W^2)/2$. For experimental metastasis, C57BL/6 mice receive retro-orbital injection of 5×105 B16F10 cells; NSG mice receive 5×104 cells. Treatments begin 24 h post-inoculation (i.p., 5 consecutive days). On Day 14, lungs are harvested, inflated with Bouin's solution (1 mL via tracheal cannulation), fixed for 24–48 h, and surface metastatic nodules are counted under stereomicroscope (10–20× magnification) by blinded observers. Humane endpoints include tumor volume >1500 mm^3, ulceration, >20% body weight loss, or distress signs. Statistical analysis employs mixed-effects analysis (REML) with Tukey's post-hoc for growth curves, Kruskal-Wallis with Dunn's test for nodule counts, and Kaplan-Meier with log-rank test for survival (GraphPad Prism v.10, significance $p < 0.05$).

Keywords B16F10 melanoma, Metastasis, Syngeneic model, Xenograft, Tumor growth inhibition

1 Introduction

Melanoma is an aggressive malignancy with a high propensity for metastasis, particularly to the lungs. The B16F10 murine melanoma-cell line is a well-established preclinical tool due to its reproducible tumorigenicity and metastatic capacity in immunocompetent (C57BL/6) and immunodeficient (NSG) mice [1]. This protocol details a comprehensive evaluation of peptide-based therapeutics (INKKI, Scramble, Mastoparan) targeting primary tumor growth and pulmonary metastasis.

Karuppusamy Arunachalam et al., *Advanced Protocols in Cancer Research*, Springer Protocols Handbooks,
https://doi.org/10.1007/978-1-0716-5348-7_29,

2 Aim

To quantitatively assess the antitumor efficacy (primary tumor growth inhibition) and antimetastatic activity (reduction in lung metastatic burden) of INKKI peptide compared to scramble control and mastoparan in both syngeneic and xenograft models of B16F10 melanoma.

3 Materials

3.1 Animals

- C57BL/6 mice (female, 6–8 weeks old, ~20–25 g). *Justification:* Syngeneic host for evaluating therapy in an intact immune context.
- **NOD.Cg**-Prkdc*scid Il2rg*tm1Wjl/SzJ (NSG) mice (female, 6–8 weeks old, ~20–25 g). *Justification:* Highly immunodeficient host for evaluating therapy-independent of adaptive immunity.
- Housing: Specific Pathogen-Free (SPF) conditions, 12 h light/dark cycle, ***ad libitum*** access to autoclaved food and water. Acclimatize for at least 7 days prior to experimentation.

3.2 Cell Line

- B16F10 murine melanoma cells (ATCC® CRL-6475). Maintain in RPMI-1640 medium supplemented with 10% heat-inactivated Fetal Bovine Serum (FBS) and 1% Penicillin-Streptomycin at 37°C, 5% CO_2. Use cells between passages 5–15.

3.3 Reagents & Compounds

- INKKI peptide: Lyophilized. Prepare a 1 mg/mL stock solution in sterile PBS (pH 7.4). Aliquot and store at −80°C. Thaw on ice before use. Working dose: 2.5 mg/kg.
- Scramble control peptide: Prepare identically to INKKI. Working dose: 2.5 mg/kg.
- Mastoparan: Prepare a 2 mg/mL stock in PBS. Working dose: 5 mg/kg.
- Vehicle Control: Sterile, endotoxin-free Phosphate-Buffered Saline (PBS).
- Trypsin-EDTA (0.25%), DPBS without Ca^2+/Mg^2+, RPMI-1640 (serum-free).

3.4 Equipment

- Laminar flow hood (Class II Biosafety Cabinet).
- CO_2 incubator, centrifuge, water bath (37°C).
- Inverted phase-contrast microscope, hemocytometer.
- Digital caliper (0.01 mm resolution).
- Dissection tools (autoclaved fine scissors, forceps).

- Insulin syringes (29G, for s.c. injections), 1 mL syringes (27 G, for i.p. and retro-orbital injections).
- Stereomicroscope with 20× magnification and integrated camera.
- Analytical balance, 4% Paraformaldehyde (PFA), Bouin's solution.
- CO_2 euthanasia chamber.

3.5 Software

- ImageJ/Fiji (for metastatic nodule analysis), GraphPad Prism v.10 (for statistical analysis and graphing).

4 Detailed Experimental Procedures

4.1 Tumor Cell Preparation and Animal Implantation

- Principle: Consistent preparation of a single-cell suspension with high viability is critical for reproducible tumor take and metastatic seeding [2].
- Step-by-Step:

1. **Cell Harvest:** Culture B16F10 cells to ~80% confluence. Aspirate medium, wash once with 5 mL DPBS. Add 2 mL of pre-warmed 0.25% Trypsin-EDTA and incubate at 37°C for 3–4 min. Neutralize with 4 mL of complete medium.
2. **Washing**: Transfer cell suspension to a 15 mL conical tube. Centrifuge at 300×*g* for 5 min at 4°C. Aspirate supernatant completely.
3. **Resuspension and Viability Check:** Resuspend the pellet in 5 mL of cold, serum-free RPMI-1640. Perform a cell count using a hemocytometer and Trypan Blue exclusion. **Critical**: Cell viability must be >97%. Adjust concentration with serum-free RPMI-1640. Keep cells on ice at all times to prevent clumping and adhesion.
4. **Animal Randomization:** Weigh and ear-tag mice. Randomly assign them to experimental groups (n = 5–8, as per power calculation) using a random number generator to minimize cage and litter bias.
5. **Subcutaneous Implantation (C57BL/6, Primary Tumor Model)**:
   - Load a 29G insulin syringe with a suspension containing 1 × 105 viable B16F10 cells in 100 μL of ice-cold PBS.
   - Restrain the mouse gently. Disinfect the right dorsal flank with 70% ethanol.

- Pinch the skin to tent it, and insert the needle subcutaneously. Inject the cell suspension slowly to form a visible, transient wheal. Withdraw the needle and apply gentle pressure.

6. **Retro-orbital Implantation (Metastasis Models):**
   - Anesthetize the mouse briefly using 3% isoflurane in an induction chamber until loss of righting reflex.
   - Load a 27G needle with the appropriate cell suspension:
     - C57BL/6 (Experimental Metastasis): 5 × 105 cells in 100 μL PBS.
     - NSG (Experimental Metastasis): 5 × 104 cells in 100 μL PBS.
   - Gently proptose the eye using a sterile gloved finger. Direct the needle into the retro-orbital sinus at a 45° angle and inject smoothly. Apply gentle pressure with a sterile gauze after withdrawal. Monitor until fully recovered.

4.2 Evaluation of Antitumor Effects in the Syngeneic Model

- **Principle:** Serial caliper measurements allow for non-invasive monitoring of tumor growth kinetics [3].
- **Step-by-Step:**

1. **Initiation of Monitoring**: Begin daily monitoring of the injection site from Day 7 post-implantation. Palpate for small nodules.
2. **Tumor Measurement**: When tumors become palpable (~Day 10–12), measure with a digital caliper every other day. Measure the longest diameter (Length, L) and the perpendicular shorter diameter (Width, W) in millimeters.
3. **Tumor Volume Calculation**: Use the modified ellipsoid formula:
   - Volume (mm^3) = ($L \times W^2$) / 2
   - Record measurements for each mouse in a dedicated log.
4. **Humane Endpoints**: Euthanize any mouse immediately if:
   - Tumor volume exceeds 1500 mm^3 (primary endpoint).
   - Tumor ulcerates or interferes with mobility.
   - Body weight loss >20% from baseline.
   - Signs of significant distress (hunching, lethargy, piloerection).
5. **Terminal Analysis**: At endpoint, euthanize by CO_2 asphyxiation followed by cervical dislocation. Excise tumors, weigh them, and photograph them next to a scale. Fix

one half in 10% Neutral Buffered Formalin for histology and snap-freeze the other half in liquid nitrogen for molecular analysis.

4.3 Quantitative Evaluation of Lung Metastatic Burden

- **Principle**: Ex vivo quantification of surface lung nodules provides a direct measure of metastatic colonization [4].
- **Step-by-Step**:

1. **Euthanasia and Lung Harvest:** On Day 14 post-inoculation, euthanize mice as above. Make a midline incision, open the thoracic cavity, and carefully excise the entire lung bloc (trachea, heart, lungs) using fine scissors.
2. **Lung Inflation and Fixation**: Cannulate the trachea with a blunt 22G needle attached to a 1 mL syringe. Slowly instill 1 mL of Bouin's solution to inflate the lungs fully. Submerge the entire bloc in Bouin's solution for 24–48 h. *Bouin's fixation turns metastatic melanoma nodules black, providing high contrast against the yellow lung parenchyma.*
3. **Nodule Counting**: After fixation, carefully separate the lungs from the heart and trachea. Place lobes on a white dissection plate. Using a stereomicroscope at 10–20× magnification, count all surface metastatic nodules (both micro- and macro-metastases) by an observer blinded to the treatment groups.
4. Documentation and Analysis: Capture digital images of each lung lobe. Report data as Total Nodule Count per Lung and Nodule Incidence (% of mice with >10 nodules).

5 Detailed Treatment Protocols

5.1 Treatment of Established Cutaneous Melanoma (C57BL/6)

- Groups (n = 8): (1) Vehicle (PBS), (2) INKKI (2.5 mg/kg), (3) Scramble (2.5 mg/kg).
- Procedure: When the mean tumor volume in the vehicle group reaches ~100 mm^3 (typically Day 10–12), initiate treatment.
- Administer compounds via intraperitoneal (i.p.) injection in a volume of 100 μL per 20 g mouse for 5 consecutive days.
- Continue monitoring tumor volume as in 4.2 until endpoint.

5.2 Prophylactic Treatment of Experimental Lung Metastasis (C57BL/6)

- Groups (n = 7): (1) Vehicle (PBS), (2) INKKI (2.5 mg/kg), (3) Scramble (2.5 mg/kg).
- Procedure: Begin treatment 24 h post retro-orbital inoculation of 5 × 105 B16F10 cells.

- Administer compounds via i.p. injection (100 μL/20 g mouse) for 5 consecutive days.
- Euthanize all mice on Day 14 for lung metastasis analysis as per Sect. 4.3.

5.3 Treatment of Metastasis in an Immunodeficient Host (NSG)

- **Groups (n = 7)**: (1) Vehicle (PBS), (2) INKKI (2.5 mg/kg).
- **Procedure**: Retro-orbitally inoculate NSG mice with 5 × 104 B16F10 cells. Begin i.p. treatment 24 h later for 5 consecutive days.
- Euthanize on Day 14 for lung analysis. *This model isolates the direct anti-metastatic effect of INKKI from adaptive immune mechanisms.*

5.4 Local Therapy with Mastoparan (C57BL/6)

- **Groups (n = 6)**: (1) Vehicle (PBS), (2) Mastoparan (5 mg/kg).
- **Procedure**: Once tumors reach ~100 mm^3, administer treatment via peritumoral injection.
- **Technique**: Restrain the mouse, disinfect the skin. Insert the needle at the tumor periphery (avoiding the center) and inject 50 μL of the compound solution subcutaneously around the tumor border. Treat for 5 consecutive days. Monitor for local toxicity (redness, swelling).

6 Statistical Analysis & Data Presentation

- **Sample Size**: Justify group sizes (n = 5–8) using a priori power analysis ($\alpha = 0.05$, Power = 0.8) based on expected effect sizes from pilot data.
- **Tumor Growth Curves**: Plot mean tumor volume ± Standard **Error of the Mean (SEM)** vs. time. Compare areas under the curve (AUC) between groups using Mixed-effects analysis (REML) followed by Tukey's post-hoc test.
- **Metastatic Nodule Counts**: Data are often non-parametric. Present as box-and-whisker plots (median, IQR, min-max). Use Kruskal-Wallis test with Dunn's post-hoc for multiple groups, or Mann-Whitney U test for two groups.
- **Survival Analysis**: Use the Kaplan-Meier method. Compare curves using the Log-rank (Mantel-Cox) test.
- **Significance**: Define as $p < 0.05$. Denote levels as: *$p < 0.05$, **$p < 0.01$, ***$p < 0.001$. All analyses performed in GraphPad Prism v.10.

- **Blinding**: Ensure tumor measurements and lung nodule counts are performed by an investigator blinded to treatment group allocation.
- **Reporting**: Data should be presented as means ± SEM for growth curves, and individual data points should be shown for terminal measurements (tumor weight, nodule counts).

References

1. Francia G, Cruz-Munoz W, Man S, Xu P, Kerbel RS (2011) Mouse models of advanced spontaneous metastasis for experimental therapeutics. Nat Rev Cancer 11(2):135–141
2. Tomayko MM, Reynolds CP (1989) Determination of subcutaneous tumor size in athymic (nude) mice. Cancer Chemother Pharmacol 24(3):148–154
3. Tate MC, Aghi MK (2009) Biology of angiogenesis and invasion in glioma. Neurotherapeutics 6(3):447–457
4. Workman P et al (2010) Guidelines for the welfare and use of animals in cancer research. Br J Cancer 102(11):1555–1577

Check for updates

Chapter 30

Evaluation of Isoquercetin and Rutin in a Human Colon Adenocarcinoma Xenograft Model in Balb/c Nude Mice

Abstract

This protocol describes a comprehensive in vivo evaluation of Isoquercetin (30 mg/kg) and Rutin (17 mg/kg) in a human colon adenocarcinoma xenograft model using male Balb/c-nude mice (n = 27, 7–8 weeks old) inoculated subcutaneously with 4 × 106 HT-29 cells in 40 μL Matrigel:DMEM (1:1). The study employs two treatment regimens: prophylactic (7-day pre-treatment gavage before tumor inoculation) and therapeutic (treatment initiated at ~100 mm³ tumor volume, Day 8 post-inoculation). Compounds are administered daily by oral gavage for 7 consecutive days, with vehicle controls (5% DMSO/saline, 2% Tween-80/saline). Tumor growth is monitored by digital caliper every 1–2 days using the volume formula $V = (S^2 \times L)/2$. At endpoint (Day 14–15), tumors are excised, weighed, and processed for: (1) histopathological analysis (H&E staining, differentiation/mitotic count/necrosis scoring); (2) TP53 immunohistochemistry (DO-7 antibody, 1:500, DAB development) with quantitative analysis using NIS-Elements software (TP53 expression index = DAB-positive area/total nuclear area × 100); and (3) lipid peroxidation assessment via TBARS assay (0.67% TBA, 100°C for 60 min, absorbance at 532 nm, MDA concentration normalized to protein). Statistical analysis employs one-way ANOVA with Tukey post-hoc or Kruskal-Wallis with Dunn's test ($p < 0.05$ significance) in GraphPad Prism 9.0. Humane endpoints include tumor volume >2000 mm³, ulceration, or >20% body weight loss.

Keywords Colon cancer, HT-29 xenograft, Balb/c-nude mice, Isoquercetin, Rutin, TP53

1 Introduction

Colon cancer remains a major cause of morbidity and mortality worldwide. Emerging evidence suggests that polyphenolic compounds such as Isoquercetin and Rutin exhibit anticancer properties, including pro-apoptotic, antiproliferative, and antioxidant effects. The use of immunodeficient mice xenografted with human tumor cells offers a reliable preclinical model to assess the therapeutic and prophylactic efficacy of candidate compounds. This study aims to evaluate the impact of Isoquercetin and Rutin on tumor growth, TP53 expression, and oxidative stress in a colon adenocarcinoma xenograft model [1].

Karuppusamy Arunachalam et al., *Advanced Protocols in Cancer Research*, Springer Protocols Handbooks,
https://doi.org/10.1007/978-1-0716-5348-7_30,

2 Aim

To evaluate the prophylactic and therapeutic effects of Isoquercetin and Rutin on tumor progression, TP53protein expression, and lipid peroxidation in Balb/c nude mice xenografted with HT-29 human colon adenocarcinoma cells.

3 Materials

3.1 Animals & Housing

27 male Balb/c nude mice (7–8 weeks old, ~20 g).

Individually ventilated cages, food & water ad libitum, controlled temperature/humidity, 12:12 light-dark cycle.

3.2 Cells & Reagents

- HT-29 human colon adenocarcinoma cells (ATCC HTB-38).
- DMEM, RPMI-1640, FBS, Penicillin-Streptomycin, Sodium pyruvate, Trypsin-EDTA (Gibco).
- Isoquercetin and Rutin (Sigma-Aldrich or equivalent).
- Xylazine and Ketamine.
- Formalin, paraffin, xylene, ethanol, and hematoxylin-eosin.
- Primary antibody: anti-TP53 (Clone DO-7, Dako).
- TBARS assay reagents (TCA, TBA, SDS, etc.).

3.3 Equipment

CO_2 incubator, centrifuge, laminar flow hood, semi-analytical balance, water bath, spectrophotometer, microscope with digital camera, NIS-Elements software, calipers, and Ultra-Turrax homogenizer.

4 Detailed Experimental Protocol [2–5]

4.1 Experimental Design and Animal Group Allocation

4.1.1 Rationale for Group Design

The study employs both prophylactic and therapeutic treatment regimens to evaluate preventive and interventional efficacy. Dose selection (Isoquercetin: 30 mg/kg, Rutin: 17 mg/kg) is based on prior pharmacokinetic and maximum tolerated dose studies. Group sizes account for potential mortality and provide statistical power (n = 5–12 per group).

4.1.2 Detailed Group Assignment Protocol

Day −14 to −7: Acclimatization and Baseline Measurements

1. Receive 27 male Balb/c nude mice (7–8 weeks, ~20 g) with health certificates.
2. House in individually ventilated cages (IVCs) with autoclaved bedding (max 5 mice/cage).
3. Maintain under specific pathogen-free (SPF) conditions: temperature 22 ± 2°C, humidity 50 ± 10%, 12:12 light-dark cycle.
4. Provide autoclaved chow and acidified water (pH 2.5–3.0) *ad libitum*.
5. Allow 7-day acclimatization with daily health monitoring.
6. Randomize using stratified randomization based on body weight to ensure equal distribution:

   Group 1 (Prophylactic): n = 12 mice.

   – Subgroup 1 A: Isoquercetin (30 mg/kg) n = 6.
   – Subgroup 1B: Rutin (17 mg/kg) n = 6.

   Group 2 (Control): n = 5 mice (Vehicle only).
   Group 3 (Therapeutic): n = 10 mice.

   – Subgroup 3 A: Isoquercetin (30 mg/kg) n = 5.
   – Subgroup 3B: Rutin (17 mg/kg) n = 5.

4.2 Compound Preparation and Administration

4.2.1 Compound Formulation and Quality Control

Isoquercetin Solution Preparation:

1. Weigh 15 mg Isoquercetin (purity ≥95% by HPLC) using an analytical balance.
2. Dissolve in 1 mL of 5% DMSO in saline (0.9% NaCl) with gentle vortexing.
3. Sonicate in a water bath at 40°C for 10 min until clear.
4. Prepare fresh daily to prevent degradation.
5. Verify concentration by measuring absorbance at 360 nm ($\varepsilon = 17{,}500\ M^{-1}cm^{-1}$).

Rutin Solution Preparation:

1. Weigh 8.5 mg Rutin (purity ≥94%).
2. Dissolve in 1 mL of 2% Tween-80 in saline.
3. Heat to 50°C with stirring for 20 min.
4. Filter through 0.22 μm syringe filter.
5. Store protected from light at 4°C for up to 48 h.

Vehicle Control:

- Prepare 5% DMSO in saline and 2% Tween-80 in saline separately.
- Administer vehicle matching each compound's formulation to the respective subgroups.

4.2.2 Gavage Administration Protocol

Daily Procedure:

1. **Fasting:** Withhold food 30 min before administration (water available).
2. **Preparation:**
   - Warm compounds to 37°C in a water bath.
   - Load appropriate dose (0.5 mL) into 1 mL syringe.
   - Attach a 22-gauge, 25-mm ball-tipped gavage needle.
   - Eliminate air bubbles.
3. **Administration:**
   - Restrain mouse gently using thumb and forefinger behind head.
   - Insert needle along roof of mouth, advancing to esophagus.
   - Administer slowly over 10–15 s.
   - Observe for signs of distress or regurgitation.
4. **Post-treatment:** Maintain fasting for 1 h after gavage.
5. **Schedule:** Administer at the same time daily (±1 h) for 7 consecutive days.

4.3 Cell Culture and Xenograft Preparation

4.3.1 HT-29 Cell Culture Maintenance

Complete Medium Preparation:

- DMEM supplemented with:
  - 10% heat-inactivated FBS.
  - 1% Penicillin-Streptomycin (100 U/mL, 100 μg/mL).
  - 1 mM Sodium Pyruvate.
  - 2 mM L-Glutamine.
- Filter through 0.22 μm bottle-top filter.
- Store at 4°C for ≤2 weeks.

Subculture Protocol:

1. Remove medium from 80%–90% confluent T75 flask.
2. Wash with 5 mL pre-warmed PBS.

3. Add 2 mL 0.25% Trypsin-EDTA.
4. Incubate at 37°C for 3–5 min.
5. Neutralize with 4 mL complete medium.
6. Centrifuge at 300 × *g* for 5 min.
7. Resuspend in fresh medium at 2–5 × 105 cells/mL.
8. Split 1:3 to 1:5 every 3–4 days.

4.3.2 Cell Preparation for Inoculation

Day −1 Preparation:

1. Grow HT-29 cells to 80% confluence in three T175 flasks.
2. Trypsinize as above, pool cells.
3. Count using hemocytometer with Trypan Blue:
   Viability = (Unstained cells/Total cells) × 100
   Required: ≥95% viability
4. Wash cells twice with serum-free DMEM.
5. Resuspend in ice-cold Matrigel:DMEM (1:1) at 1 × 108 cells/mL.
6. Keep on ice until inoculation (≤30 min).

4.4 Tumor Xenografting Procedure

4.4.1 Surgical Preparation

Materials Sterilization:

- Autoclave surgical instruments (forceps, scissors).
- Sterilize the work surface with 70% ethanol.
- Use sterile drapes.

Animal Preparation:

1. Anesthetize the mouse with 2% isoflurane in oxygen.
2. Place in prone position on heating pad (37°C).
3. Shave the dorsal area (~2 × 2 cm).
4. Disinfect with alternating povidone-iodine and 70% ethanol (three times).
5. Cover with sterile drape with 1 cm opening.

4.4.2 Cell Inoculation

1. Load 40 µL cell suspension (4 × 106 cells) into insulin syringe with 29G needle.
2. Pinch the dorsal skin to create a tent.
3. Insert needle bevel-up at 30° angle.
4. Inject slowly over 10 s.

5. Withdraw the needle and apply gentle pressure.
6. Monitor until recovery from anesthesia.
7. Return to the clean cage.

Post-operative Care:

- Administer 0.05 mg/kg buprenorphine SQ for analgesia.
- Monitor twice daily for 3 days.
- Record injection site appearance.

4.5 Treatment Timeline and Monitoring

4.5.1 Prophylactic Group Timeline

Day −7 to −1: Daily gavage with compounds.
Day 0: Tumor cell inoculation.
Day 1–7: No treatment.
Day 8+: Daily tumor measurement.
Day 14: Endpoint (or earlier if ethical endpoint reached).

4.5.2 Therapeutic Group Timeline

Day 0: Tumor cell inoculation.
Day 1–7: Daily tumor measurement.
Day 8: Start treatment (tumor ~100 mm^3).
Day 8–14: Daily gavage with compounds.
Day 15: Endpoint.

4.5.3 Tumor Measurement Protocol

Daily Procedure (8:00–10:00 AM):

1. Calibrate digital calipers against a standard.
2. Anesthetize briefly with 2% isoflurane.
3. Measure the longest diameter (L) and the perpendicular short diameter (S).
4. Calculate volume:
   $$\text{Volume (mm}^3) = (S^2 \times L) / 2$$
5. Record in a standardized datasheet.
6. Plot growth curves for each animal.

Response Criteria:

- Partial Response: ≥50% volume reduction.
- Progressive Disease: ≥25% volume increase.
- Stable Disease: Neither PR nor PD criteria met.

4.6 Ethical Endpoint Monitoring and Euthanasia

4.6.1 Daily Health Assessment Checklist

- **Body Weight:** Record daily; >20% loss = endpoint.
- **Tumor Size:** >2000 mm^3 or ulceration = endpoint.
- **Behavior:** Immobility, hunched posture, isolation.
- **Physical Signs:** Piloerection, labored breathing, dehydration.
- **Tumor Condition:** Ulceration, infection, necrosis.

4.6.2 Humane Endpoint Euthanasia

1. Anesthetize with ketamine (100 mg/kg) + xylazine (10 mg/kg) IP.
2. Verify lack of pedal reflex.
3. Perform cardiac puncture for blood collection (if required).
4. Cervical dislocation as a secondary method.
5. Confirm death by the absence of respiration and heartbeat.

4.7 Tissue Collection and Processing

4.7.1 Necropsy Protocol

1. Place euthanized mouse on dissecting board.
2. Make midline incision from sternum to pelvis.
3. Reflect skin to expose tumor.
4. Carefully dissect tumor from surrounding tissue.
5. Weigh tumor immediately (wet weight).
6. Photograph with scale.

4.7.2 Tissue Allocation

Approximate 500 mg tumor:
– 250 mg → 10% formalin for histology (24 h, then 70% ethanol).
– 100 mg → Snap freeze in liquid N_2 for TBARS (store at −80°C).
– 100 mg → RNA later for molecular analysis.
– 50 mg → Fresh for primary culture (if applicable).

4.8 Histopathological Analysis

4.8.1 Tissue Processing and Sectioning

1. Fix in 10% neutral buffered formalin for 24 h.
2. Transfer to 70% ethanol.
3. Process through ethanol series (80%, 95%, 100%) and xylene.
4. Embed in paraffin using oriented embedding.
5. Cut 4 μm serial sections.
6. Float on a 42°C water bath.

7. Mount on positively charged slides.
8. Dry at 60°C for 1 h.

4.8.2 H&E Staining Protocol

1. Deparaffinize:
    - Xylene I: 5 min.
    - Xylene II: 5 min.
    - 100% ethanol I: 2 min.
    - 100% ethanol II: 2 min.
    - 95% ethanol: 1 min.
    - 70% ethanol: 1 min.
    - Distilled water: 1 min.
2. Stain in Harris hematoxylin: 8 mins.
3. Rinse in running tap water: 5 min.
4. Differentiate in 0.3% acid alcohol: 10 s.
5. Blue in Scott's tap water: 30 s.
6. Counterstain in eosin: 1 min.
7. Dehydrate and mount.

4.8.3 Histopathological Scoring

Grade according to the following criteria (10 random 400× fields):

- **Differentiation:** Well, moderate, poor.
- **Mitotic Count:** Number/10 HPF.
- **Necrosis:** Percentage of total area.
- **Invasion:** Presence at margins.

4.9 TP53 Immuno-histochemistry

4.9.1 Antigen Retrieval and Staining

1. Deparaffinize and rehydrate as above.
2. **Heat-Induced Epitope Retrieval:**
    - Place in 10 mM sodium citrate buffer, pH 6.0.
    - Microwave: 5 min high, 10 min medium, 15 min cool.
    - Cool to room temperature (20 min).
3. **Peroxidase Blocking:**
    - 3% H_2O_2 in methanol: 10 min.
    - Wash 3× with PBS.
4. **Protein Blocking:**
    - 5% normal goat serum: 30 min.

5. **Primary Antibody:**
   - Anti-TP53 (DO-7) 1:500 in blocking buffer.
   - Incubate overnight at 4°C in a humid chamber.
6. **Secondary Detection:**
   - HRP-polymer secondary: 30 min.
   - DAB development: 2–5 min (monitor).
   - Stop in distilled water.
7. **Counterstaining:**
   - Hematoxylin: 30 s.
   - Blue in tap water.
   - Dehydrate, clear, mount.

4.9.2 Quantitative Analysis

1. Scan slides at 40× resolution.
2. Using NIS-Elements AR:
   - Set color threshold for brown (DAB) staining.
   - Analyze 3 representative fields (400×).
   - Calculate:

     TP53 Expression Index = (DAB-positive area / Total nuclear area) × 100
   - Score nuclear staining intensity: 0 (none), 1+ (weak), 2+ (moderate), 3+ (strong).
   - H-score = Σ (percentage of cells × intensity score).

4.10 Lipid Peroxidation Assessment (TBARS Assay)

4.10.1 Tissue Homogenization

1. Weigh 30 mg frozen tumor tissue.
2. Add to 300 μL ice-cold RIPA buffer with:
   - 1 mM PMSF.
   - 1 mM EDTA.
   - Protease inhibitor cocktail.
3. Homogenize with Ultra-Turrax (15,000 rpm, 3 × 10 s, on ice).
4. Centrifuge at 10,000 × *g*, 4°C, 10 min.
5. Collect supernatant, determine protein concentration by BCA assay.

4.10.2 TBARS Reaction

Reagent Preparation:

- **TBA Stock:** 0.67% thiobarbituric acid in 50% acetic acid.
- **SDS Solution:** 8.1% sodium dodecyl sulfate.
- **TCA Solution:** 20% trichloroacetic acid.

Procedure:

1. In 1.5 mL tube, mix:
   - 100 μL tissue supernatant.
   - 50 μL SDS solution.
   - 750 μL TCA solution.
   - 750 μL TBA stock.
2. Heat at 100°C for 60 min in heating block.
3. Cool on ice for 10 min.
4. Centrifuge at 1000 × *g* for 10 min.
5. Transfer 200 μL supernatant to 96-well plate.
6. Read absorbance at 532 nm with reference at 600 nm.

4.10.3 Standard Curve and Calculation

1. Prepare MDA standard from 1,1,3,3-tetramethoxypropane.
2. Create standards: 0, 1, 2, 5, 10, 20 μM.
3. Process standards alongside samples.
4. Calculate:
   - MDA (nmol/mg protein) = (Sample MDA concentration) / (Protein concentration in mg/mL)

4.11 Data Analysis and Statistics

4.11.1 Primary Endpoints

1. **Tumor Growth Inhibition:**
   TGI (%) = [(V_control - V_treated) / V_control] × 100
2. Time to Reach 1000 mm³.
3. Final Tumor Weight.
4. TP53 Expression Index.
5. MDA Concentration.

4.11.2 Statistical Analysis

1. Normality Test: Shapiro-Wilk test.
2. Group Comparisons:
   - One-wayANOVA with Tukey post-hoc (parametric).
   - Kruskal-Wallis with Dunn's test (non-parametric).
3. Survival Analysis: Kaplan-Meier with log-rank test.

4. Correlation: Pearson or Spearman correlation.
5. Software: GraphPad Prism 9.0.
6. Significance: $p < 0.05$.

4.11.3 Quality Control Measures

- Blinding: Technician blinded to treatment groups during measurements.
- Replicates: Technical triplicates for all assays.
- Positive Controls: Include for IHC and TBARS assays.
- Calibration: Daily calibration of all instruments.
- Documentation: Maintain a detailed laboratory notebook with all raw data.

References

1. Bachelard H et al (2015) Optimization of flavonoid extraction for in vivo studies. J Pharmacol Methods 72:45–52
2. Geran RI et al (1972) Protocols for screening chemical agents and natural products against animal tumors and other biological systems. Cancer Chemother Rep 3(2):1–103
3. Livak KJ, Schmittgen TD (2001) Analysis of relative gene expression data using real-time quantitative PCR. Methods 25(4):402–408
4. Ohkawa H et al (1979) Assay for lipid peroxides in animal tissues by thiobarbituric acid reaction. Anal Biochem 95(2):351–358
5. Workman P et al (2010) Guidelines for the welfare and use of animals in cancer research. Br J Cancer 102(11):1555–1577

Part VI

Integrated Preclinical Platforms

Chapter 31

Comprehensive Preclinical Evaluation of Anticancer Compounds: Cytotoxicity, Apoptosis Induction, and In Vivo Efficacy

Abstract

This protocol describes a comprehensive preclinical evaluation pipeline for metal-based anticancer compounds, integrating in vitro cytotoxicity screening, mechanistic apoptosis studies in BxPC-3 pancreatic adenocarcinoma cells, and in vivo toxicity/efficacy assessment in Balb/c nude mice. Initial screening employs MTT assays (48 h exposure) across 12 human cancer cell lines and normal PBMCs to determine IC_{50} values and selectivity indices (SI = IC_{50} PBMCs/IC_{50} cancer cells). Mechanistic studies in BxPC-3 cells include: (1) cell cycle analysis by propidium iodide (PI) staining (50 µg/mL, RNase A 1 mg/mL) with sub-G_1 quantification via flow cytometry; (2) mitochondrial membrane potential ($\Delta\Psi m$) assessment using JC-1 dye (2.5 µg/mL, 15 min incubation) with red/green fluorescence ratio measurement; (3) caspase activity assays (caspase-3, -6, -8, -9) using colorimetric substrates (Ac-DEVD-pNA, VEID-pNA, IETD-pNA, LEHD-pNA) at 405 nm; and (4) ROS detection by DCFH-DA (10 µM, 30 min) with/without NAC (5 mM) pre-treatment. In vivo, acute toxicity (LD_{50}) is determined by a single i.p. injection (10–100 mg/kg, n = 6/group, 15-day monitoring). Antitumor efficacy uses BxPC-3 xenografts (1×10^6 cells intradermally) in Balb/c nude mice (n = 6/group, 3 M/3 F) treated weekly i.p. with vehicle, compound (8 and 33 mg/kg), or cisplatin (3.3 mg/kg). Tumor volume is monitored by caliper ($V = L \times W^2/2$) until humane endpoint (>1500 mm^3). Statistical analysis employs one-way/two-way ANOVA with Bonferroni post-hoc or Kaplan-Meier with log-rank test (GraphPad Prism, $p < 0.05$ significance).

Keywords Metal-based compounds, BxPC-3 xenograft, Apoptosis, Mitochondrial membrane potential, In vivo toxicity

1 Introduction

Transition metal complexes, particularly those of copper, represent a promising class of anticancer agents with mechanisms distinct from traditional platinum-based drugs like cisplatin. Their potential to overcome resistance and exhibit selective toxicity is of significant interest. This protocol details a multidisciplinary strategy to characterize candidate metal complexes, beginning with broad-spectrum cytotoxicity screening to identify sensitive cell lines and calculate a selectivity index (SI). Subsequent mechanistic studies are concentrated on a sensitive model (BxPC-3 pancreatic cells) to investigate

Karuppusamy Arunachalam et al., *Advanced Protocols in Cancer Research*, Springer Protocols Handbooks, https://doi.org/10.1007/978-1-0716-5348-7_31,

apoptotic hallmarks, including cell cycle arrest, loss of mitochondrial membrane potential ($\Delta\Psi m$), caspase activation, and ROS dysregulation [1]. Finally, the protocol outlines steps to translate in vitro findings into an in vivo context, determining acute toxicity (LD_{50}) and evaluating antitumor activity in a xenograft model, thereby providing a holistic preclinical assessment [2, 3]. This protocol aims to establish a sequential pipeline for the in vitro and in vivo evaluation of metal based The objectives are to: (1) determine their cytotoxic profile and selectivity across a panel of human cancer cell lines versus healthy peripheral blood mononuclear cells (PBMCs); (2) elucidate their primary mechanism of action, focusing on the induction of apoptosis via reactive oxygen species (ROS) generation, mitochondrial dysfunction, and caspase activation in the sensitive BxPC-3 pancreatic adenocarcinoma cell line; and (3) assess the acute toxicity and antitumor efficacy of the lead complex in vivo using a BxPC-3 xenograft model in Balb/c nude mice.

2 Aim

This protocol aims to establish a sequential pipeline for the in vitro and in vivo evaluation of metal-based compounds.

3 Materials

- **Cell Lines:** A panel of 12 human cancer lines: MCF-7, MDA-MB231 (breast); NCI-H460, A549 (lung); THP-1 (leukemia), U937 (lymphoma), Molt-4 (leukemia); Colo 205 (colon); SkMel-5 (melanoma); PC3 (prostate); BxPC-3 (pancreas); and murine B16F10 (melanoma).
- **Primary Control Cells:** Peripheral blood mononuclear cells (PBMCs) isolated from healthy donors.
- **Culture Media:** DMEM-F12 for adherent cancer lines; RPMI 1640 for suspension lines and PBMCs. Both were supplemented with 10% Fetal Bovine Serum (FBS) and 20 μg/mL gentamicin.
- **Test Compounds:** 1, 2, 3; their respective organic ligands; copper salt (e.g., $CuCl_2$).
- **Controls:** Cisplatin (positive cytotoxic control); N-acetylcysteine **(NAC)** (antioxidant control).
- **Key Assay Reagents:**
  - MTT (3-(4,5-dimethylthiazol-2-yl)-2,5-diphenyltetrazolium bromide).
  - Propidium Iodide (PI), RNase A.

- JC-1JC-1 (5,5′,6,6′-tetrachloro-1,1′,3,3′-tetraethylbenzimidazolylcarbocyanine iodide) dye.
- Caspase substrates: Ac-DEVD-pNA (caspase-3), VEID-pNA (caspase-6), IETD-pNA (caspase-8), LEHD-pNA (caspase-9).
- DCFH-DA (2′,7′-dichlorodihydrofluorescein diacetate) fluorescent probe.
- Ficoll-Paque for PBMC isolation.

- **Animals**: Male and female Balb/c nude mice (6–8 weeks old).
- **Software**: GraphPad Prism (v5.01 or later) for statistical analysis and IC_{50}/LD_{50} calculation; FlowJo or WinMDI for flow cytometry data analysis.

4 Methods

4.1 *In Vitro* Cytotoxicity and Selectivity Profiling

4.1.1 Cell Viability Assay (MTT)

1. **Cell Seeding:** Seed adherent cancer cells in 96-well plates at 2×10^4 cells/well in 100 μL complete medium. For PBMCs, seed at 1×10^5 cells/well. Incubate for 4–6 h (37°C, 5% CO_2) to allow adherence/recovery.
2. **Compound Treatment:** Prepare serial dilutions of test compounds (Compound 1 & 2: 0–50 μM; Compound 3, ligands, copper salt: 0–200 μM) and cisplatin (0–50 μM) in fresh medium. Aspirate seeding medium and add 100 μL of compound solution to respective wells. Include vehicle control wells (medium with equivalent DMSO/solvent). Incubate for 48 h.
3. **MTT Development:** Add 20 μL of MTT solution (5 mg/mL in PBS) to each well. Incubate for 4 h at 37°C.
4. **Formazan Solubilization:** Carefully aspirate the medium. Add 100 μL of acidified isopropanol (0.04% HCl in isopropanol) to each well to dissolve the formazan crystals. Shake gently for 10 min.
5. **Absorbance Measurement:** Read the absorbance at 570 nm using a microplate reader.
6. **Data Analysis:** Calculate cell viability as a percentage of the vehicle control. Use non-linear regression (log(inhibitor) vs. response) in GraphPad Prism to determine the $\mathbf{IC_{50}}$ value for

each compound-cell line pair. Calculate the **Selectivity Index (SI)**) = IC_{50} (PBMCs) / IC_{50} (Cancer Cell Line) [1].

4.1.2 Apoptosis Assessment by Cell Cycle Analysis (PI Staining)

1. **Treatment:** Seed BxPC-3 cells (5×10^5 cells/well) in 6-well plates. After 6 h, treat with Complex 1 (3.5 & 7.0 μM), Complex 2 (4.5 & 9.0 μM), or cisplatin (22 μM) for 48 h.
2. **Cell Harvest and Fixation:** Harvest cells by trypsinization, pool with floating cells, and centrifuge (800 × *g*, 5 min). Wash pellet with PBS. Fix cells by resuspending in 1 mL of ice-cold 70% ethanol and incubating at −20°C for ≥1 h.
3. **Staining:** Centrifuge fixed cells, wash with PBS, and resuspend in 500 μL of staining solution (50 μg/mL PI, 1 mg/mL RNase A, 0.2% Triton X-100 in PBS). Incubate in the dark at 37°C for 30 min.
4. **Flow Cytometry:** Analyze 10,000 events per sample on a flow cytometer using the FL2 channel. Gate out aggregates using pulse processing (FSC-A vs. FSC-H).
5. **Data Analysis:** Use software (e.g., WinMDI, FlowJo) to model cell cycle phases (G0/G1, S, G2/M). Quantify the percentage of cells with sub-G1 DNA content (apoptotic population) [2].

4.2 Mechanistic Studies on Apoptosis in BxPC-3 Cells

4.2.1 Evaluation of Mitochondrial Membrane Potential ($\Delta\Psi m$)

1. **Treatment and Staining:** Treat BxPC-3 cells as in) as in Sect. 4.3. Harvest cells and resuspend in 1 mL complete medium containing 2.5 μg/mL JC-1 dye. Incubate at 37°C, 5% CO_2 for 15 min in the dark.
2. **Washing and Analysis:** Wash cells twice with warm PBS. Resuspend in 500 μL PBS and analyze immediately by flow cytometry.
3. **Data Interpretation:** JC-1 aggregates in healthy mitochondria (high ΔΨm) emit red fluorescence (585/42 nm, FL2). JC-1 monomers in depolarized mitochondria emit green fluorescence (530/30 nm, FL1). Calculate the red/green fluorescence ratio. A decrease indicates loss of ΔΨm, a hallmark of early apoptosis [3].

4.2.2 Caspase Activity Assay (Colorimetric)

1. **Cell Lysis:** BxPC-3 cells with Complex 1 (7.0 μM) or cisplatin (22 μM) for 12 and 24 h. Harvest 3–5×10^6 cells, wash with PBS, and lyse in 100 μL ice-cold lysis buffer for 30 min on ice. Centrifuge (10,000 × *g*, 1 min, 4°C).

2. **Protein Quantification:** Determine protein concentration in the supernatant (e.g., Bradford assay).
3. **Reaction Setup:** In a 96-well plate, add 50 μL of cell lysate (adjust to 1–4 mg/mL protein) to 50 μL of reaction buffer. Add 5 μL of the respective 4 mM caspase substrate (Ac-DEVD-pNA for caspase-3, etc.) to initiate the reaction. Include a blank (lysis buffer + substrate).
4. **Incubation and Measurement:** Incubate plate at 37°C for 1 h. Measure the absorbance at 405 nm in a microplate reader.
5. **Data Analysis:** Subtract blank absorbance. Express caspase activity as the fold-increase in absorbance relative to the untreated control lysate [4].

4.2.3 Evaluation of Reactive Oxygen Species (ROS) Generation

1. **Constitutive ROS & NAC Inhibition:** Seed BxPC-3 cells. Treat) with NAC (1.25, 2.5, 5.0 mM) or vehicle for 3 or 48 h.
2. **ROS Detection in Treated Cells:** Seed BxPC-3 cells. Pre-treat one set with NAC (5.0 mM) for 2 h. Then, treat all cells with Complex 1 (3.5, 7.0 μM), cisplatin (22 μM), or vehicle for 48 h.
3. **Staining and Analysis (Common for both):** Harvest cells, wash with PBS, and incubate with 10 μM **DCFH-DA** in PBS at 37°C for 30 min in the dark. Wash cells, resuspend in 500 μ L PBS, and analyze fluorescence intensity in the FL1 channel of a flow cytometer (10,000 events). Increased mean fluorescence intensity (MFI) indicates higher intracellular ROS ROS) levels [5].

4.3 In Vivo Toxicity and Efficacy Studies

4.3.1 In Vivo Experimentation

Ethics Note: All procedures must be approved by an Institutional Animal Care and Use Committee.

4.3.2 Determination of Acute Toxicity (LD_5 ₀)

1. **Dosing Groups:** Randomly group healthy Balb/c nude mice (n=6 per dose, 3M/3F). Prepare doses of Complex 1 (10, 25, 50, 75, 100 mg/kg) in vehicle (ultrapure water + DMSO).
2. **Administration and Monitoring:** Administer a single intraperitoneal (i.p.) injection to each group. Monitor animals daily for 15 days for signs of toxicity (lethargy, weight loss >20%, moribund state) and record survival.
3. **Calculation:** At the end of the observation period, use the survival data and a non-linear regression model (log(inhibitor) vs. response) in GraphPad Prism) to calculate the median lethal dose (LD_{50}) [6].

4.3.3 Evaluation of Antitumor Activity in a Xenograft Model

1. **Tumor Induction:** Anesthetize mice (i.p. xylazine 10 mg/kg + ketamine 85 mg/kg). Inoculate 1×10^6 BxPC-3 cells in 50 μ L PBS intradermally into the dorsal flank.
2. **Randomization and Treatment:** Once palpable tumors form (~50-100 mm³), randomize mice into four groups (n=6, 3 M/3 F):
   - Group 1: Vehicle control (i.p., weekly).
   - Group 2: Compound 1, low dose (e.g., 8 mg/kg, i.p., weekly).
   - Group 3: Compound 1, high dose (e.g., 33 mg/kg, i.p., weekly).
   - Group 4: Cisplatin (3.3 mg/kg, i.p., weekly).
3. **Tumor Monitoring:** Measure tumor length (L) and width (W) with calipers two to three times weekly. Calculate tumor volume: **V (mm³) = (L × W²) / 2.**
4. **Endpoint:** Euthanize mice by CO_2 inhalation at a predefined humane endpoint (e.g., tumor volume >1500 mm³ or significant body condition loss). Plot mean tumor volume over time for each group [7].

4.3.4 Statistical Analysis

- Express all data as mean ± standard deviation (SD).
- For multiple group comparisons (e.g., dose-response, different treatments), use one-way or two-way ANOVAtwo-way ANOVA followed by Bonferroni's post-hoc test.
- For survival analysis (LD_{50} study), use the Kaplan-Meier method and log-rank test.
- Perform all analyses in GraphPad Prism. Denote significance as: $*p<0.05$, $**p<0.01$, $***p<0.001$.

References

1. Mosmann T (1983) Rapid colorimetric assay for cellular growth and survival: Application to proliferation and cytotoxicity assays. J Immunol Methods 65(1-2):55–63
2. Nicoletti I et al (1991) A rapid and simple method for measuring thymocyte apoptosis by propidium iodide staining and flow cytometry. J Immunol Methods 139(2):271–279
3. Cossarizza A et al (1993) Mitochondrial modifications during rat thymocyte apoptosis: a study at the single cell level. Exp Cell Res 214(1):323–330
4. Thornberry NA, Lazebnik Y (1998) Caspases: enemies within. Science 281(5381):1312–1316
5. Wang H, Joseph JA (1999) Quantifying cellular oxidative stress by dichlorofluorescein assay using microplate reader. Free Radic Biol Med 27(5-6):612–616
6. Tsirmoula S, Dimas K, Hatziapostolou M, Lamprou M, Ravazoula P, Papadimitriou E (2012) Implications of pleiotrophin in human PC 3 prostate cancer cell growth in vivo. Cancer Sci 103(10):1826–1832
7. Perše M (2021) Cisplatin mouse models: treatment, toxicity and translatability. Biomedicines. 9(10):1406

Chapter 32

Comprehensive Protocol for In Vitro and In Vivo Antitumor Evaluation of Phytocompounds in the Ehrlich Ascites Tumor Model

Abstract

This protocol describes a comprehensive in vitro and in vivo evaluation of phytocompounds' antitumor activity using the Ehrlich Ascites Tumor (EAT) model in female Swiss albino mice (6–8 weeks, 25–30 g). In vitro cytotoxicity is assessed by MTT assay (48 h exposure, 545 nm absorbance) against EAC cells and normal L929 fibroblasts to determine IC_{50} values and selectivity indices ($SI = IC_{50}$ L929 / IC_{50} EAC; $SI \geq 3$ considered selective). For in vivo studies, mice are inoculated intraperitoneally with 6×10^6 viable EAC cells (Day 0) and treated daily for 7 consecutive days (Days 1–7) with test compounds (2 and 6 mg/kg, i.p.), cisplatin (3 mg/kg, i.p. positive control), or saline (negative control). Antitumor efficacy is evaluated by body weight and abdominal circumference measurements (Days 1 and 8) with percentage inhibition calculated, and survival analysis by the Kaplan–Meier method. Genotoxicity is assessed via alkaline comet assay on peripheral blood (24 h and 48 h post-treatment) with 100 nucleoids/sample scored for damage index (0–400). Apoptosis/necrosis in ascitic cells is quantified by Annexin V-FITC/PI flow cytometry (10,000 events/sample). Systemic toxicity is evaluated through hematological parameters (TLC, RBC, Hb, HCT, PLT), serum biochemistry (ALT, AST, ALP, BUN, creatinine, LDH), and organ indices (liver, kidney, spleen, heart, lungs) calculated as (organ weight/final body weight) × 100. Statistical analysis employs one-way/two-way ANOVA with appropriate post-hoc tests ($p < 0.05$ significance) in GraphPad Prism.

Keywords Ehrlich ascites tumor, MTT assay, Comet assay, Annexin V/PI

1 Introduction

Phytocompounds have shown potential as anticancer agents due to their redox properties, DNA-binding capacity, and selective cytotoxicity. The Ehrlich Ascites Tumor (EAT) model, both in vitro and in vivo, provides a valuable system to assess the efficacy, mechanism of action, and toxicity profile of investigational compounds. This protocol outlines the detailed steps for evaluating the antiproliferative activity of phytocompounds, including in vitro cytotoxicity (MTT assay), in vivo tumor progression, genotoxicity (comet assay), apoptosis and necrosis (Annexin V-FITC/PI flow cytometry), and hematological/biochemical toxicity.

Karuppusamy Arunachalam et al., *Advanced Protocols in Cancer Research*, Springer Protocols Handbooks,
https://doi.org/10.1007/978-1-0716-5348-7_32,

2 Aim

To comprehensively evaluate the antiproliferative, genotoxic, apoptotic, and systemic toxic effects of RuMet and RuTrp ruthenium(II)/amino acid complexes using in vitro cell-based assays and the in vivo EATmodel in Swiss mice.

3 Materials and Reagents

- **Cell Lines:** Ehrlich Ascites Carcinoma (EAC) cells (maintained *in vivo*), L929 murine fibroblast cells (ATCC® CCL-1™).
- **Animals:** Female Swiss albino mice, 6–8 weeks old, 25–30 g. (Note: Weight range adjusted to standard).
- **Media & Supplements:**
  - RPMI-1640 Medium (for EAC culture *ex vivo*).
  - DMEM Medium (for L929 cells).
  - Fetal Bovine Serum (FBS), heat-inactivated, 10% (v/v).
  - Penicillin-Streptomycin solution (100 U/mL penicillin, 100 μg/mL streptomycin).
  - Phosphate-Buffered Saline (PBS), pH 7.4, sterile.
- **Test & Control Compounds:**
  - Compounds (stock solutions prepared in DMSO for in vitro and saline for in vivo).
  - Positive Control: Cisplatin (stock in saline).
  - Vehicle Controls: 0.9% sterile saline (for in vivo), DMSO (final conc. ≤0.5% for in vitro).
- **Assay-Specific Reagents:**
  - **MTT Assay**: Thiazolyl Blue Tetrazolium Bromide (MTT, 5 mg/mL in PBS, filter-sterilized), Sodium Dodecyl Sulfate (SDS, 10% w/v in 0.01 N HCl).
  - **Viability**: 0.4% Trypan Blue solution.
  - **Comet Assay**: Normal Melting Point Agarose (NMPA, 1.5%), Low Melting Point Agarose (LMPA, 0.5%), Lysis Buffer (2.5 M NaCl, 100 mM EDTA, 10 mM Tris, 1% Triton X-100, pH 10; add 10% DMSO fresh), Alkaline Electrophoresis Buffer (300 mM NaOH, 1 mM EDTA, pH >13), Neutralization Buffer (0.4 M Tris-HCl, pH 7.5), Ethidium Bromide (20 μg/mL) or alternative DNA stain (e.g., SYBR® Gold).

- **Apoptosis/Necrosis**: Annexin V-FITC Apoptosis Detection Kit (e.g., BD Pharmingen™ Cat. No. 556547) containing Annexin V-FITC, Propidium Iodide (PI), and 10X Binding Buffer.
- **Anesthesia**: Ketamine (80–100 mg/kg) and Xylazine (5–10 mg/kg) mixture in saline.

- **Equipment:**
  - **Cell Culture**: Class II Biosafety Cabinet, CO_2 incubator, inverted microscopeinverted microscope, centrifuge.
  - **Assays**: Microplate reader (545 nm filter), flow cytometer (e.g., BD FACSCalibur™ with CellQuest Pro software), electrophoresis tank and power supply.
  - **Imaging**: Fluorescence microscope with appropriate filters for Ethidium Bromide (Ex/Em ~518/605 nm).
  - **Animal**: Precision balance, vernier caliper, microhematocrit tubes, sterile surgical tools.
  - **Clinical Pathology**: Automated hematology analyzer (e.g., Beckman Coulter Ac•T diff™), automated biochemistry analyzer (e.g., Vitalab Flexor®).

4 Detailed Experimental Protocols

4.1 Animal Housing, Acclimatization, and Ethics

1. House mice in groups of 3–5 in individually ventilated cages (IVCs) under a controlled 12-h light/dark cycle, temperature (22 ± 2°C), and humidity (55 ± 10%).
2. Provide standard rodent chow and autoclaved water *ad libitum*.
3. Acclimatize animals to the facility for a minimum of 7 **days** prior to any procedure.
4. All procedures must be reviewed and approved by an Institutional Animal Care and Use Committee or equivalent ethics board, following ARRIVE guidelines [1].

4.2 Maintenance and Harvest of Ehrlich Ascites Carcinoma (EAC) Cells

1. Maintain EAC cells in vivo by serial intraperitoneal (i.p.) passage in healthy Swiss mice every 7–10 days.
2. For harvest, euthanize a tumor-bearing mouse (7 days post-inoculation) via cervical dislocation under deep anesthesia (ketamine/xylazine).
3. Aseptically inject 5–10 mL of sterile, ice-cold PBS into the peritoneal cavity. Gently massage the abdomen.
4. Carefully aspirate the peritoneal fluid containing ascites cells using an 18G needle. Transfer to a 15 mL conical tube on ice.

5. Centrifuge at 300 × *g* for 10 min at 4°C. Wash cell pellet twice with cold PBS.
6. Resuspend cells in RPMI-1640 or PBS. Determine cell concentration and viability using the Trypan Blue Exclusion Method:
   - Mix 10 μL of cell suspension with 10 μL of 0.4% Trypan Blue.
   - Load onto a hemocytometer. Count unstained (viable) and blue-stained (non-viable) cells in the four corner quadrants.
   - Viability (%) = [Total Viable Cells / (Total Viable + Non-viable Cells)] × 100.
   - Proceed only if viability is ≥90%. Adjust cell density as required for subsequent assays.

4.3 In Vitro Cytotoxicity Assessment (MTT Assay)

4.3.1 Cell Seeding and Treatment

1. Culture L929 fibroblasts in DMEM + 10% FBS, and maintain EAC cells ex vivo in RPMI-1640 + 10% FBS. Incubate at 37°C, 5% CO_2.
2. Harvest cells in the logarithmic growth phase. Prepare a single-cell suspension and count.
3. Seed cells in 96-well flat-bottom tissue culture plates:
   - EAC cells: 1×10^5 cells/well in 100 μL medium.
   - L929 cells: 2×10^4 cells/well in 100 μL medium.
4. Incubate plates for 24 h to allow cell adherence (L929) and adaptation.
5. Prepare serial dilutions of compounds and cisplatin in complete medium from DMSO stocks. Ensure final DMSO concentration is ≤0.5%.
6. Aspirate old medium from wells and add 100 μL of fresh medium containing the test compounds (e.g., 0.2, 2, 20, 100, 200 μM). Include vehicle control (medium with 0.5% DMSO) and blank control (medium only). Use n = 6 replicates per concentration.
7. Incubate plates for 48 h.

4.3.2 MTT Incubation and Quantification

1. After 48 h, carefully add 10 μL of MTT solution (5 mg/mL) directly to each well. Swirl the plate gently.
2. Incubate for 3–4 h at 37°C in the dark. Purple formazan crystals will form in metabolically active cells.

3. Carefully aspirate the medium without disturbing the formazan crystals.
4. Add 100 μL of SDS solubilization solution (10% SDS in 0.01 N HCl) to each well to dissolve the crystals.
5. Cover plate and incubate overnight at 37°C in a humidified chamber to ensure complete dissolution.
6. Read absorbance at 545 nm (reference 690 nm) using a microplate reader.

4.3.3 Data Analysis

1. Calculate the mean absorbance for each treatment group. Subtract the mean absorbance of the blank control (wells with medium and MTT/SDS but no cells).
2. Cell Viability (%) = [(Mean $Abs_{treatment}$ − Mean Abs_{empty}) / (Mean $Abs_{vehiCle}$ − Mean Abs_{empty})] × 100.
3. Plot % Viability vs. Log_{10}(Concentration). Determine the IC_{50} (concentration causing 50% growth inhibition) using non-linear regression analysis (log(inhibitor) vs. response—Variable slope (four parameters)) in GraphPad Prism® v9.0+.
4. Calculate Selectivity Index (SI): SI = IC_{50} (L929) / IC_{50} (EAC). Compounds with SI ≥3.0 are typically considered selectively cytotoxic toward the cancer cells [2].

4.4 In Vivo Experimental Design and Treatment

4.4.1 Tumor Induction

1. Randomly divide acclimatized Swiss mice into six groups (n=8/group): Group I: Normal (no tumor, saline only); Group II: EAC Control (tumor + saline); Group III: EAC + Cisplatin (3 mg/kg, positive control); Groups IV & V: EAC + compound (2 & 6 mg/kg); Groups VI & VII: EAC + compound (2 & 6 mg/kg).
2. For tumor-bearing groups (II-VII), inject 6×10^6 viable EAC cells in 0.2 mL sterile PBS intraperitoneally (i.p.) on Day 0.

4.4.2 Treatment Administration

1. Commence treatment 24 h post-tumor inoculation (Day 1).
2. Prepare fresh solutions of compounds and cisplatin in sterile 0.9% saline daily.
3. Administer treatments via i.p. injection in a volume of 10 mL/kg body weight (e.g., 0.2 mL for a 20 g mouse) for 7 consecutive days (Day 1 to Day 7).
4. Monitor animals daily for signs of toxicity (lethargy, piloerection, weight loss >20%, abnormal posture), tumor ascites development (abdominal distension), and mortality.

4.5 Evaluation of Antitumor Efficacy

4.5.1 Body Weight and Abdominal Circumference

1. Measure individual mouse body weight and abdominal circumference (at the largest point around the abdomen) using a digital balance and a flexible measuring tape, respectively. Record daily.
2. Calculate Percentage Inhibition for each treated group:

   - For Body Weight Gain: % Inhibition = [1 - (Mean ΔBW_{treate}d / Mean ΔBW_{tumor} c_{ontrol})] × 100.
   - For Ascites Development (Circumference): % Inhibition = [1 - (Mean ΔAC_{treate}d / Mean ΔAC_{tumor} c_{ontrol})] × 100.
   - Where Δ = (Measurement on Day 8 - Measurement on Day 1).

4.5.2 Survival Analysis (Optional Extension)

1. For a subset of animals (n=6/group), continue observation post-treatment without euthanasia on Day 8.
2. Record date of death or humane endpoint (severe ascites, moribund state).
3. Plot Kaplan-Meier survival curves and compare using the Log-rank (Mantel-Cox) testLog-rank (Mantel-Cox) test.

4.6 Assessment of Genotoxicity (Alkaline Comet Assay)

4.6.1 Blood Collection and Slide Preparation

1. At 24 h and 48 h after the first treatment dose, collect ~20 μL of peripheral blood from the retro-orbital plexus of anesthetized mice (one group per time point) into heparinized microtubes.
2. **Pre-coat slides:** Dip clean frosted microscope slides in melted 1.5% NMPA, wipe back, and dry completely. Label.
3. Mix 10 μL of whole blood with 90 μL of 0.5% LMPA (at 37°C). Quickly pipette 80 μL of this mixture onto a pre-coated slide. Immediately place a coverslip on top. Place the slide on a cold metal plate (4°C) for 10 min to solidify the agarose.
4. Gently remove coverslip.

4.6.2 Lysis and Electrophoresis

1. Immerse slides in freshly prepared, chilled Lysis Buffer in a Coplin jar. Protect from light. Incubate at 4°C for a minimum of 1 h (or overnight).
2. Carefully remove slides and place them side-by-side in a horizontal electrophoresis tank filled with fresh, cold Alkaline Electrophoresis Buffer (pH >13) to a level ~0.25 cm above the slides.

3. Allow DNA to unwind for 20 min in the dark at 4°C.
4. Turn on power supply: 25 V (~0.74 V/cm) for 30 min. Adjust time/voltage to achieve a comet tail length of ~1–2× the head diameter in the positive control.
5. Gently remove slides and neutralize by washing 3 × 5 min with Neutralization Buffer. Air-dry slides.

4.6.3 Staining and Analysis

1. Stain slides with 50 µL of Ethidium Bromide (20 µg/mL) or SYBR® Gold for 10–15 min in the dark.
2. Rinse gently with distilled water, and apply a coverslip.
3. Visualize using a fluorescence microscope (20× objective) with a green excitation filter. Capture images of 100 randomly selected nucleoids per sample (50 from each of two replicate slides).
4. Analyze comet images using software (e.g., OpenComet). Report results as % Tail DNA or Tail Moment. Alternatively, use a manual Damage Index (DI) scoring system (0=no damage to 4=severe damage): DI = Σ(Class Frequency × Class Number) / 100. Max score = 400 [3].

4.7 Analysis of Apoptosis and Necrosis by Flow Cytometry

1. On Day 8, euthanize mice and harvest ascitic fluid as in Sect. 4.2.
2. Wash EAC cells twice with cold PBS. Count and adjust concentration to 1×10^6 cells/mL in cold PBS.
3. Transfer 100 µL of cell suspension (1×10^5 cells) to a flow cytometry tube.
4. Add 5 µL of Annexin V-FITC and 5 µL of Propidium Iodide (PI) from the detection kit.
5. Gently vortex and incubate for 15 minat room temperature (25°C) in the dark.
6. Add 400 µL of 1× Annexin Binding Buffer to each tube within 1 h of analysis.
7. Acquire data on a flow cytometer (e.g., BD FACSCalibur™). Collect at least 10,000 events per sample.
8. Set up quadrants on an Annexin V-FITC (FL1) vs. PI (FL2 or FL3) dot plot:
   - Lower Left (LL): Annexin V^- / PI^- (Viable cells).
   - Lower Right (LR): Annexin V^+ / PI^- (Early Apoptotic cells).
   - Upper Right (UR): Annexin V^+ / PI^+ (Late Apoptotic/ Necrotic cells).
   - Upper Left (UL): Annexin V^- / PI^+ (Primary Necrotic cells).

9. Report the percentage of cells in each quadrant for statistical comparison [4].

4.8 Assessment of Systemic Toxicity [5,6]

4.8.1 Hematological Analysis

1. On Day 8, collect blood via cardiac puncture under deep anesthesia into two tubes: an EDTA-coated tube (for hematology) and a plain tube (for serum).
2. Analyze EDTA-blood within 3 h using an automated hematology analyzer. Key parameters: Total Leukocyte Count (TLC), Red Blood Cell Count (RBC), Hemoglobin (Hb), Hematocrit (HCT), Platelet Count (PLT), and Differential Leukocyte Count.

4.8.2 Serum Biochemical Analysis

1. Allow blood in the plain tube to clot for 30 min at room temperature.
2. Centrifuge at 2000 × *g* for 15 min at 4°C.
3. Carefully aspirate the supernatant (serum) and store in aliquots at −80°C until analysis.
4. Use an automated analyzer to assess:
   - Liver Function: Alanine Aminotransferase (ALT), Aspartate Aminotransferase (AST), Alkaline Phosphatase (ALP), Total Bilirubin.
   - Renal Function: Blood Urea Nitrogen (BUN), Creatinine.
   - General Metabolism/Tissue Damage: Lactate Dehydrogenase (LDH), Total Protein.

4.8.3 Organ Index and Gross Pathology

1. After blood collection, euthanize the mice and perform a gross necropsy.
2. Excise vital organs: liver, kidneys, spleen, heart, and lungs. Rinse in ice-cold saline, blot dry on filter paper.
3. Weigh each organ to the nearest 0.1 mg using an analytical balance.
4. Calculate the Relative Organ Weight (Organ Index):
   - Organ Index (%) = [Organ Weight (g) / Final Body Weight (g)] × 100.
5. Compare indices of treated groups to both tumor control and normal groups to differentiate tumor-related changes from compound-induced toxicity [5,6].

References

1. Percie du Sert N et al (2020) The ARRIVE guidelines 2.0: updated guidelines for reporting animal research. PLoS Biol 18(7):e3000410
2. Duan YC et al (2016) Design, synthesis and anticancer activity of novel quinazoline derivatives. Eur J Med Chem 112:130–138.
3. Singh NP, McCoy MT, Tice RR, Schneider EL (1988) A simple technique for quantitation of low levels of DNA damage in individual cells. Exp Cell Res 175(1):184–191
4. Vermes I, Haanen C, Steffens-Nakken H, Reutelingsperger C (1995) A novel assay for apoptosis. flow cytometric detection of phosphatidylserine expression on early apoptotic cells using fluorescein labelled Annexin V. J Immunol Methods 184(1):39–51
5. Gerlier D, Thomasset N (1986) Use of MTT colorimetric assay to measure cell activation. J Immunol Methods 94(1-2):57–63
6. Freshney RI (2010) Culture of animal cells: a manual of basic technique and specialized applications, 6th edn. Wiley-Blackwell

Part VII

Immuno-Oncology and Inflammation Assays

Check for updates

Chapter 33

In Vivo Assay for Leukocyte Migration, Exudation, and Myeloperoxidase (MPO) Activity Using the Murine Air Pouch Model

Abstract

This protocol describes the murine air pouch model for evaluating the anti-inflammatory effects of test compounds (Me-NFM and NFM, 100–400 μM) on leukocyte migration, exudate formation, and myeloperoxidase (MPO) activity following carrageenan-induced inflammation. Air pouches are generated in male mice (25–30 g) by subcutaneous injection of sterile air (5 mL on Day 0, 2.5 mL on Days 2 and 4). On Day 6, inflammation is induced by injecting 1 mL of 1% carrageenan into the pouch. Test compounds or vehicle are administered intraperitoneally 30 min prior to carrageenan. After 24 h (Day 7), mice are euthanized, pouches are lavaged with 2 mL PBS containing heparin (20 IU/mL), and exudate is collected. Total leukocyte counts are performed using a Neubauer chamber with trypan blue exclusion; differential counts (neutrophils, lymphocytes, monocytes) are determined on May-Grünwald-Giemsa-stained cytospin preparations (200 cells/slide, 1000× oil immersion). MPO activity in lavage fluid supernatant is quantified by colorimetric assay (450 nm) using hydrogen peroxide substrate, with results expressed as mU/mL (1 Unit = oxidation of 1 μmol H_2O_2/min). Data are presented as mean ± SEM, with statistical significance determined by one-way ANOVA followed by Dunnett's post-hoc test ($p < 0.05$).

Keywords Air pouch model, Leukocyte migration, Myeloperoxidase, Carrageenan, Inflammation

1 Introduction

The murine air pouch model is a widely accepted method to study inflammation in vivo, enabling quantification of leukocyte infiltration and pro-inflammatory enzyme activities such as myeloperoxidase (MPO). This model mimics synovial-like cavities and provides a reproducible environment to assess the anti-inflammatory potential of test compounds [1].

Karuppusamy Arunachalam et al., *Advanced Protocols in Cancer Research*, Springer Protocols Handbooks,
https://doi.org/10.1007/978-1-0716-5348-7_33,

2 Aim

To evaluate the effect of Me-NFM and NFM on leukocyte migration, inflammatory exudate formation, and MPO activity in a carrageenan-induced air pouch inflammation model in mice.

3 Materials

3.1 Animals

- Healthy male mice (25–30 g).
- Standard housing conditions with free access to food and water.

3.2 Reagents and Chemicals

- Sterile air (for air pouch induction).
- Carrageenan (1% w/v in saline).
- Me-NFM and NFM (100–400 μM).
- Sterile 0.9% NaCl solution.
- Heparin (20 IU/mL).
- Phosphate-buffered saline (PBS, pH 7.6; NaCl 137 mM, KCl 2.7 mM, phosphate buffer salts 10 mM).
- May-Grünwald-Giemsa stain.
- Myeloperoxidase (MPO) assay reagents.
- Hydrogen peroxide (H_2O_2).
- ELISA plate reader (450 nm).
- Neubauer chamber.
- Cytospin apparatus.
- Ether (for euthanasia).

4 Experimental Groups

Group	Treatment Description
1	Positive control (Cg 1% only)
2	Negative control (0.9% saline only)
3	Me-NFM (100–400 μM, i.p.) + Cg
4	NFM (100–400 μM, i.p.) + Cg

5 Methods

5.1 Animal Preparation and Air Pouch Induction [1, 2]

1. **Animal Selection**
   - Select healthy male mice (25–30 g, 6–8 weeks old).
   - House them under standard conditions (22 ± 2°C, 12 h light/dark cycle) with food and water ad libitum.
   - Acclimate animals for at least 5 days before starting the experiment.
2. **Air Pouch Formation**
   - Day 0: Inject 5 mL of sterile air subcutaneously into the dorsal region of each mouse using a sterile syringe and a 25G needle.
   - Day 2 and Day 4: Re-inflate the pouch by injecting 2.5 mL of sterile air into the same location to maintain cavity volume.

5.2 Induction of Inflammation

1. **Carrageenan Injection (Day 6)**
   - Prepare a 1% carrageenan solution in sterile 0.9% saline.
   - Inject 1 mL of this solution subcutaneously into the air pouch to induce localized inflammation.

5.3 Drug Treatment

1. **Treatment with Test Compounds**
   - Prepare Me-NFM and NFM solutions in sterile saline at concentrations of 100, 200, and 400 μM.
   - Administer the test compounds intraperitoneally (i.p.) 30 min before carrageenan injection:
     - Group 1: Carrageenan only (positive control).
     - Group 2: Saline only (negative control).
     - Group 3: Me-NFM (100–400 μM) + Carrageenan.
     - Group 4: NFM (100–400 μM) + Carrageenan.
   - Maintain dosage volume constant (e.g., 0.1 mL/10 g body weight).

5.4 Sample Collection (Day 7)

1. **Euthanasia and Fluid Collection**
   - At 24 h after carrageenan injection, euthanize animals via ether overdose in a well-ventilated chamber.
   - Fix the animals on a dissection board in a supine position.
   - Make a midline dorsal incision to expose and carefully open the air pouch.

- Lavage the air pouch by injecting 2 mL of sterile PBS (pH 7.6) containing heparin (20 IU/mL) into the cavity using a syringe.
- Gently massage the pouch for 30 s to allow cell detachment.
- Aspirate the lavage fluid with the same syringe and transfer it into sterile microcentrifuge tubes.
- Keep samples on ice until analysis.

5.5 Leukocyte Migration Analysis

1. **Total Leukocyte Count**
   - Mix 10 μL of the lavage fluid with 10 μL of trypan blue (0.4%).
   - Load onto a Neubauer hemocytometer.
   - Count viable (unstained) leukocytes under a light microscope (100× magnification).
2. **Differential Leukocyte Count**
   - Centrifuge 200 μL of lavage fluid at 1000 rpm for 10 min.
   - Resuspend the pellet in 50 μL of PBS.
   - Prepare cytospin slides and fix them with methanol for 5 min.
   - Stain with May-Grünwald-Giemsa.
   - Identify and count at least 200 cells per slide under oil immersion (1000× magnification), categorizing as neutrophils, lymphocytes, or monocytes.

5.6 Myeloperoxidase (MPO) Activity Assay (Fig. 1)

1. **Sample Preparation for MPO**
   - Centrifuge lavage fluid at 3000 rpm for 10 min at 4°C.
   - Collect supernatant and store at −20°C until analysis.
   - Use the method described by Rao et al. for MPO quantification.
2. **MPO Assay Procedure**
   - In a 96-well ELISA plate, prepare the reaction mixture:
   - 100 μL of sample.
   - 100 μL of reaction buffer containing hydrogen peroxide (H_2O_2) and a chromogenic substrate such as TMB (tetramethylbenzidine).
   - Incubate at 37°C for 15 min in the dark.
   - Stop the reaction with 50 μL of 2 N H_2SO_4 (if TMB is used).
   - Read absorbance at 450 nm using a microplate reader.

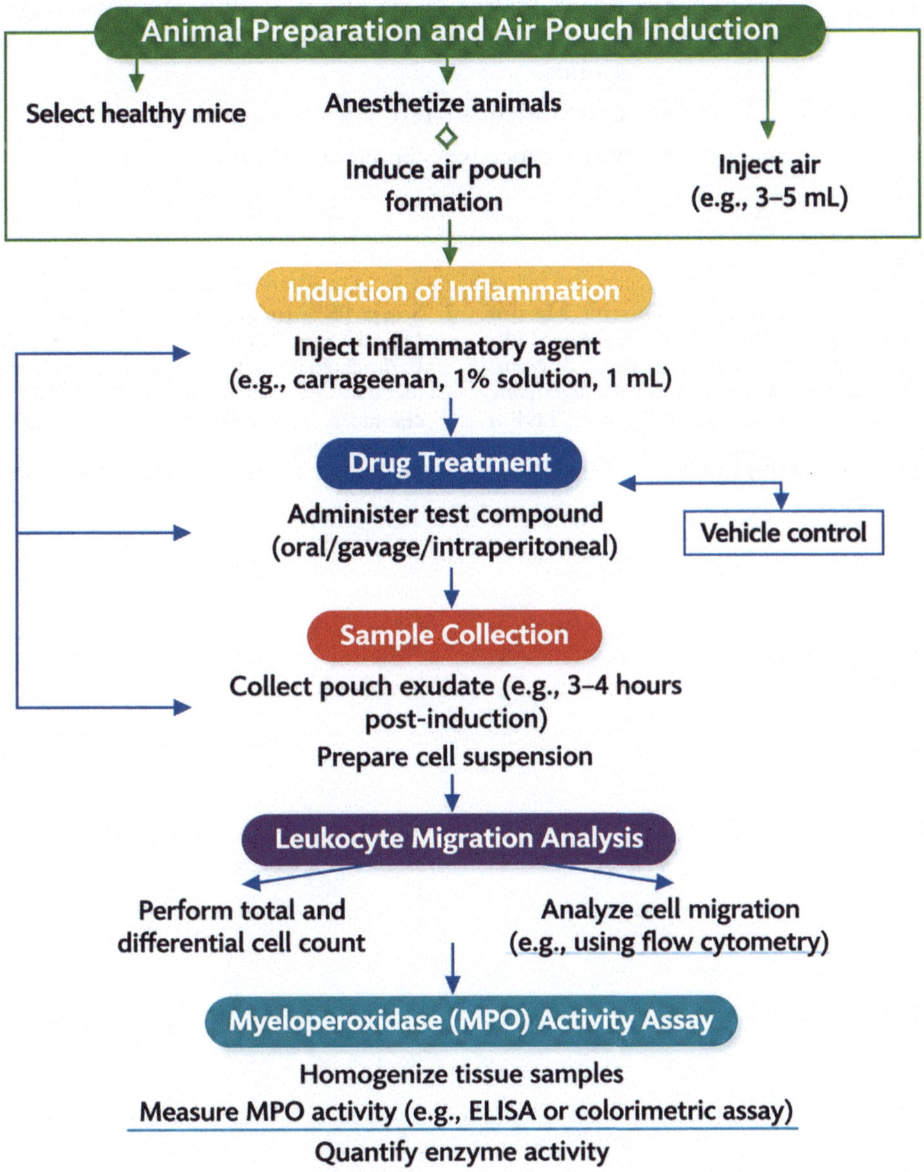

Fig. 1 Graphical representation of in vivo assay for leukocyte migration, exudation, and myeloperoxidase (MPO) activity using the murine air pouch model

- Calculate MPO activity using a standard curve and express as mU/mL.
- 1 Unit of MPO = oxidation of 1 μmol of H_2O_2/min.

5.7 Statistical Analysis

1. **Data Recording and Analysis**
   - Express data as mean ± SEM.

- Analyze statistical significance using one-way ANOVA, followed by Dunnett's post hoc test for comparisons to control groups.
- Use Student's t-test when comparing two groups.
- Significance is accepted at $p < 0.05$.

References

1. Silva DNPB, Adriana F, de Oliveira Martins DT, Borges QI, Lindote MVN, Zoratti MTR, Damazo AS (2021) Methanolic extract of cariniana rubra gardner ex miers stem bark negatively regulate the leukocyte migration and TNF-α and up-regulate the annexin-A1 expression. J Ethnopharmacol 270:113778
2. Sreeja PS, Arunachalam K, de Oliveira Martins DT, da Silva Lima JC, Balogun SO, Pavan E, Parimelazhagan T (2018) Sphenodesme involucrata var. paniculata (CB Clarke) Munir.: chemical characterization, anti-nociceptive and anti-inflammatory activities of methanol extract of leaves. J Ethnopharmacol 225:71–80

Chapter 34

Isolation and In Vitro Differentiation of Bone Marrow-Derived Macrophages (BMDMs)

Abstract

This protocol describes the isolation and in vitro differentiation of primary murine bone marrow-derived macrophages (BMDMs) from C57BL/6 mice, providing a gold-standard model for studying primary macrophage biology. Bone marrow is aseptically harvested from femurs and tibias of 6–8 week old mice by flushing with Complete L Medium (RPMI-1640, 20% heat-inactivated FBS, 30% L929-conditioned medium as source of M-CSF, 1% penicillin/streptomycin, 2 mM L-glutamine). The resulting single-cell suspension is cultured in non-tissue culture-treated Petri dishes at 1 × 106 cells/mL for 7 days at 37°C, 5% CO_2, with fresh medium added on Day 4. Differentiated BMDMs are harvested on Day 7 by scraping with ice-cold PBS, yielding 5–10 × 106 cells per mouse with >95% viability. Quality control includes flow cytometric analysis showing >90% CD11b+F4/80+ double-positive cells and phase-contrast microscopic confirmation of characteristic large, spread, vacuolated morphology. This protocol generates pure, terminally differentiated primary macrophages suitable for polarization, phagocytosis, cytokine production, and host-pathogen interaction studies.

Keywords Bone marrow-derived macrophages, Primary cell culture, M-CSF, L929-conditioned medium, Hematopoietic progenitors

1 Introduction

Bone Marrow-Derived Macrophages (BMDMs) are a gold-standard model for studying primary macrophage biology. Unlike immortalized cell lines, BMDMs retain the phenotypic and functional plasticity of native macrophages, making them ideal for investigating polarization, phagocytosis, cytokine production, and host-pathogen interactions [1]. This protocol outlines the sterile extraction of bone marrow from C57BL/6 mice and its differentiation over 7 days in the presence of M-CSF, which is provided by L929-conditioned medium [2]. The resulting cells are >90% pure macrophages (CD11b+ F4/80+).

Karuppusamy Arunachalamet al., *Advanced Protocols in Cancer Research*, Springer Protocols Handbooks,
https://doi.org/10.1007/978-1-0716-5348-7_34,

2 Aim

To generate a pure, terminally differentiated population of primary murine macrophages from bone marrow progenitors, using L929-cell conditioned medium as a source of Macrophage Colony-Stimulating Factor (M-CSF).

3 Materials

- **Animals:** C57BL/6 mice, 6–8 weeks old.
- **Reagents & Media:**
  - Complete L Medium: RPMI-1640, 20% Heat-Inactivated Fetal Bovine Serum (FBS), 30% L929-Conditioned Medium, 1% Penicillin/Streptomycin (100 U/mL & 100 μg/mL), 2 mM L-glutamine. Filter sterilize (0.22 μm). Pre-warm to 37°C.
  - Sterile 1× Phosphate Buffered Saline (PBS), pH 7.4.
  - 70% Ethanol in a spray bottle.
- **Supplies:**
  - Sterile surgical tools: Fine dissecting scissors (two pairs), forceps (serrated and fine), bone cutters.
  - 10 mL syringes with 25-gauge (25G) needles.
  - 100 mm × 20 mm non-tissue culture treated (Optilux) Petri dishes.
  - 70 μm cell strainers.
  - 15 mL and 50 mL conical tubes.
  - Cell scrapers.
  - Hemocytometer or automated cell counter.
  - Trypan Blue solution (0.4%).
- **Equipment:**
  - Biosafety cabinet (Class II).
  - CO_2 incubator (37°C, 5% CO_2).
  - Centrifuge.
  - Water bath (37°C).

4 Detailed Protocol [2, 3]

4.1 Day 0: Bone Marrow Harvest and Primary Culture Setup

1. **Preparation:**
   - Sterilize all dissection tools by autoclaving or immersion in 70% ethanol.
   - Spray the interior of the biosafety cabinet with 70% ethanol and turn on the UV light for 15 min.
   - Pour 5–10 mL of sterile PBS into a 100 mm Petri dish. Label it "Wash."
   - Prepare a second, empty 100 mm Petri dish. Label it "Marrow Collection."
   - Pre-warm a full bottle of Complete L Medium in a 37°C water bath.
2. **Euthanasia and Dissection:**
   - Euthanize the mouse by CO_2 asphyxiation followed by cervical dislocation, following approved institutional protocols.
   - Lay the mouse dorsally and thoroughly spray the abdomen and hind limbs with 70% ethanol.
   - Using sterile forceps and scissors, make an incision in the skin around the mid-abdomen. Peel the skin downward to fully expose both hind legs.
   - Carefully dissect away the muscle tissue from the femurs and tibias using forceps and scissors. Be meticulous to avoid cutting the bones or severing the femur from the hip ball joint.
   - At the hip and ankle joints, sever the tendons to free the entire femur and tibia from each leg. Place the bones into the "Wash" dish with PBS.
3. **Bone Marrow Flushing:**
   - Transfer one femur to the empty "Marrow Collection" dish.
   - Using sterile scissors, trim approximately 1–2 mm from each end of the bone to fully open the marrow cavity.
   - Fill a 10 mL syringe fitted with a 25G needle with 5–10 mL of pre-warmed Complete L Medium.
   - Insert the needle into one end of the bone and forcefully flush the marrow into the dish. The pink marrow plug should be ejected. Repeat from the opposite end if necessary.
   - Repeat steps for all bones (2 femurs, 2 tibias per mouse).

4. **Generating a Single-Cell Suspension:**
   - Using a 10 mL pipette, vigorously aspirate and dispense the marrow plugs and medium to dissociate the tissue. Pipette up and down 20–30 times until no visible clumps remain.
   - Pass the cell suspension through a 70 μm cell strainer into a 50 mL conical tube to remove bone fragments and any remaining aggregates.
   - Centrifuge the filtrate at 300 × *g* for 5 min at room temperature (RT).
   - Aspirate the supernatant. Resuspend the pellet in 10 mL of fresh Complete L Medium.
5. **Primary Culture Initiation:**
   - Count the cells using a hemocytometer with Trypan Blue exclusion. Expect 15–30 × 106 nucleated cells per mouse.
   - Adjust the cell concentration to 1 × 106 cells/mL with Complete L Medium.
   - Gently pipette 10 mL of the cell suspension (containing 10 × 106 cells) into a 100 mm non-tissue culture-treated Petri dish.
   - Label the dish with date, cell type, and passage (P0).
   - Place the dish in a 37°C, 5% CO_2 incubator.

4.2 Day 4: Medium Refresh

1. On day 4 of culture, carefully add 10 mL of fresh, pre-warmed Complete L Medium directly to the existing medium in the dish. Do not disturb or remove the semi-adherent cells. Gently swirl the dish to mix. Return to the incubator.

4.3 Day 7: Harvesting Differentiated BMDMs

1. Remove Non-Adherent Cells: Carefully aspirate and discard all medium from the dish. This contains non-adherent progenitors, granulocytes, and debris.
2. Wash: Gently add 10 mL of room-temperature PBS to the dish, swirl, and aspirate to remove any loosely adherent cells.
3. **Detach Macrophages:**
   - Add 5 mL of ice-cold PBS to the dish.
   - Using a sterile cell scraper, firmly but gently scrape the bottom of the dish to dislodge the adherent macrophages. They will detach as sheets or clusters.
   - Tilt the dish and pipette the cell suspension into a 15 mL conical tube.

4. **Wash and Count:**

- Centrifuge at 300 × *g* for 5 min at 4°C.
- Aspirate the supernatant. Resuspend the pellet in 10 mL of RPMI-1640 + 10% FBS.
- Centrifuge again as before.
- Resuspend in 5–10 mL of desired culture medium and perform a cell count. Expect a yield of 5–10 × 10^6 BMDMs per mouse.
- Assess viability via Trypan Blue exclusion; it should be >95%.

5 Quality Control

- Flow Cytometry: Stain 1 × 105 cells with anti-CD11b (APC) and anti-F4/80 (FITC) antibodies. Differentiated BMDMs should be >90% double-positive.
- Morphology: Observe under a phase-contrast microscope. Differentiated BMDMs are large, spread, and highly vacuolated.

References

1. Zhang X, Goncalves R Mosser DM (2008) The isolation and characterization of murine macrophages. Current Protocols in Immunology, 83(1):14.1.1-14.1.14. https://currentprotocols.onlinelibrary.wiley.com/doi/abs/10.1002/0471142735.im1401s83 Accessed 28 Jun 2026
2. Murray PJ, Allen JE, Biswas SK, Fisher EA, Gilroy DW, Goerdt S, Gordon S, Hamilton JA, Ivashkiv LB, Lawrence T, Locati M, Mantovani A, Martinez FO
3. Mege JL, Mosser DM, Natoli G, Saeij JP, Schultze JL, Shirey KA, Wynn TA (2014) Macrophage activation and polarization: nomenclature and experimental guidelines. Immunity 41(1):14–20. https://doi.org/10.1016/j.immuni.2014.06.008

Chapter 35

Macrophage Activation Quantified via Nitric Oxide (NO) Griess Assay

Abstract

This protocol describes the quantification of nitric oxide (NO) production by activated macrophages using the Griess reaction, a standard readout for pro-inflammatory (M1) macrophage activation. Differentiated bone marrow-derived macrophages (BMDMs) are seeded in 24-well plates at 5×105 cells/well and allowed to adhere for 6 h. Cells are stimulated with 100 U/mL IFN-γ and 200 ng/mL LPS (positive control) in the presence or absence of test compounds (e.g., peptides at 0.2–200 μM) for 24–72 h. Culture supernatants are collected and mixed 1:1 with freshly prepared Griess reagent (1% sulfanilamide in 2.5% phosphoric acid combined 1:1 with 0.1% N-(1-Naphthyl)ethylenediamine dihydrochloride). Following 10–15 min incubation at room temperature, absorbance is measured at 550 nm using a microplate reader. A sodium nitrite standard curve (0–100 μM) enables quantification of nitrite concentration (μM), which is directly proportional to NO production. Results are expressed as μM NO_2^- or fold-change relative to vehicle control, with statistical analysis by one-way ANOVA. This assay provides a quantitative measure of macrophage inflammatory activation and enables evaluation of immunomodulatory compound effects.

Keywords Nitric oxide, Griess assay, Macrophage activation, iNOS, IFN-γ, LPS

1 Introduction

Activated macrophages, particularly the M1 phenotype, upregulate inducible nitric oxide synthase (iNOS), which produces nitric oxide (NO) from L-arginine. NO is a critical effector molecule with antimicrobial and immunoregulatory functions. In solution, NO rapidly oxidizes to stable nitrite (NO_2^-) [1]. The Griess reaction quantifies nitrite by a diazotization reaction, producing a purple azo dye measurable at 550 nm. This assay is a standard readout for macrophage pro-inflammatory activation.

Karuppusamy Arunachalam et al., *Advanced Protocols in Cancer Research*, Springer Protocols Handbooks,
https://doi.org/10.1007/978-1-0716-5348-7_35,

2 Aim

To measure the production of nitric oxide, a key inflammatory mediator, by BMDMs in response to stimulation with interferon-gamma (IFN-γ) and lipopolysaccharide (LPS), and to test the inhibitory effect of the peptide.

3 Materials

- **Cells:**
- **Reagents:**
  - Complete Assay Medium: RPMI-1640 + 10% FBS (no antibiotics).
  - Recombinant Murine IFN-γ (stock: 105 U/mL in PBS + 0.1% BSA).
  - Lipopolysaccharide (LPS, stock: 1 mg/mL in sterile water).
  - Peptide (stock: 10 mM in PBS or DMSO; note vehicle control).
  - Griess Reagent: *Solution A:* 1% (w/v) sulfanilamide in 2.5% (v/v) phosphoric acid. *Solution B:* 0.1% (w/v) N-(1-Naphthyl)ethylenediamine dihydrochloride (NEDD) in water. Store separately at 4°C, protected from light. Combine equal volumes immediately before use.
  - Sodium Nitrite Standard: Prepare a 100 μM stock in complete assay medium. Generate a standard curve (0, 2, 5, 10, 20, 40, 60, 80, 100 μM) by serial dilution.
- **Supplies:**
  - 24-well tissue culture plates.
  - 96-well clear flat-bottom plates.
  - Multichannel pipette.
- **Equipment:** Microplate reader capable of measuring absorbance at 550 nm.

4 Detailed Protocol [1, 2]

4.1 Day 1: Cell Plating and Treatment

1. **Cell Seeding:**
   - Harvest and count BMDMs as in Protocol 3.15.

- Resuspend cells at 1 × 106 cells/mL in Complete Assay Medium.
- Seed 500 μL (5 × 105 cells) per well in a 24-well plate.
- Incubate for 6 h at 37°C, 5% CO_2 to allow for adherence.

2. **Treatment Preparation:**
   - Prepare all treatment solutions at 2× final concentration in Complete Assay Medium.
     - Vehicle Control: Medium only.
     - Positive Control: 200 U/mL IFN-γ + 400 ng/mL LPS.
     - Experimental Groups: 2× IFN-γ/LPS + varying 2× concentrations of Peptide (e.g., 0.2, 2, 20, 200 μM).
   - *Important:* Include a "No Cell" background control well with medium only.
3. **Treatment Application** [3, 4]:
   - After the 6-h adherence period, carefully aspirate the medium from each well.
   - Immediately add 500 μL of the 2× treatment solutions to the corresponding wells, resulting in the desired 1× final concentrations.
   - Gently swirl the plate to mix. Return the plate to the incubator.

4.2 Day 2/3/4: Supernatant Collection & Griess Reaction (Time-Course)

1. For each time point (e.g., 24, 48, 72 h), use a separate plate.
2. At the designated time, remove the plate from the incubator.
3. Carefully collect 100 μL of supernatant from each well, avoiding disturbance of the cell monolayer. Transfer to a labeled microcentrifuge tube.
4. *Optional:* Centrifuge supernatants at 10,000 × *g* for 2 min to pellet any cellular debris.
5. **Griess Reaction:**
   - Pipette 50 μL of each supernatant (and sodium nitrite standards) in duplicate into a 96-well plate.
   - Add 50 μL of freshly prepared Griess Reagent (1:1 mix of Solutions A & B) to each well.
   - Incubate the plate at room temperature, protected from light, for 10–15 min.
   - Measure the absorbance at 550 nm using the plate reader.

5 Data Analysis

1. Calculate the average absorbance for each duplicate.
2. Subtract the average absorbance of the "No Cell" background control from all sample values.
3. Generate a standard curve by plotting the absorbance (y-axis) against the known sodium nitrite concentration (x-axis). Perform linear regression to obtain the equation ($y = mx + c$).
4. Calculate the nitrite concentration for each sample using the standard curve equation: $[NO_2^-]$ (μM) = (Sample OD - c) / m.
5. Express data as μM of NO_2^- or as fold-change relative to the vehicle control.
6. Perform statistical analysis (e.g., one-way ANOVA with post-hoc test) comparing experimental groups to the positive control.

6 Troubleshooting

- High Background: Ensure all reagents and media are nitrate/nitrite-free. Filter supernatants through a 0.22 μm membrane before assay.
- Low Signal: Increase cell seeding density to 1 × 106 cells/well. Confirm the activity of IFN-γ and LPS stocks. Extend stimulation time.
- Poor Standard Curve Linearity: Prepare fresh sodium nitrite stock and Griess reagent. Ensure accurate pipetting for serial dilutions.

References

1. Green LC, Wagner DA, Glogowski J, Skipper PL, Wishnok JS, Tannenbaum SR (1982) Analysis of nitrate, nitrite, and [^{15}N]nitrate in biological fluids. Anal Biochem 126(1):131–138. https://doi.org/10.1016/0003-2697(82)90118-x
2. MacMicking J, Xie QW, Nathan C (1997) Nitric oxide and macrophage function. Annu Rev Immunol 15:323–350. https://doi.org/10.1146/annurev.immunol.15.1.323
3. Lichtman JW, Conchello JA (2005) Fluorescence microscopy. Nat Methods 2(12):910–919. https://doi.org/10.1038/nmeth817
4. Erazo-Oliveras A, Muthukrishnan N, Baker R, Wang TY, Pellois JP (2012) Improving the endosomal escape of cell-penetrating peptides and their cargos: strategies and challenges. Pharmaceuticals 5(11):1177–1209. https://doi.org/10.3390/ph5111177

Check for updates

Chapter 36

Cellular Internalization and Localization of Fluorescein Isothiocyanate (FITC)-Labeled Peptide via Confocal Microscopy

Abstract

This protocol describes the visualization and quantification of intracellular uptake and subcellular localization of FITC-conjugated peptides using confocal microscopy. B16F10-Nex2 murine melanoma cells are seeded on sterile glass coverslips in 24-well plates at 1×10^4 cells/well and cultured overnight to 60%–70% confluence. Cells are treated with FITC-labeled peptide (500 μM in serum-free medium) for 1–24 h at 37°C, 5% CO_2 in the dark. Following treatment, cells are washed with PBS, fixed with 4% paraformaldehyde for 15 min at room temperature, and optionally permeabilized with 0.1% Triton X-100 for 10 min. Nuclear counterstaining is performed with DAPI (100 ng/mL) for 10 min. Coverslips are mounted on slides using ProLong™ Gold Antifade mounting medium and cured overnight. Confocal microscopy is performed using 63× oil immersion objective with sequential scanning: 488 nm laser for FITC (emission 500–550 nm) and 405 nm laser for DAPI (emission 410–480 nm). Z-stacks are acquired at 0.5 μm steps. Image analysis using ImageJ/Fiji includes maximum intensity projection, mean fluorescence intensity measurement in nuclear and cytoplasmic regions, and calculation of nuclear/cytoplasmic ratios. This protocol enables visualization of peptide trafficking and subcellular destination.

Keywords Peptide internalization, Confocal microscopy, FITC conjugate, Subcellular localization, Z-stack imaging, B16F10-Nex2 cells

1 Introduction

Understanding the cellular entry mechanism and intracellular fate of therapeutic peptides is crucial for elucidating their mechanism of action. Fluorescent labeling with Fluorescein Isothiocyanate (FITC) allows direct visualization of peptide internalization using confocalmicroscopy. This protocol details the steps for preparing cells, treating with peptide -FITC, fixation, nuclear counterstaining, and high-resolution imaging to distinguish between membrane-bound, cytosolic, and nuclear localization over time [1].

Karuppusamy Arunachalam et al., *Advanced Protocols in Cancer Research*, Springer Protocols Handbooks,
https://doi.org/10.1007/978-1-0716-5348-7_36,

2 Aim

To visualize and quantify the intracellular uptake, trafficking, and subcellular localization of FITC-conjugated peptide in B16F10-Nex2 melanoma cells.

3 Materials

- **Cell Line:** melanoma) cells.
- **Reagents:**
  - Complete Growth Medium: DMEM + 10% FBS.
  - Peptide-FITC conjugate: 500 µM stock in PBS or DMSO (aliquot and store at −20°C, protected from light).
  - Serum-free medium (for treatment).
  - 4% Paraformaldehyde (PFA) in PBS, pH 7.4 (freshly prepared or aliquoted, store at −20°C).
  - Permeabilization Buffer: 0.1% Triton X-100 in PBS.
  - Blocking Buffer: 1% Bovine Serum Albumin (BSA) in PBS.
  - DAPI (4′,6-diamidino-2-phenylindole): 10 µg/mL stock solution in PBS.
  - ProLong™ Gold Antifade Mountant.
  - Sterile 1× PBS.
- **Supplies:**
  - 12 mm diameter #1.5 thickness glass coverslips.
  - 24-well tissue culture plates.
  - Forceps for coverslip handling.
  - Parafilm.
  - Humidified chamber (e.g., Petri dish with damp paper towel).
  - Microscope slides.
- **Equipment:**
  - Confocal Laser Scanning Microscope (e.g., Zeiss LSM 780/880, Leica SP8).
  - 63× oil immersion objective (NA 1.4).
  - CO_2 incubator (37°C, 5% CO_2).
  - Aluminum foil (for light protection).

4 Detailed Protocol

4.1 Day 1: Cell Seeding and Coverslip Preparation

1. **Coverslip Sterilization:**
   - Place coverslips in a glass beaker.
   - Rinse with 70% ethanol, then with absolute ethanol.
   - Flame-sterilize or autoclave. Alternatively, use pre-sterilized coverslips.
2. **Cell Seeding:**
   - Using sterile forceps, place one coverslip in the bottom of each well of a 24-well plate.
   - Trypsinize and count B16F10-Nex2 cells.
   - Resuspend cells at 2×10^4 cells/mL in complete growth medium.
   - Seed 500 μL (~1×10^4 cells) directly onto each coverslip.
   - Gently swirl the plate to ensure even distribution.
   - Incubate overnight (16–18 h) at 37°C, 5% CO_2 to achieve 60%–70% confluence.

4.2 Day 2: Peptide Treatment and Fixation

1. **Treatment Preparation:**
   - Warm serum-free medium to 37°C.
   - Dilute the Peptide-FITC stock to 500 μM in serum-free medium. Protect from light.
   - Prepare a vehicle control (serum-free medium with matching DMSO/PBS concentration).
2. **Treatment:**
   - Carefully aspirate the complete medium from the wells.
   - Wash cells gently once with 500 μL pre-warmed, serum-free medium.
   - Add 250 μL of the 500 μM Peptide-FITC solution or vehicle control to the appropriate wells.
   - Incubate for the desired time points (e.g., 1 h for short-term uptake, 24 h for long-term localization) at 37°C, 5% CO_2 in the dark (wrap plate in foil).
3. **Fixation:**
   - After incubation, aspirate the treatment medium.
   - Wash cells three times, gently but thoroughly, with 500 μL of room-temperature PBS.

- Add 500 μL of 4% PFA to each well. Incubate for 15 min at room temperature.
- Aspirate PFA (dispose as hazardous waste) and wash 3 × 5 min with PBS.

4.3 Permeabilization, Staining, and Mounting

1. **Permeabilization and Blocking (Optional but recommended for cytoplasmic signal clarity):**
   - Add 500 μL of 0.1% Triton X-100 in PBS. Incubate for 10 min at room temperature.
   - Wash 2 × 5 min with PBS.
   - Add 500 μL of 1% BSA in PBS. Incubate for 30 min at room temperature to block non-specific binding.
   - Wash 1 × 5 min with PBS.
2. **Nuclear Staining:**
   - Prepare a working solution of DAPI (1:1000 dilution from stock = ~100 ng/mL) in PBS.
   - Add 300 μL of DAPI solution to each well. Incubate for 10 min at room temperature, protected from light.
   - Wash 3 × 5 min with PBS to remove excess DAPI.
3. **Mounting:**
   - Place a 20–30 μL drop of ProLong™ Gold Antifade Mountant onto a clean microscope slide.
   - Using fine forceps, carefully remove a coverslip from the well. Hold by the edge and blot the excess liquid by touching the edge to a clean Kimwipe.
   - Invert the coverslip (cell-side down) onto the droplet of mounting medium. Avoid bubbles.
   - Gently press down. Remove any excess mounting medium with a Kimwipe.
   - Allow the slides to cure in the dark, at room temperature, for at least 4 h (preferably overnight) before imaging. Seal edges with nail polish for long-term storage (at −20°C).

4.4 Confocal Imaging and Analysis

1. **Microscope Setup:**
   - Turn on the confocal system, lasers, and software (e.g., ZEN, LAS X). Allow the system to stabilize.
   - Select the 63× oil immersion objective. Apply a drop of immersion oil to the objective.

2. **Parameter Settings:**
   - Laser Lines: 488 nm Argon laser for FITC (Ex: 488 nm, Em: 500–550 nm). 405 nm Diode laser for DAPI (Ex: 405 nm, Em: 410–480 nm).
   - Set detector gain and offset using control samples (untreated and vehicle-treated) to avoid pixel saturation. Use sequential scanning mode to eliminate bleed-through.
   - Set the pinhole to 1 Airy Unit for optimal optical sectioning.
3. **Image Acquisition:**
   - Find a cell of interest. Focus on the DAPI signal to locate the nucleus.
   - Acquire a single optical section or, for precise localization, acquire a Z-stack. Set the top and bottom of the cell using the software's Z-stack function. Use a step size of 0.5 μm.
   - Acquire images for at least 10–15 representative cells per condition.
4. **Image Analysis (using ImageJ/Fiji):**
   - Open the Z-stack file.
   - Image > Stacks > Z-project to create a Maximum Intensity Projection.
   - To quantify signal intensity:
     - Draw Regions of Interest (ROIs) around the nucleus (based on DAPI) and the cytoplasm.
     - Analyze > Measure to get mean fluorescence intensity (MFI) for FITC in each compartment.
     - Calculate Nuclear/Cytoplasmic ratio: N/C Ratio = (MFI_nucleus - Background) / (MFI_cytoplasm - Background).
   - For co-localization analysis (if using a second organelle marker):
     - Install the "JACoP" or "Coloc 2" plugin.
     - Analyze > Colocalization to calculate Pearson's Correlation Coefficient (PCC) or Manders' Overlap Coefficient (MOC).
5. **Troubleshooting**
   - High Background Fluorescence: Increase the number of PBS washes post-fixation. Include a BSA blocking step. Ensure antibodies (if used) are titrated.

- Weak or Faded FITC Signal: Protect all steps from light. Use fresh peptide-FITC conjugate. Increase peptide concentration or treatment time.
- Cells Detaching from Coverslip: Be extremely gentle during washes. Ensure coverslips are properly coated if needed (e.g., with poly-L-lysine). Fix cells before they become over-confluent.

Reference

1. Zhang X, Goncalves R, Mosser DM (2008) The isolation and characterization of murine macrophages. Curr Protoc Immunol 83(1): 14.1.1–14.1.14. https://doi.org/10.1002/0471142735.im1401s83

Chapter 37

Annexin V-FITC/Propidium Iodide (PI) Flow Cytometry Apoptosis Assay

Abstract

This protocol describes quantitative analysis of apoptosis and necrosis by flow cytometry using Annexin V-FITC and propidium iodide (PI) dual staining. B16F10-Nex2 cells are seeded in 6-well plates at 5×10^5 cells/well and treated with peptide (165 μM) or vehicle control for 12 h at 37°C, 5% CO_2. Both adherent and floating cells are collected, washed with ice-cold PBS, and resuspended in 100 μL of 1× Annexin V Binding Buffer (0.1 M HEPES, 1.4 M NaCl, 25 mM $CaCl_2$, pH 7.4). Cells are stained with 5 μL Annexin V-FITC and 2 μL PI (1 mg/mL) for 15 min at room temperature in the dark. After adding 400 μL binding buffer, samples are filtered through 40 μm strainers and analyzed within 1 h on a flow cytometer with 488 nm laser, acquiring 10,000 events per sample. Unstained and single-stained controls are used for compensation and quadrant gating. Populations are distinguished as: viable (Annexin V^-/PI^-), early apoptotic (Annexin V^+/PI^-), late apoptotic (Annexin V^+/PI^+), and necrotic (Annexin V^-/PI^+). Total apoptosis is calculated as the sum of early and late apoptotic percentages. This method provides robust quantification of cell death pathways induced by therapeutic compounds.

Keywords Apoptosis, Necrosis, Annexin V, Propidium iodide, Flow cytometry, Phosphatidylserine externalization, Cell death quantification, Peptide

1 Introduction

During early apoptosis, phosphatidylserine (PS) translocates from the inner to the outer leaflet of the plasma membrane. Annexin V, a calcium-dependent phospholipid-binding protein, has high affinity for PS. Propidium Iodide (PI) is a DNA intercalating dye excluded by intact plasma membranes. Dual staining allows discrimination: Viable (Annexin V^-/PI^-), Early Apoptotic (Annexin V^+/PI^-), Late Apoptotic (Annexin V^+/PI^+), and Necrotic (Annexin V^-/PI^+). Flow cytometry provides a statistically robust, quantitative analysis of these populations [1].

Karuppusamy Arunachalam et al., *Advanced Protocols in Cancer Research*, Springer Protocols Handbooks,
https://doi.org/10.1007/978-1-0716-5348-7_37,

2 Aim

To quantitatively distinguish and enumerate viable, early apoptotic, late apoptotic, and necrotic/necroptotic cells in a population by simultaneously detecting the loss of plasma membrane asymmetry (phosphatidylserine externalization) and loss of membrane integrity.

3 Materials

- **Cell Line:** B16F10-Nex2 cells.
- **Reagents:**
  - **Annexin V Binding Buffer (10×):** 0.1 M HEPES, 1.4 M NaCl, 25 mM $CaCl_2$, pH 7.4. Dilute to 1× with deionized water before use. Store at 4°C.
  - **Annexin V-FITC:** Commercial kit component or purified protein (e.g., BioLegend, BD Pharmingen). Dilute as per manufacturer's instructions (typically 1:100).
  - **Propidium Iodide (PI) Stock:** 1 mg/mL in PBS. Store at 4°C in the dark.
  - **Treatment:** Peptide (165 μM working concentration in complete medium).
  - **Controls:**

    Unstained: Cells only.

    Single Stain FITC: Cells + Annexin V-FITC.

    Single Stain PI: Cells + PI (may require mild fixation or permeabilization with 70% ethanol on ice for 5 min).

    Positive Control: Cells treated with 1 μM Staurosporine for 4–6 h.
  - Trypsin-EDTA (0.25%), Complete Growth Medium, sterile PBS.
- **Supplies:**
  - 6-well tissue culture plates.
  - 5 mL polystyrene round-bottom FACS tubes.
  - 40 μm cell strainer caps for FACS tubes.
  - Ice bucket and ice.
- **Equipment:**
  - Flow cytometer equipped with 488 nm laser and filters for FITC (530/30 nm) and PI (610/20 nm or 585/42 nm).

- Centrifuge with cooling capability (4°C).
- FlowJo or FCS Express software for analysis.

4 Detailed Protocol [1, 2]

4.1 Day 1: Cell Treatment

1. Seed B16F10-Nex2 cells at 5×10^5 cells/well in 6-well plates in 2 mL complete medium. Incubate overnight (~70% confluence).
2. Prepare fresh 165 μM peptide in complete medium. Aspirate old medium and add 2 mL of treatment or vehicle control to respective wells. Incubate for 12 h at 37°C, 5% CO_2.

4.2 Day 2: Cell Harvesting and Staining (Perform Steps on Ice or at 4°C Where Possible)

1. **Cell Collection:** Gently collect both adherent and floating cells.
   - Transfer the supernatant (containing detached cells) to a 15 mL conical tube.
   - Wash the well with 1 mL of ice-cold PBS and add to the same tube.
   - Add 0.5 mL of trypsin-EDTA to the well, incubate 2–3 min at 37°C to detach remaining adherent cells.
   - Neutralize with 1.5 mL of complete medium and pool with the cells in the conical tube.
2. **Washing:**
   - Centrifuge at 400 × *g* for 5 min at 4°C.
   - Aspirate supernatant completely. Resuspend pellet in 2 mL of ice-cold PBS.
   - Repeat centrifugation. Aspirate supernatant.
3. **Staining:**
   - Resuspend the cell pellet gently in 100 μL of 1× Annexin V Binding Buffer.
   - Add 5 μL of Annexin V-FITC and 2 μL of PI stock (1 mg/mL) to the cell suspension.
   - Mix gently by tapping. Incubate for 15 min at room temperature in the dark (NOT on ice, as Annexin V binding is Ca^{2+} and temperature dependent).
4. **Analysis Preparation:**
   - After incubation, immediately add 400 μL of 1× Annexin V Binding Buffer to each tube.
   - Keep samples on ice and in the dark.

- Optional but highly recommended: Filter cells through a 40 µm strainer cap into a FACS tube just before acquisition to remove aggregates.

5. **Flow Cytometry Acquisition:**

- Set up the flow cytometer. Use unstained and single-stained controls to set voltages and perform spectral compensation.
- Create an FSC-A vs. SSC-A plot to gate on the main cell population, excluding debris.
- Create a pulse geometry gate (FSC-A vs. FSC-H) to select single cells.
- On the gated single cells, create a dot plot of FITC-A (Annexin V) vs. PI-A.
- Adjust quadrant positions using the unstained (double negative) and single-stained controls.
- Acquire at least 10,000 events within the single-cell gate for each sample. Use a low flow rate.

5 Data Analysis

1. **Gating Strategy:**
   - Q1 (LR): PI^+ / Annexin V^- → Necrotic cells.
   - Q2 (UR): PI^+ / Annexin V^+ → Late apoptotic/secondary necrotic cells.
   - Q3 (LL): PI^- / Annexin V^- → Viable cells.
   - Q4 (UL): PI^- / Annexin V^+ → Early apoptotic cells.
2. Quantification: Calculate the percentage of cells in each quadrant.
3. Reporting: Total Apoptosis = % Early Apoptotic (Q4) + % Late Apoptotic (Q2). Report values as mean ± SEM from triplicate experiments.

6 Troubleshooting

- Excessive PI^+ staining (Necrosis): Reduce treatment intensity/duration. Ensure cells are processed quickly and kept cold. Avoid vortexing.

- Low Annexin V signal: Ensure $CaCl_2$ is present in the binding buffer. Increase incubation time to 20 min. Check reagent activity.
- High background in unstained control: Check for autofluorescence of treatment compound. Ensure thorough washing post-treatment.

References

1. Vermes I, Haanen C, Steffens-Nakken H, Reutelingsperger C (1995) A novel assay for apoptosis Flow cytometric detection of phosphatidylserine expression on early apoptotic cells using fluorescein labelled Annexin V. J Immunol Methods 184(1):39–51. https://doi.org/10.1016/0022-1759(95)00072-i
2. Rieger AM, Nelson KL, Konowalchuk JD, Barreda DR (2011) Modified annexin V/propidium iodide apoptosis assay for accurate assessment of cell death. J Vis Exp 50:e2597. https://doi.org/10.3791/2597

Chapter 38

Transmission Electron Microscopy (TEM) for Ultrastructural Analysis of Apoptosis

Abstract

This protocol describes transmission electron microscopy (TEM) methodology for visualizing ultrastructural hallmarks of apoptosis at nanometer resolution. Treated cells are fixed in situ with Karnovsky's fixative (2.5% glutaraldehyde, 4% paraformaldehyde in 0.1 M sodium cacodylate buffer, pH 7.4) for 2 h at 4°C. Cells are scraped, pelleted by centrifugation (800 ×*g*, 10 min), and washed three times with cacodylate buffer. Secondary fixation is performed with 1% osmium tetroxide (OsO_4) for 1 h at 4°C in the dark. Following buffer washes, samples are dehydrated through a graded ethanol series (30%, 50%, 70%, 90%, 100% anhydrous; 10 min each) and infiltrated with epoxy resin (e.g., Epon 812) using sequential ethanol:resin mixtures (1:1, 1:3, then 100% resin). Pellets are embedded in beam capsules and polymerized at 60°C for 48 h. Ultrathin sections (70 nm) are cut using an ultramicrotome with a diamond knife, collected on Formvar/carbon-coated copper grids, and double-stained with 2% uranyl acetate (10 min) and Reynolds' lead citrate (5 min). Imaging is performed on a transmission electron microscope (e.g., Jeol JEM-1400) at 10,000–30,000× magnification. Key apoptotic features documented include chromatin condensation and margination, nuclear fragmentation, cytoplasmic condensation, intact organelles, and apoptotic body formation.

Keywords Transmission electron microscopy, Apoptosis, Ultrastructure, Chromatin condensation, Osmium tetroxide, Glutaraldehyde fixation

1 Introduction

Transmission Electron Microscopy(TEM) remains the definitive method for identifying apoptosis based on cellular morphology. It provides unparalleled detail of subcellular changes. This protocol involves chemical fixation to preserve structure, dehydration, resin embedding, ultrathin sectioning, and heavy metal staining to generate contrast. The resulting images reveal key features such as marginated chromatin, apoptotic bodies, and intact plasma membranes until late stages, distinguishing apoptosis from necrosis [1].

Karuppusamy Arunachalam et al., *Advanced Protocols in Cancer Research*, Springer Protocols Handbooks,
https://doi.org/10.1007/978-1-0716-5348-7_38,

2 Aim

To visualize and document the characteristic ultrastructural hallmarks of apoptotic cell death at nanometer resolution, including chromatin condensation, nuclear fragmentation, cytoplasmic vacuolization, and organelle integrity.

3 Materials

Caution: Many reagents are highly toxic. Use in a fume hood with appropriate PPE.

- **Fixatives (prepare in fume hood):**
  - Primary Fixative (Karnovsky's): 2.5% Glutaraldehyde + 4% Paraformaldehyde in 0.1 M Sodium Cacodylate Buffer, pH 7.4. Store at 4°C.
  - Secondary Fixative: 1% Osmium Tetroxide (OsO_4) in 0.1 M Sodium Cacodylate Buffer. Prepare from crystalline OsO_4 or a sealed ampoule. Store wrapped in foil at 4°C.
- Buffers and Washes: 0.1 M Sodium Cacodylate Buffer, pH 7.4 (alternative: 0.1 M Phosphate Buffer).
- Dehydration Series: Ethanol (30%, 50%, 70%, 90%, 100% anhydrous) or Acetone.
- Embedding Resin: Epoxy resin (e.g., Epon 812, Agar 100) with hardener (DDSA, MNA) and accelerator (DMP-30). Prepare according to manufacturer's instructions.
- Stains:
  - Uranyl Acetate: 2% aqueous solution or saturated solution in 50% ethanol. Radioactive—handle with care.
  - Reynolds' Lead Citrate: Prepare fresh to avoid carbonate precipitation.
- **Supplies:**
  - Cell scrapers.
  - 1.5 mL microcentrifuge tubes (preferably low-binding).
  - Beam capsules or flat embedding molds.
  - Diamond knife (for ultrathin sectioning).
  - Formvar/Carbon-coated 200-mesh copper grids.
  - Filter paper.
- Equipment: Ultramicrotome, Transmission Electron Microscope (e.g., Jeol JEM-1400).

4 Detailed Protocol [1, 2]

4.1 Fixation and Embedding (Perform in Fume Hood)

1. **In Situ Primary Fixation:**
   - After treatment, quickly aspirate medium from the culture dish (e.g., 6-well plate).
   - Immediately flood the cells with 2 mL of ice-cold Primary Fixative.
   - Incubate at 4°C for 2 h (or overnight for convenience).
2. **Cell Scraping and Pellet Formation:**
   - Gently scrape the fixed, adherent cells using a cell lifter.
   - Transfer the cell suspension (cells + fixative) to a labeled 1.5 mL microcentrifuge tube.
   - Centrifuge at 800 × *g* for 10 min at 4°C to form a firm pellet.
   - Carefully remove the supernatant (toxic waste) without disturbing the pellet.
3. **Washing:** Resuspend the pellet in 1 mL of 0.1 M Cacodylate Buffer. Centrifuge as before. Repeat three times, 10 min each.
4. **Post-Fixation (Secondary Fixation) with Osmium:**
   - Resuspend the pellet in 1 mL of 1% Osmium Tetroxide solution.
   - Incubate for 1 h at 4°C in the dark (wrap tube in foil). This step adds electron density to membranes.
   - Centrifuge. Wash pellet 3 × 10 min with cacodylate buffer.
5. **Dehydration (Gradual Water Removal):**
   - Resuspend pellet in 30% Ethanol, incubate 10 min. Centrifuge.
   - Repeat sequentially with 50%, 70%, 90% ethanol (10 min each).
   - Perform three changes of 100% anhydrous ethanol, 10 min each.
6. **Resin Infiltration and Embedding:**

- Transition solvent: Use Propylene Oxide (PO) or a 1:1 mix of Ethanol:Resin.
  - Step 1: 1:1 Ethanol:Resin mix for 1 h.
  - Step 2: 1:3 Ethanol:Resin mix for 1 h (or overnight).
  - Step 3: 100% Resin for 2–4 h (change resin once).

- Embedding: Transfer the pellet to a fresh tube or beam capsule filled with fresh 100% resin. Orient the pellet if possible.
- Polymerization: Place in a 60°C oven for 48 h to harden the resin completely.

4.2 Sectioning and Staining

1. **Trimming:** Using a razor blade and trimmer, carefully trim the resin block around the cell pellet to create a small trapezoidal face (~0.5 mm × 0.5 mm).
2. **Ultrathin Sectioning:**
    - Mount the block in the ultramicrotome.
    - Using a glass knife, cut 1 μm "semi-thin" sections. Stain with Toluidine Blue to locate the cell pellet under a light microscope.
    - Switch to a diamond knife. Fill the knife boat with ultra-pure water.
    - Cut 70 nm thick "ultrathin" sections. The interference colors should be silver-gold.
    - Carefully pick up sections on Formvar/carbon-coated copper grids. Allow to dry on filter paper.
3. **Contrast Staining:**
    - Place grids, section-side down, on a drop of 2% Uranyl Acetate in a petri dish lined with parafilm. Stain for 10 min.
    - Rinse thoroughly with several drops of distilled water, then blot.
    - Place grids on a drop of Reynolds' Lead Citrate. Stain for 5 min in a CO_2-free environment (use a dish with NaOH pellets).
    - Rinse thoroughly with distilled water and allow to dry completely.

4.3 TEM Imaging

1. Load the grid into the TEM holder.
2. Insert into the microscope and evacuate the column.
3. Begin imaging at low magnification (e.g., 2000×) to locate cells.
4. Increase magnification to 10,000×–30,000× to observe ultrastructural details.
5. **Key Apoptotic Features to Document:**
    - Early: Chromatin condensation and margination along the nuclear envelope.
    - Mid: Nuclear fragmentation, cytoplasmic condensation, intact organelles.

- Late: Formation of membrane-bound apoptotic bodies containing nuclear and cytoplasmic material.
- Mitochondria: Look for swelling or cristae disruption (may indicate intrinsic pathway involvement).

5 Troubleshooting

- Poor Pellet Formation: Increase cell number. Add a drop of warm liquid agarose to the pellet after primary fixation to encase cells before processing.
- Soft Resin/Incomplete Polymerization: Ensure resin components are mixed thoroughly and accurately. Check oven temperature.
- Poor Contrast: Ensure uranyl acetate and lead citrate are fresh. Staining times may need optimization. Check that OsO_4 fixation was effective.

References

1. Kerr JF, Wyllie AH, Currie AR (1972) Apoptosis: a basic biological phenomenon with wide-ranging implications in tissue kinetics. Br J Cancer 26(4): 239–257. https://doi.org/10.1038/bjc.1972.33
2. Hayat MA (2000) Principles and techniques of electron microscopy: biological applications, 4th edn. Cambridge University Press

Check for updates

Chapter 39

Detection of Intracellular Superoxide Anion Production Using Dihydroethidium (DHE)

Abstract

This protocol describes the detection and semi-quantification of intracellular superoxide anion (O_2^-) production using the oxidation-sensitive fluorescent probe dihydroethidium (DHE). B16F10-Nex2 cells are seeded in glass-bottom 24-well plates at $5\text{–}\times 10^4$ cells/well and cultured overnight. Following treatment with peptide (165 μM) for 3–6 h, cells are loaded with 5 μM DHE (diluted from 5 mM DMSO stock in serum-free HBSS) for 30 min at 37°C, 5% CO_2 in the dark. After incubation, cells are washed twice with warm HBSS and immediately imaged using an epifluorescence or confocal microscope equipped with TRITC/Cy3 filter set (excitation 518–550 nm, emission 560–605 nm). For quantitative analysis, images from ≥5 random fields per condition are captured with identical acquisition settings. Using ImageJ/Fiji, the background is subtracted, cellular regions are thresholded, and mean fluorescence intensity (MFI) per cell is measured. Results are expressed as fold increase over untreated control. Positive controls (menadione 50–100 μM or antimycin A 1–10 μM) and negative controls (N-acetylcysteine 5 mM pre-treatment) validate assay specificity. This protocol enables real-time assessment of oxidative stress in live cells and implicates superoxide-mediated mechanisms in compound-induced cytotoxicity.

Keywords Superoxide, Dihydroethidium, Reactive oxygen species, Oxidative stress, Fluorescence microscopy

1 Introduction

Superoxide anion is a key ROS produced in mitochondria and by NADPH oxidases during cellular stress, immune response, and apoptosis. DHE is non-fluorescent until it crosses cell membranes and is oxidized by O_2^- to form 2-hydroxyethidium, which intercalates into DNA, emitting bright red fluorescence. This assay provides a real-time, qualitative, and semi-quantitative measure of superoxide levels. It is critical to note that other oxidants can also oxidize DHE to ethidium, which has a similar fluorescence signature, making this a general ROS indicator with a preference for superoxide [1].

Karuppusamy Arunachalam et al., *Advanced Protocols in Cancer Research*, Springer Protocols Handbooks, https://doi.org/10.1007/978-1-0716-5348-7_39,

2 Aim

To detect and semi-quantify the generation of superoxide anion (O_2^-), a primary reactive oxygen species (ROS), in live cells using the cell-permeable, oxidation-sensitive fluorescent probe Dihydroethidium (DHE).

3 Materials

- **Cell Line:** B16F10-Nex2 cells.
- **Reagents:**
  - Dihydroethidium (DHE): 5 mM stock in anhydrous DMSO. Aliquot and store at −20°C, protected from light and moisture. Desiccate.
  - Positive Control: Menadione (50–100 μM) or Antimycin A (1–10 μM). *Alternatively:*)).
  - Negative Control: N-acetylcysteine (NAC, 5 mM) pre-treatment for 1 h.
  - Treatment: Peptide (165 μM).
  - Hanks' Balanced Salt Solution (HBSS) or phenol-red free imaging medium.
  - Serum-free medium.
- **Supplies:**
  - 24-well plates with glass-bottom inserts or chambered coverslips for live imaging.
  - Aluminum foil.
- **Equipment:**
  - Epifluorescence or Confocalmicroscope equipped with a TRITC/Cy3 filter set (Ex: ~518–550 nm, Em: ~560–605 nm).
  - Environmental chamber to maintain 37°C and 5% CO_2 during live imaging (optional but recommended).

4 Detailed Protocol [1, 2]

4.1 Day 1: Cell Seeding

1. Seed B16F10-Nex2 cells at 5×10^4 cells/well in a glass-bottom 24-well plate in 500 μL complete medium. Incubate overnight to reach ~60% confluence.

4.2 Day 2: Treatment and Staining (All Steps Protected from Light)

1. **Pre-treatment (Optional–for inhibitor studies):** Aspirate medium. Add medium containing ROS scavenger (e.g., 5 mM NAC) or vehicle. Incubate for 1 h at 37°C.
2. **Peptide Treatment:**
   - Aspirate medium (or inhibitor medium).
   - Add pre-warmed serum-free medium containing 165 μM peptide or vehicle control.
   - Incubate for desired time points (e.g., 3 h and 6 h) at 37°C, 5% CO_2.
3. **DHE Loading:**
   - During the last 30 min of peptide treatment, prepare the DHE working solution.
   - Dilute the 5 mM DHE stock in warm, serum-free HBSS or imaging medium to a final concentration of 5 μM. Mix well by vortexing.
   - Aspirate the treatment medium from the wells.
   - Immediately add 250 μL of the 5 μM DHE solution to each well.
   - Return the plate to the incubator for exactly 30 min.
4. **Washing and Imaging:**
   - After incubation, quickly aspirate the DHE solution.
   - Wash cells gently but thoroughly twice with 500 μL of pre-warmed, serum-free HBSS.
   - Add 500 μL of fresh HBSS or imaging medium to each well.
   - Proceed to imaging immediately. Do not allow cells to sit for extended periods.

4.3 Image Acquisition and Analysis

1. **Microscope Settings:**
   - Use a TRITC filter set (e.g., Ex: 540/25 nm, Em: 605/55 nm).
   - Use a 20× or 40× objective.
   - Set exposure time, gain, and laser power using the untreated control to establish a baseline, ensuring no pixel saturation in treated samples.
   - Keep settings identical for all samples and replicates.
2. **Acquisition:**
   - For each well, capture images from at least five random, non-overlapping fields of view.
   - If using a live-cell chamber, take a time-course (e.g., every 10 min for 1 h).

3. **Quantitative Analysis with ImageJ/Fiji:**
   - Open an image.
   - Process > Subtract Background (rolling ball radius = 50 pixels).
   - Set a threshold to define the cellular area: Image > Adjust > Threshold. Adjust until cells are selected. Convert to a mask (Process > Binary > Convert to Mask).
   - Use the mask to measure fluorescence intensity only within cells:
     - Analyze > Set Measurements → Check "Mean Gray Value" and "Area".
     - Analyze > Analyze Particles to measure each cell.
   - Record the **Mean Fluorescence Intensity (MFI)** per cell.
   - Calculate the average MFI for all cells in all fields for a given condition.
   - Normalize data: Fold Increase = (Avg MFI_treated) / (Avg MFI_untreated control).
4. **Qualitative Analysis:** Visually assess the pattern: diffuse cytoplasmic vs. punctuate (mitochondrial) vs. nuclear fluorescence.

5 Troubleshooting

- **Rapid Photobleaching:** Minimize light exposure. Use lower light intensity and faster acquisition settings.
- **High Background/Non-specific staining:** Ensure thorough washing after DHE incubation. Use serum-free medium during staining, as serum esterases can affect DHE. Prepare fresh DHE stock.
- **No Signal:** Confirm DHE stock is viable (should be colorless to pale yellow). Check filter set alignment. Try a higher concentration (up to 10 μM) or longer loading time (up to 45 min).

References

1. Zhao H, Kalivendi S, Zhang H, Joseph J, Nithipatikom K, Vásquez-Vivar J, Kalyanaraman B (2003) Superoxide reacts with hydroethidine but forms a fluorescent product that is distinctly different from ethidium: potential implications in intracellular fluorescence detection of superoxide. Free Radic Biol Med 34(11):1359–1368. https://doi.org/10.1016/S0891-5849(03)00142-4
2. Kalyanaraman B, Darley-Usmar V, Davies KJ, Dennery PA, Forman HJ, Grisham MB, Mann GE, Moore K, Roberts 2ndLJ, Ischiropoulos H (2012) Measuring reactive oxygen and nitrogen species with fluorescent probes: challenges and limitations. Free Radic Biol Med 52(1):1–6. https://doi.org/10.1016/j.freeradbiomed.2011.09.030

Chapter 40

MTT Cell Viability Assay to Test Protective Effect of N-Acetylcysteine (NAC)

Abstract

This protocol describes the MTT (3-(4,5-dimethylthiazol-2-yl)-2,5-diphenyltetrazolium bromide) colorimetric assay for assessing cell viability and evaluating the cytoprotective effect of the antioxidant N-acetylcysteine (NAC) against peptide-induced cytotoxicity. B16F10-Nex2 cells are seeded in 96-well plates at 1×10^4 cells/well and cultured overnight. Cells are pre-treated with or without 4 mM NAC for 4 h, followed by the addition of peptide (15.6–500 μM final concentration) with or without 2 mM NAC for 24 h at 37°C, 5% CO_2. After treatment, 20 μL of MTT solution (5 mg/mL in PBS) is added to each well and incubated for 3 h. Medium is carefully aspirated, and formazan crystals are solubilized with 100 μL of 10% SDS in 0.01 M HCl (or acidified isopropanol/DMSO) with shaking for 10–15 min. Absorbance is measured at 570 nm with reference filter at 630–690 nm using a microplate reader. Cell viability is calculated as a percentage of the vehicle control after background subtraction. Rescue of viability by NAC pre-treatment (significant increase in viability compared to peptide-only treatment) implicates oxidative stress in the cytotoxic mechanism. All conditions are tested in triplicate or quadruplicate with appropriate controls (cell-only, background, vehicle). Data are analyzed using one-way ANOVA with post-hoc tests ($p < 0.05$ significance).

Keywords MTT assay, Cell viability, N-acetylcysteine, Oxidative stress, Cytoprotection

1 Introduction

The MTT (3-(4,5-dimethylthiazol-2-yl)-2,5-diphenyltetrazolium bromide) assay measures cellular metabolic activity via mitochondrial reductase enzymes, which convert the yellow tetrazolium salt MTT into purple formazan crystals. A reduction in formazan production correlates with loss of cell viability, mitochondrial dysfunction, or decreased cell number. This protocol uses NAC, a precursor to glutathione and a potent ROS scavenger, to test if oxidative stress is a primary mechanism of peptide-induced cell death. Rescue of viability by NAC would implicate ROS in the cytotoxic pathway [1].

Karuppusamy Arunachalam et al., *Advanced Protocols in Cancer Research*, Springer Protocols Handbooks,
https://doi.org/10.1007/978-1-0716-5348-7_40,

2 Aim

To determine if pre-treatment with the antioxidant N-acetylcysteine (NAC) rescues B16F10-Nex2 cells from peptide-induced cytotoxicity, using the MTT assay as a measure of metabolically active cells.

3 Materials

- **Cell Line:** B16F10-Nex2 cells.
- **Reagents:**
  - MTT Reagent: 5 mg/mL MTT in sterile PBS. Filter sterilize (0.22 μm). Store at 4°C in the dark for up to 2 weeks or at −20°C for longer.
  - Solubilization Solution: 10% SDS in 0.01 M HCl. Alternatively, use acidified isopropanol (0.04 N HCl in isopropanol) or DMSO.
  - N-Acetylcysteine (NAC): 1 M stock in sterile water or PBS, adjust pH to 7.0–7.4. Filter sterilize. Prepare fresh or aliquot and store at -20°C.
  - Peptide: Prepare a serial dilution in complete medium to achieve final concentrations from 15.6 μM to 500 μM.
  - Complete growth medium, sterile PBS.
- Supplies: 96-well flat-bottom tissue culture plates, multichannel pipette, plate shaker.
- Equipment: Microplate reader capable of measuring absorbance at 570 nm with a reference filter at 630–690 nm.

4 Detailed Protocol [1, 2]

4.1 Day 1: Cell Seeding and NAC Pre-Treatment

1. Harvest and count B16F10-Nex2 cells.
2. Resuspend cells in complete medium at a density of 1×10^5 cells/mL.
3. Seed 100 μL of cell suspension (~1×10^4 cells) into each well of a 96-well plate. Include control wells:
   - Cell-only Control (CC): Cells + medium (for 100% viability).
   - Background Control (BC): Medium only, no cells (for background subtraction).
4. Incubate plate overnight at 37°C, 5% CO_2 to allow cell adherence.

4.2 Day 2: NAC Pre-Treatment and Peptide Challenge

1. **NAC Pre-Treatment:**
   - Prepare complete medium containing 4 mM NAC (final concentration in well).
   - Aspirate medium from the wells designated for the "+NAC" groups.
   - Add 100 μL of the 4 mM NAC medium to these wells.
   - For the "−NAC" groups, simply add 100 μL of fresh complete medium.
   - Incubate the plate for 4 h at 37°C, 5% CO_2.

2. **Peptide Treatment:**
   - After the 4-hpre-treatment, do not aspirate the medium.
   - Prepare 2× concentrations of peptide in complete medium (e.g., 31.2–1000 μM). For NAC groups, prepare these solutions also containing 4 mM NAC.
   - Carefully add 100 μL of the 2× peptide solutions directly to the existing 100 μL of medium in the corresponding wells. This results in a 1:1 dilution, giving the final desired concentrations (15.6–500 μM peptide, with or without 2 mM NAC).
   - For the CC (no drug) and BC wells, add 100 μL of fresh medium (with or without 2 mM NAC as matched to the treatment groups).
   - Include triplicate or quadruplicate wells for each condition.
   - Return plate to incubator for 24 h.

4.3 Day 3: MTT Assay

1. After 24 h, carefully remove the plate from the incubator.
2. Add 20 μL of the 5 mg/mL MTT solution directly to each well (including BC wells). Final MTT concentration is ~0.5 mg/mL.
3. Return the plate to the incubator for 3 h. Protect from light.
4. After incubation, carefully remove all medium and MTT solution from the wells using a multichannel pipette. Avoid disturbing the purple formazan crystals at the bottom of the wells.
5. Add 100 μL of the solubilization solution (10% SDS in 0.01 M HCl) to each well.
6. Place the plate on a plate shaker for 10–15 min at low speed to ensure complete
7. L929-Conditioned Medium Preparation: Culture L929 cells in RPMI-1640 + 10% FBS until confluent and overgrown for 5–7 days. Collect supernatant, filter (0.22 μm), and store at −20°C. Titrate for optimal BMDM differentiation (typically 20%–30% final concentration).

References

1. Mosmann T (1983) Rapid colorimetric assay for cellular growth and survival: application to proliferation and cytotoxicity assays. J Immunol Methods 65(1-2):55–63. https://doi.org/10.1016/0022-1759(83)90303-4
2. Zafarullah M, Li WQ, Sylvester J, Ahmad M (2003) Molecular mechanisms of N-acetylcysteine actions. Cell Mol Life Sci 60(1):6–20. https://doi.org/10.1007/s000180300001

Part VIII

Translational and Clinical Research Protocols

Chapter 41

Lymphocyte Isolation Protocol from Human Peripheral Blood

Abstract

The extraction of lymphocytes from peripheral blood is a crucial technique in fields such as immunology, molecular diagnostics, and translational research. Peripheral blood mononuclear cells (PBMCs), which consist of lymphocytes (T cells, B cells, NK cells) and monocytes, are typically isolated through density gradient centrifugation. This protocol outlines a standardized method using Ficoll for the density gradient separation of lymphocytes from human plasma or whole blood. The process guarantees high cell viability and purity, making it appropriate for various applications, including flow cytometry, RNA/DNA extraction, cell culture, and functional assays.

Keywords Lymphocytes, PBMC, Ficoll, Density gradient centrifugation, Immunology

1 Introduction

Lymphocytes play a vital role in both the adaptive and innate immune systems, comprising T lymphocytes, B lymphocytes, and natural killer cells. The separation of these cells is important for immunophenotyping, cytokine analysis, proliferation assays, and molecular research.

The use of Ficoll-Paque in density gradientcentrifugation effectively separates mononuclear cells according to differences in density. After centrifugation, PBMCs form a distinct interface layer (buffy coat), which can be collected carefully and processed further [1–3].

2 Materials

2.1 Reagents

1. Fresh human peripheral blood (collected in EDTA or heparin tubes).
2. Phosphate-buffered saline (PBS), sterile.
3. Ficoll-Paque gradient medium.
4. Red blood cell (RBC) lysis buffer (optional).
5. Trypan blue solution (for viability assessment).

Karuppusamy Arunachalam et al., *Advanced Protocols in Cancer Research*, Springer Protocols Handbooks,
https://doi.org/10.1007/978-1-0716-5348-7_41,

2.2 Equipment

1. Centrifuge with swing-bucket rotor.
2. 15 mL and 50 mL conical tubes.
3. Pipettes and sterile tips.
4. Hemocytometer or automated cell counter.
5. Biosafety cabinet.
6. Inverted microscope.

3 Methods

1. Collect 5–10 mL of peripheral blood in an anticoagulant tube and ensure that the samples are processed within 2–4 h of collection to maintain cell integrity.
2. Dilute the collected blood in a 1:1 ratio with sterile phosphate-buffered saline (PBS) (e.g., mix 5 mL of blood with 5 mL of PBS) to reduce viscosity and facilitate proper separation during centrifugation.
3. Carefully layer the diluted blood over Ficoll-Paque in a 15 mL tube, for instance, placing 8 mL of diluted blood on top of 4 mL of Ficoll, taking care not to disturb the interface and mix between the layers.
4. Centrifuge the tubes at 400 × g for 30 min at room temperature without applying the brake during deceleration and observe the formation of four distinct layers consisting of plasma at the top, the peripheral blood mononuclear cell (PBMC) layer or buffy coat immediately below, the Ficoll layer as the third, and red blood cells at the bottom.
5. Carefully remove the top plasma layer and aspirate the PBMC layer carefully using a sterile pipette and transfer it to a new 15 mL tube, then add PBS to achieve a total volume of 10–15 mL and wash the cells by centrifuging at 300 × g for 10 min, discarding the supernatant and repeating the wash step once again with 1× PBS to remove residual Ficoll and plasma components.
6. If red blood cell contamination is present, resuspend the cell pellet in 1–2 mL of red blood cell lysis buffer and incubate for 15 min at room temperature, then add PBS and centrifuge at 300 × g for 5 min.
7. After centrifugation, discard the supernatant and resuspend the cells in an appropriate buffer or culture medium.
8. Mix 10 μL of the cell suspension with 10 μL of Trypan blue, count the cells using a hemocytometer, and confirm that cell

viability is greater than 95% before proceeding to downstream applications.

9. For cell culture applications, resuspend the cells in complete RPMI medium; for DNA or RNA extraction, proceed immediately or store the cells at −80°C; and for long-term cryopreservation, freeze the cells in a solution of 90% fetal bovine serum (FBS) and 10% dimethyl sulfoxide (DMSO) at −80°C for 24 h and transfer to liquid nitrogen for long-term storage.

References

1. Böyum A (1968) Isolation of mononuclear cells and granulocytes from human blood. Scand J Clin Lab Invest Suppl 97:77–89.
2. Freshney RI (2016) Culture of animal cells: a manual of basic technique and specialized applications. Wiley-Blackwell
3. Maecker HT, McCoy JP, Nussenblatt R (2012) Standardizing immunophenotyping for the human immunology project. Nat Rev Immunol 12:191–200

Check for updates

Chapter 42

Circulating Tumor Cell (CTC) Isolation Protocol

Abstract

Circulating tumor cells (CTCs), rare cancer cells, are shed from primary or metastatic sites and enter the bloodstream. They play a vital role as biomarkers for cancer diagnosis, prognosis, and treatment monitoring. Since the frequency of CTCs is very low (1–100 cells per 10^9 blood cells), isolation requires highly sensitive and specific methods. This protocol provides a standardized approach for isolating CTCs by immunomagnetic enrichment of epithelial cell adhesion molecule (EpCAM)-positive cells, followed by immunofluorescence detection. This method is applicable for further molecular analysis of isolated cells by PCR and sequencing.

Keywords Circulating tumor cells, Liquid biopsy, EpCAM, Immunomagnetic separation, Cancer biomarkers

1 Introduction

Liquid biopsy techniques have transformed the field of cancer by allowing non-invasive monitoring of tumors. Of these techniques, CTC analysis offers real-time data on the spread and metastatic properties of cancer.

CTCs are usually isolated based on one of the following three principles:

1. Immunoaffinity-based capture (using EpCAM-targeted magnetic beads).
2. Size-based filtration systems.
3. Microfluidic chip technology.

The immunomagnetic technique is still employed because of its specificity and reproducibility. EpCAM-positive cells are isolated using antibody-coated magnetic beads in the presence of a magnetic field. The isolated cells are then characterized by their positivity for cytokeratin and negativity for CD45 [1–3].

Karuppusamy Arunachalam et al., *Advanced Protocols in Cancer Research*, Springer Protocols Handbooks,
https://doi.org/10.1007/978-1-0716-5348-7_42,

2 Materials

2.1 Reagents

1. Peripheral blood sample (7.5–10 mL) collected in EDTA tube.
2. Phosphate-buffered saline (PBS).
3. Ficoll-Paque or density gradient medium.
4. Anti-EpCAM magnetic beads.
5. Blocking buffer (PBS + 1% BSA).
6. Cytokeratin antibody (fluorescent-labeled).
7. Anti-CD45 antibody (fluorescent-labeled).
8. DAPI or nuclear stain.
9. Fixation buffer (4% paraformaldehyde).
10. Permeabilization buffer (0.1% Triton X-100).

2.2 Equipment

1. Centrifuge (room temperature).
2. Magnetic separation rack.
3. Fluorescencemicroscope.
4. Hemocytometer or automated cell counter.
5. 15 mL and 50 mL conical tubes.
6. Pipettes and sterile tips.

3 Methods

1. Collect 7.5–10 mL of peripheral blood into EDTA tubes and gently invert the tubes multiple times immediately after collection to ensure thorough mixing of the anticoagulant and to prevent clot formation.
2. Process the collected blood samples within 4 h of collection to maintain cell viability and preserve cellular integrity throughout downstream procedures.
3. Dilute the blood at a 1:1 ratio by adding an equal volume of 1× phosphate-buffered saline (1× PBS) to the blood sample and mix gently to obtain a homogeneous cell suspension without inducing shear stress.
4. Carefully layer the diluted blood suspension over the Ficoll density gradient medium, ensuring that the blood–PBS mixture is added slowly along the tube wall so that the interface remains clearly defined and the phases do not mix.

5. Centrifuge the tubes at 400 × *g* for 30 min at room temperature without applying the brake, allowing efficient separation of blood components based on density and the formation of distinct layers.
6. After centrifugation, carefully aspirate the mononuclear cell layer (buffy coat) located at the plasma–Ficoll interface, taking care not to disturb the plasma layer above or the granulocyte and erythrocyte layers below.
7. Wash the collected mononuclear cells by resuspending them gently in PBS and centrifuging at 300 × *g* for 10 min, then carefully discard the supernatant to remove residual Ficoll and plasma proteins.
8. Resuspend the resulting cell pellet thoroughly in an appropriate volume of PBS to reduce nonspecific antibody and bead binding during the immunomagnetic enrichment step.
9. Add anti-EpCAMmagnetic beads to the cell suspension according to the manufacturer's recommended bead-to-cell ratio, and mix gently but thoroughly to ensure uniform bead distribution.
10. Incubate the bead–cell suspension for 30 min at room temperature with gentle rotation or mixing to allow optimal binding of magnetic beads to EpCAM-positive cells.
11. Place the tube onto a magnetic rack for approximately 5 min, ensuring the tube remains undisturbed to allow complete separation of bead-bound cells from unbound cells.
12. Carefully remove and discard the supernatant without disturbing the bead-bound cell fraction retained against the tube wall by the magnetic field.
13. Wash the bead-bound cells twice with PBS by gently resuspending the cells, returning the tube to the magnetic rack, and removing the supernatant each time to eliminate unbound cells and debris.
14. Fix the enriched bead-bound cells by resuspending them in 4% paraformaldehyde and incubating for 10 min at room temperature to preserve cellular morphology and antigenicity.
15. Wash the fixed cells with PBS to remove residual paraformaldehyde, using centrifugation or magnetic separation as appropriate for the sample format.
16. Permeabilize the cells by incubating them in 0.1% Triton X-100 for 5 min, handling the samples gently to maintain cell structure and bead attachment.
17. Prepare an antibody staining cocktail containing anti-cytokeratin antibody, anti-CD45 antibody, and DAPI at the

recommended concentrations, and add it to the permeabilized cells with thorough but gentle mixing.

18. Incubate the cells in the staining solution for 30 min at room temperature in the dark to prevent photobleaching and to ensure optimal antibody and nuclear dye binding.
19. Wash the stained cells with PBS to remove unbound antibodies and excess DAPI, preparing the samples for downstream analysis.
20. Identify circulating tumor cells as DAPI-positive cells with cytokeratin expression, absence of CD45 staining, and intact cellular morphology under microscopic observation.
21. Enumerate circulatingtumor cells using fluorescencemicroscopy by systematically scanning the entire stained preparation and recording the number of cells that meet all defined CTC criteria.

4 Quality Control

1. Include healthy donor blood as a negative control.
2. Include a spiked cancer cell line as a positive control.
3. Record recovery efficiency.
4. Store isolated cells appropriately for downstream molecular assays.

References

1. Alix-Panabières C, Pantel K (2014) Challenges in circulating tumour cell research. Nat Rev Cancer 14:623–631
2. Cristofanilli M et al (2004) Circulating tumor cells, disease progression, and survival in metastatic breast cancer. N Engl J Med 351:781–791
3. Yu M, Bardia A, Wittner BS et al (2013) Circulating breast tumor cells exhibit dynamic changes in epithelial and mesenchymal composition. Science 339:580–584

Check for updates

Chapter 43

Exosome Isolation Protocol from Blood

Abstract

Exosomes are tiny extracellular vesicles (30–150 nm) found in plasma and serum. They are promising biomarkers for liquid biopsy applications. Because blood samples are complex, careful pre-clearing and sequential centrifugation steps are necessary to obtain high-purity exosomes. This protocol outlines a standardized differential ultracentrifugation method tailored for human plasma and serum samples. The process includes removing cells and debris, getting rid of large vesicles, pelleting exosomes using ultracentrifugation, and washing steps to enhance purity. The isolated vesicles are suitable for downstream DNA, RNA, proteomic, and functional analyses.

Keywords Exosomes, Plasma, Serum, Extracellular vesicles, Ultracentrifugation, Liquid biopsy

1 Introduction

Exosomes from plasma and serum are increasingly used in cancer diagnostics, cardiovascular research, and studies of inflammatory diseases. However, blood contains many proteins (such as albumin and immunoglobulins) and lipoproteins that might contaminate exosome preparations.

Differential ultracentrifugation is a well-accepted and reproducible method for isolating exosomes from plasma and serum. Following standardized pre-analytical handling is crucial for reproducibility and adherence to extracellular vesicle research guidelines.

2 Materials

2.1 Reagents

1. Human peripheral blood collected in EDTA tubes (for plasma).
2. Serum collection tubes (for serum samples).
3. Phosphate-buffered saline (PBS), sterile and 0.22 μm filtered.
4. Protease inhibitor cocktail (optional).
5. 0.22 μm syringe filters.

Karuppusamy Arunachalam et al., *Advanced Protocols in Cancer Research*, Springer Protocols Handbooks,
https://doi.org/10.1007/978-1-0716-5348-7_43,

2.2 Equipment

1. Refrigerated centrifuge.
2. Ultracentrifuge with fixed-angle or swinging-bucket rotor.
3. Ultracentrifuge tubes (polypropylene).
4. 1.5 mL DNase/RNase-free microcentrifuge tubes.
5. Pipettes and sterile filtered tips.
6. Vortex mixer.

3 Methods [1–3]

1. Collect whole blood in EDTA tubes, making sure to mix gently immediately after collection to prevent coagulation and keep plasma quality.
2. Centrifuge the blood at 300 × *g* for 10 min at 4°C to separate plasma from cellular components.
3. Carefully transfer the plasma supernatant to a new sterile tube without disturbing the cell pellet.
4. Centrifuge the transferred plasma at 2000 × *g* for 10 min at 4 °C to eliminate any remaining cellular debris and platelets.
5. For serum preparation, let whole blood clot undisturbed for 30 min at room temperature to ensure complete coagulation.
6. Centrifuge the clotted blood at 2000 × *g* for 10 min at 4°C to separate serum from the clot.
7. Carefully move the clear serum supernatant to a new sterile tube, avoiding disruption of the clot.
8. Centrifuge the clarified plasma or serum at 10,000 × *g* for 30 min at 4 °C to remove large vesicles, apoptotic bodies, and remaining debris.
9. Carefully transfer the resulting supernatant into a clean ultracentrifuge tube without disturbing the pellet formed during centrifugation.
10. Filter the supernatant through a 0.22 μm syringe or vacuum filter to eliminate large vesicles and particulate contaminants.
11. Ultracentrifuge the filtered plasma or serum at 100,000 × *g* for 70 min at 4°C to pellet small extracellular vesicles, including exosomes.
12. Carefully discard the supernatant after ultracentrifugation, making sure the exosome pellet at the bottom of the tube is undisturbed.

13. Resuspend the exosome pellet gently in an equal volume of sterile phosphate-buffered saline (PBS) to wash and remove soluble protein contaminants.
14. Perform a second ultracentrifugation step at 100,000 × g for 70 min at 4°C to re-pellet the exosomes and improve sample purity.
15. Remove the supernatant carefully and resuspend the final exosome pellet in 50–200 μL of sterile PBS, adjusting the volume based on downstream applications.
16. Store the isolated exosome preparation at −80°C to maintain vesicle stability and integrity during long-term storage.
17. Avoid repeated freeze–thaw cycles, as these can affect exosome structure and cargo composition.
18. Proceed with DNA or RNA extraction as soon as possible to minimize degradation and ensure optimal nucleic acid quality.

4 Quality Control and Characterization

1. Perform nanoparticle tracking analysis (NTA) to determine the size distribution and particle concentration of the isolated exosome preparation.
2. Use transmission electron microscopy(TEM) to visually confirm vesicle shape and check for intact, cup-shaped exosomes.
3. Conduct Western blot analysis to verify exosome identity by detecting known exosomal markers, including CD9, CD63, and CD81.
4. Measure the total protein content of the exosome samples using the bicinchoninic acid (BCA) assay to evaluate sample yield and consistency [1–3].

References

1. Théry C, Amigorena S, Raposo G, Clayton A (2006) Isolation and characterization of exosomes from biological fluids. Curr Protoc Cell Biol 30:3.22.1–3.22.29
2. Raposo G, Stoorvogel W (2013) Extracellular vesicles: exosomes, microvesicles, and friends. JCell Biol 200:373–383
3. Théry C, Witwer KW, Aikawa E et al (2018) Minimal information for studies of extracellular vesicles 2018 (MISEV2018). J Extracell Vesicles 7:1535750

Subject Index

Karuppusamy Arunachalam et al., *Advanced Protocols in Cancer Research*, Springer Protocols Handbooks,
https://doi.org/10.1007/978-1-0716-5348-7,

The manufacturer's authorised representative in the EU is Springer Nature Customer Service Centre GmbH, Europaplatz 3, 69115 Heidelberg, Germany. If you have any concerns regarding our products, please contact ProductSafety@springernature.com

Printed and bound by CPI Group (UK) Ltd, Croydon, CR0 4YY
22/09/2026
02220961-0019